To Anne and Florian
Youth – Power – New goals

P.J. Frosch and A.M. Kligman (Eds.)

Noninvasive Methods for the Quantification of Skin Functions

An Update on Methodology and Clinical Applications

With 33 Tables and 210 Illustrations

Springer-Verlag
Berlin Heidelberg New York London Paris
Tokyo Hong Kong Barcelona Budapest

Prof. Dr. med. Peter J. Frosch
Hautklinik der Städtischen Kliniken Dortmund
Lehrstuhl Dermatologie der
Universität Witten/Herdecke
Beurhausstr. 40
4600 Dortmund 1
Germany

Albert M. Kligman, M.D.
Department of Dermatology
University of Pennsylvania
School of Medicine
Philadelphia, PA 19104-6142
USA

ISBN-13:978-3-642-78159-9 e-ISBN-13:978-3-642-78157-5
DOI: 10.1007/978-3-642-78157-5

Softcover reprint of the hardcover 1st edition 1993

Typesetting: FotoSatz Pfeifer GmbH, Gräfelfing
23/3145-543210 – Printed on acid-free paper

Foreword

More than 10 years ago, I had the chance to visit the university hospital in Münster, Germany. At the outpatient clinic there, I accidently met a young dermatologist who was devoted to the study of the quantification of irritated skin during his busy daily clinical work. I sensed immediately that this Dr. P. Frosch was conducting his research with the ideals and enthusiasm which were so familiar to me. Soon we found that we shared a similar past experience; we both had begun our careers in dermatological investigation with the same mentor. For me it was more than 25 years ago that I first met Dr. Kligman, Professor at the University of Pennsylvania in Philadelphia, USA. I reminisced that I had been greatly shocked by his initial question "As a dermatologist, do you want to study living or dead skin?" because, at that time and even today, whenever we cannot collect enough information about the skin with the naked eye, it is common practice to histologically examine a skin sample that is invasively removed from living tissue. Many dermatologists still would never think of studying the living intact skin itself noninvasively with the aid of existing advanced technologies to assess its structural and functional properties. At that time Dr. Kligman intended to build up a system of evaluating the skin from various aspects, using methods that had been unduly neglected in the past and introducing various technological instruments. He used to say that such a system would eventually make it possible for a blind person to be a dermatologist. Greatly influenced by his enthusiasm, many young researchers engaged in intensive research activities with him, later to become successful in various places in the world. Therefore, after achieving great many things with his ardent academic mind, it is quite natural for Prof. Peter Frosch, who is now flourishing in this field, to edit such a unique book with AMK.

We are now able to evaluate the living skin with various established technological methodologies as fully described in the part I of this book; they are now available anywhere in the world. In many fields they far exceed even immunohistochemical techniques in their ability to provide precise and profound information about the skin's funktions. In fact, recently numerous important findings have emerged for applications of these techniques in the study of both healthy and diseased skin, as extensively described in the part II. These sections will certainly serve to facilitate the design and analysis of the future investigations of eager readers.

Almost 15 years have passed since the Society for Bioengineering and the Skin was founded by Prof. R. Marks in Cardiff. In the fall of 1992, we organized its 9th International Symposium in Sendai, a city in northern Japan. To our great surprise, more than 400 people from all over the world came to the far end of Asia to attend this meeting. We will never forget our confusion on the first morning at the reception desk, faced with such an unexpectedly large number of participants. Of course, we ran out of printed programs and had to hastily copy more to meet the demand.

Thus, I think that many of us are now greatly in need of an additional breakthrough. Although these new noninvasive methodologies are still a rapidly developing field, they hold great promise in the future, as predicted by Dr. Kligman. Any dermatologists or scientists who study the skin and who eagerly hope to make further progress in their clinical and basic studies should become familiar with these techniques. I think that this is a book that will provide them with fresh information.

Hachiro Tagami, M.D.
The president of the 9th International Symposium on Bioengineering and the Skin
Professor of Dermatology and Chairman of the Department of Dermatology
Tohoku University, Sendai, Japan

Contents

List of Authors

Agner, T., Department of Dermatology A, Bispebjerg Hospital, 2400 Copenhagen, Denmark

Altmeyer, P., Dermatologische Klinik der Ruhr-Universität, Gudrunstraße 56, 4630 Bochum, FRG

Auer, T., Dermatologische Klinik der Ruhr-Universität, Gudrunstraße 56, 4630 Bochum, FRG

Böhler, U., Dermatologische Phlebologie, Hautklinik der Medizinischen Fakultät der RWTH Aachen, Pauwelsstraße 30, 5100 Aachen, FRG

Coenraads, P.-J., Occupational Dermatology Unit, State University Hospital, PO Box 30.001, 9700 RB Groningen, The Netherlands

Corcuff, P., Laboratoires de Recherche de L'Oreal, Departement de Biophysique, 1, Avenue Eugène Schueller, 93600 Aulnay sous Bois, France

Cua, A.B., Department of Dermatology, University of California, San Francisco, CA, USA

Czernielewski, J., Centre International de Recherches Dermatologiques Galderma (CIRD Galderma), 635 Route des Lucioles, Sophia Antipolis, 06565 Valbonne Cedex, France

Duteil, L., Centre International de Recherches Dermatologiques Galderma (CIRD Galderma), 635 Route des Lucioles, Sophia Antipolis, 06565 Valbonne Cedex, France

el-Gammal, S., Dermatologische Klinik der Ruhr-Universität, Gudrunstraße 56, 4630 Bochum, FRG

Ermert, H., Institut für Hochfrequenztechnik der Ruhr-Universität Bochum, Universitätsstraße 150 IC6, 4630 Bochum, FRG

Frödin, T., Department of Dermatology, University Hospital, 581 85 Linköping, Sweden

Frosch, P.J., Hautklinik, Städtische Kliniken Dortmund, Beurhausstraße 40, 4600 Dortmund 1, FRG

Gaßmüller, J., Humanpharmakologie II, Schering AG, 1000 Berlin, FRG

Gloor, M., Hautklinik des Städtischen Klinikums Karlsruhe, Moltkestraße 18, 7500 Karlsruhe, FRG

Hammentgen, R., Herzzentrum Nordrhein-Westfalen, Ruhr-Universität Bochum, Georgstraße 11, 4970 Bad Oeynhausen, FRG

Herpens, A., Beiersdorf AG, Forschungszentrum, Unnastr. 48, 2000 Hamburg 20, FRG

Hoffmann, K., Dermatologische Klinik der Ruhr-Universität, Gudrunstraße 56, 4630 Bochum, FRG

Hoppe, U., Beiersdorf AG, Forschungszentrum, Unnastraße 48, 2000 Hamburg 20, FRG

Kietzmann, M., Hautklinik Linden, Medizinische Hochschule Hannover, Ricklinger Straße 5, 3000 Hannover 91, FRG

Kligman, A.M., Department of Dermatology, University of Pennsylvania, School of Medicine, Philadelphia, PA 19104-6142, USA

Kurte, A., Hautklinik, Städtische Kliniken Dortmund, Beurhausstraße 40, 4600 Dortmund 1, FRG

Lentner, A., Dermatologische Phlebologie, Hautklinik der Medizinischen Fakultät der RWTH Aachen, Pauwelsstraße 30, 5100 Aachen, FRG

Leveque, J.L., Laboratoires de Recherche de L'Oreal, Departement de Biophysique, 1, Avenue Eugène Schueller, 93600 Aulnay sous Bois, France

Lubach, D., Hautklinik Linden, Medizinische Hochschule Hannover, Ricklinger Straße 5, 3000 Hannover 91, FRG

Lunderstädt, R., Universität der Bundeswehr, Hostenhofstraße 35, 2000 Hamburg, FRG

Maibach, H.I., Department of Dermatology, University of California, San Francisco, CA, USA

Manning, S., Biosearch Inc., 3408-50 "B" Street, Philadelphia, PA 19134, USA

Matthes, U., Dermatologische Klinik der Ruhr-Universität, Gudrunstraße 56, 4630 Bochum, FRG

Nater, J.P., Occupational Dermatology Unit, State University Hospital, PO Box 30.001, 9700 RB Groningen, The Netherlands

Neumann, G., Hautklinik Linden, Medizinische Hochschule Hannover, Ricklinger Straße 5, 3000 Hannover 91, FRG

Oyoun-Niepel, N., Dermatologische Phlebologie, Hautklinik der Medizinischen Fakultät der RWTH Aachen, Pauwelsstraße 30, 5100 Aachen, FRG

Piérard, G.E., Department of Dermatopathology, University of Liège, CHU du Sart Tilman, 4000 Liège, Belgium

Piérard-Franchimont, C., Department of Dermatopathology, University of Liège, CHU du Sart Tilman, 4000 Liège, Belgium

Pilz, B., Hautklinik, Städtische Kliniken Dortmund, Beurhausstraße 40, 4600 Dortmund 1, FRG

Pinnagoda, J., Occupational Dermatology Unit, State University Hospital PO Box 30.001. 9700 RB Groningen, The Netherlands

Queille-Roussel, C., Centre International de Recherches Dermatologiques Galderma (CIRD Galderma), 635 Route des Lucioles, Sophia Antipolis, 06565 Valbonne Cedex, France

Sauermann, G., Beiersdorf AG, Forschungszentrum, Unnastraße 48, 2000 Hamburg 20, FRG

Schaefer, H., Centre de Pharmacologie Clinique Appliquée à la Dermatologie (CPCAD), Hôpital Pasteur, 06000 Nice, France

Schatz, H., Department of Dermatology, University of Pennsylvania, School of Medicine, Philadelphia, PA 19104-6142, USA

Serup, J., Department of Dermatology A, Bispebjerg Hospital, 2400 Copenhagen, Denmark

Steiert, P., Dermatologische Klinik der Ruhr-Universität, Gudrunstraße 56, 4630 Bochum, FRG

Stoudemayer, T., Biosearch Inc., 3408-50 "B" Street, Philadelphia, PA 19134, USA

Triebskorn, A., Hautklinik des Städtischen Klinikums Karlsruhe, Moltkestraße 18, 7500 Karlsruhe, FRG

Tupker, R.A., Occupational Dermatology Unit, State University Hospital, PO Box 30.001, 9700 RB Groningen, The Netherlands

Vogel, H.G., Hoechst AG, Geschäftsbereich Pharma, Postfach 80 03 20, 6230 Frankfurt/Main 80, FRG

Wienert, V., Dermatologische Phlebologie, Hautklinik der Medizinischen Fakultät der RWTH Aachen, Pauwelsstraße 30, 5100 Aachen, FRG

Wilhelm, K.-P., Klinik für Dermatologie und Venerologie, Medizinische Universität zu Lübeck, Ratzeburger Allee 160, 2400 Lübeck, FRG und Department of Dermatology, University of California, San Francisco, CA, USA

Preface

Until recently dermatology was a purely "visual field" – skin lesions were described in a beautiful way with much love for morphologic details. This descriptive phase in the evolution of dermatology has lost its dominance with the introduction of modern quantitative techniques in every field, from microbiology to immunology. Molecular biology has provided stunning insights into the pathogenesis of skin diseases.

On the other hand, cutaneous physiology has been a stepchild in investigative dermatology for many years. Measurements of skin temperature, sebum production and transepidermal water loss were crude and used techniques which were complicated, expensive, and time-consuming. Lack of reproducibility was an inevitable result. The literature was confusing and contradictory. It is only in the last decade or so that quantitative instrumentation has become available. Perhaps the seminal event was the introduction of the evaporimeter by Nilsson for the measurement of transepidermal water loss. Initially developed to monitor water loss in premature infants, the convenience and reliability of this tool was quickly realized by investigators everywhere. This development spearheaded the age of noninvasive techniques whereby the skin is not perturbed by the measuring probe. Evaporimetry has many applications: assessment of skin damaged induced by detergents and irritants, impairment of the barrier function in chronic diseases such as psoriasis, monitoring of wound healing, response to treatments and many others.

New instruments have rapidly appeared which will change the way dermatologists study disease processes. We now have an impressive set of tools to study skin functions: skin blood flow by Laser-Doppler velocimetry, visualization of the compartments of skin by ultrasound techniques, determination of skin elasticity by a variety of devices which measure the skin's ability to restore itself after deformations, quantification of erythema by colorimetry, sebum pore patterns, etc. Great advances have been made in the characterization of the surface relief using image analysis. Dry skin, a disagreeable burden to the patient in cold weather, can finally be quantified by a simple but effective technique of applying adhesive discs to remove scales. In addition to Laser-Doppler other methods can complement studies of the microcirculation such as measurement of transcutaneous oxygen pressure, heat flow colorimetry or imaging by fluorescence. Some of these techniques are still investigational and not commercially available. However, it is only a matter of time until these will be in the hands of investigators everywhere. Moreover, these procedures will soon reach the bedside for monitoring patients.

This book provides a broad survey of current techniques which are having a strong impact on dermatological investigation. Readers who have not followed the bio-engineering literature will surely be impressed by the variety of instruments now available to evaluate skin functions. The time has passed where looking at and feeling the skin were our sole means of deciding whether it was normal or abnormal.

One of us (AMK) not so long ago prophesized that the day would come when ingenious instrumentation would make it possible for a blind man to become a dermatologist. That goal is still to be attained but there is no doubt that all of us are "seeing" a good deal more than was thought possible a short while ago.

P. J. Frosch
A. M. Kligman

Part I: The Basics: Methodology

The Surface of the Skin – The Microrelief

J. L. LEVEQUE AND P. CORCUFF*

Introduction

The surface of a body is by definition its outer part which limits it in any direction. More importantly, it is the visible covering of the body. This simple fact has considerable sociological importance, which immediately justifies the interest that researchers have taken in studying the skin for the past 10 years or so. First of all, the surface of the skin is largely what we perceive of others, and this type of received information will be, at first, the basis of judgements concerning a whole series of related criteria (pleasant or unpleasant, young or old, healthy or sick, aggressive or not, etc). In addition to the olfactory aspects of an encounter between two individuals, contact can be established by touch, which is a highly developed sense. Very little is yet known about its physiology, but it involves physical contact of two surfaces which, as we shall see later, have a very complex organization. The very important part played by appearance, and hence by the skin surface, in social relations has now been acknowledged and scientifically described [1]. It gives additional significance and responsibility to dermatology and cosmetology.

From the physiological point of view, the notion of surface is often synonymous with that of exchanges. The surface of the skin is the frontier where the often contradictory demands of two media are resolved – the biological medium and the external environment. The principal function of the skin, and in particular of its outer layer, the stratum corneum (SC), is to attenuate external stresses (climatic variations, physical, chemical, and bacteriological attack, etc.) and, of course, to limit loss of substances from the internal environment, whatever the conditions are. What particular role does cutaneous relief play in this process? As a matter of fact, this question has hardly been studied.

In the following chapter, a description of cutaneous relief and of what is known, or rather assumed, about its function will be given. A short review of methods for both the study and objective measurement of the skin pattern will follow. The different aspects of cutaneous microrelief according to anatomical sites will then be discussed. Finally, the way these aspects can be changed, in the course of aging or exposure to the sun and in different pathologies and cosmetic conditions, will be explained.

* Laboratoires de Recherche de L'OREAL, Departement de Biophysique, 1, Avenue Eugène Schueller, 93600 Aulnay sous Bois, France

Description of Cutaneous Relief

The skin surface is not flat but contains a number of more or less rectilinear grooves which can be classified according to their depth and hence to the magnification which is required to describe them easily. The most visible are *wrinkles* which are between 100 μm and several mm deep, depending on age and environmental factors. They are found in specific areas, e.g., expression lines on the face and plicatures at joints.

At low magnification (x10), the surface of the skin shows a network which is known as microrelief or texture. Parallel rectilinear furrows cross others to form rectangles, squares, lozenges, trapeziums, and triangles. Hashimoto [2] has proposed a classification into four groups of lines. *Primary lines* are wide, from 20 to 100 μm deep, depending on site and age (see below). They criss-cross to form parallelograms, rectangles, and squares, except fingerprints, which are particular formations located on fingers and toes (dermatoglyphism). *Secondary lines* are finer (5–40 μm). They branch off from the primary lines, forming diagonals of the primary lines. Primary and secondary lines generally (but not always) cross one another at the outlets of pilosebaceous or sweat ducts. Under stronger magnification (x100), which excludes any direct visual examination, the *tertiary lines* are the limits of the corneocytes, and the *quaternary lines* feature the corneocytes. A view of the different lines is reproduced in Fig. 1.

Cutaneous Relief – Physiological Aspects

The first consequence of this complex network of lines of varying depth is to increase the actual surface area of the human body compared with its apparent area. Depending on the body site and on age, the actual area would seem to be between 10% and 50% greater than it appears to the naked eye (see below). Thus the interface between biological medium and environment is increased. This promotes exchanges such as those occurring in certain animals, (e.g., batrachians) in which a very high percentage of respiration (50%) is assumed through the skin. Under certain circumstances requiring intense gaseous exchanges, for instance, for batrachians living in high-altitude lakes (e.g., Titicaca), the skin forms folds or numerous dermal papillae so that the total area greatly increases [3]. For humans, however, respiration through the skin is less than 5%. From this point of view it is possible that human cutaneous relief has a vestigial evolutionary function.

Regarding heat exchanges, nothing definite is known, but certain changes in skin microrelief depending on the season have been reported [4].

Another approach has been to consider the skin lines as channels for draining sweat and sebum over long distances in order to preserve an ideal moisture level on the skin surface [2]. This hypothesis is based on the fact that the lines often meet at the outlet of a pilosebaceous or sweat duct.

According to another hypothesis, the network of lines may play a role in the extensibility of the skin. We must go back to Dupuytren's observations in 1836 and then to Langer's studies [5] to understand the essential role of skin texture in relation to the elastic properties of dermis. These studies proposed the first full anatomical map of

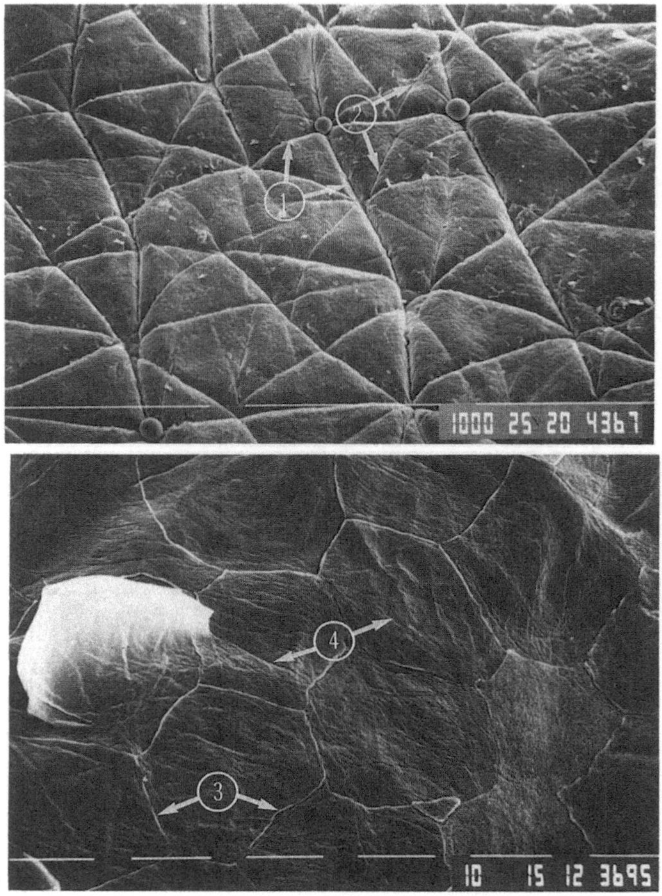

a

b

Fig. 1a, b. Scanning electron micrograph of the skin surface showing a primary (*1*) and secondary (*2*) lines b tertiary (*3*) and quaternary (*4*) lines

skin anisotropy. The parallelism between the direction of Langer's lines and the principal orientations of the primary lines is striking. It is obvious on the back [6], where anisotropy is particularly marked but also applies to the upper arms, forearms [7], legs, and abdomen [8].

The relationship between the organization of collagen fibres in papillary dermis and cutaneous relief has been shown by Pierard et al. [9, 10], who demonstrated that skin patterns correspond perfectly to certain groups of dermal papillae (Fig. 2). The plexus pattern of the skin could constitute a reserve of tissue preventing damage to the epidermis and stratum corneum, which are less extensible than the dermis [11].

The structure of these papillae is reinforced by a "candelabra" of elastic fibers (oxytalan), which form branches perpendicular to the dermoepidermal junction. Total or partial destruction of this elastic network (through UV radiation, aging, etc.) could flatten papillae and cause changes in the cutaneous relief (see below).

The relationship between the microrelief and skin extensibility has been partly docu-

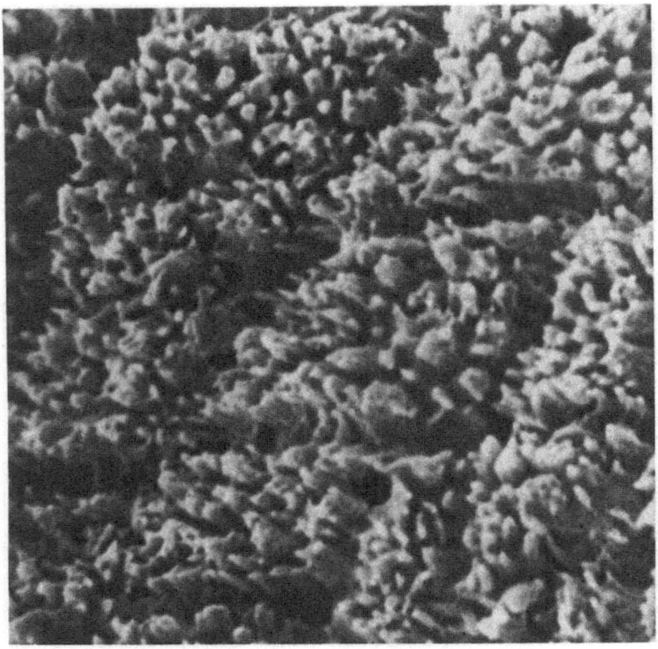

Fig. 2. Primary lines imprinted on the surface of the papillary dermis after removal of the epidermis. Lines isolate groups of papillae. (Courtesy Dr. G.E. Pierard)

mented [12–14]. To conclude, we also have to mention the optical properties of the skin. The lattice of microplateaus might play some part in diffusion and light reflection but objective data are not available.

Methods of Study

Skin topography can be studied in vivo under low magnification. For reasons of convenience and because of the presence of the translucent stratum corneum, which disturbs optical observations (reflection, diffraction, etc.), almost all studies are conducted with casts. Silicone dental rubbers are preferred, since they provide a very faithful negative reproduction of the skin surface. The most widely used resin is Silflo (Flexico Ltd., England). Observations can be made either from this negative impression or from a positive Araldite cast, which allows observations under transmitted light and from scanning electron microscopy after gold coating. These visual methods of evaluation are very common and qualitative.

The oldest method of measurement and still the most widely used nowadays is profilometry. It was primarily used to measure the roughness of metallic surfaces, so that measurement instruments have had to be adapted for skin; these include Surfcom [15], Surfometer [16], Talysurf [17], Anaglyphographe [18], and Perth-O-Meter [19]. The basic principle involves moving a stylus over the surface along a straight line and plotting the profile followed by the tip (Fig. 3). A series of sweeps is needed in order to obtain an average profile representative of the surface under study.

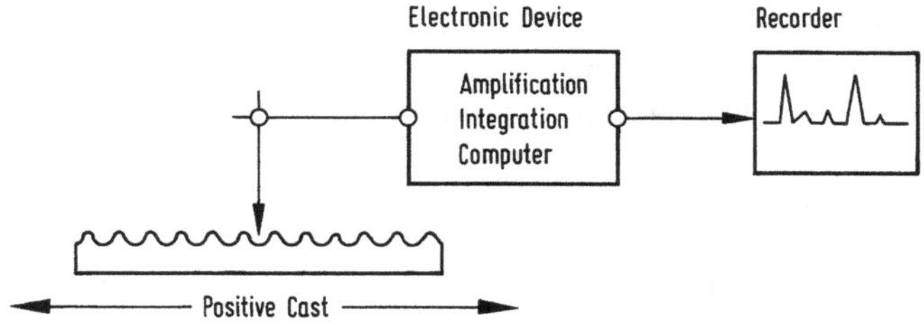

Fig. 3. The profilometric method

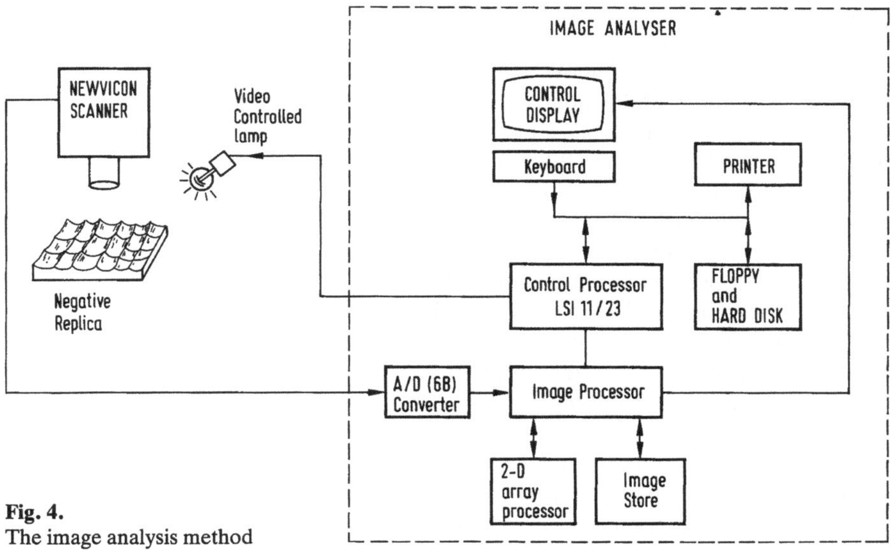

Fig. 4.
The image analysis method

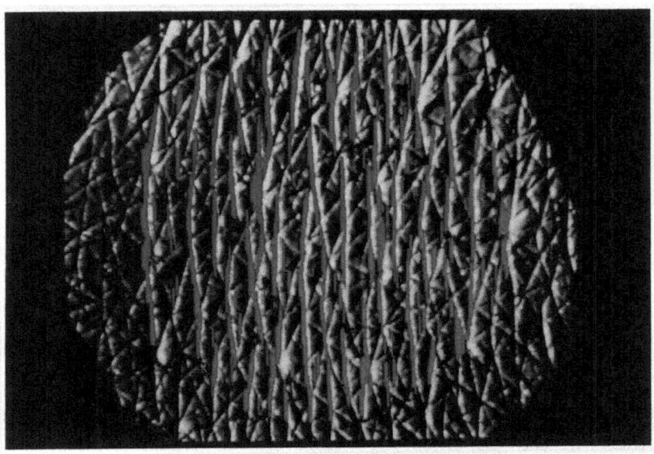

Fig. 5. The skin replica is displayed and analyzed through the monitor of the image analyzer. *Red features* correspond to shadowed areas.

The description of these profiles results in more than ten calculation parameters, which are obtained with a computer. Some of these parameters, defined for metallurgy, are often difficult to interpret in terms of cutaneous relief. The best review on the method has been reported by T. Cook [20].

Profilometry is a time-consuming and delicate mechanical method which gives a two-dimensional picture of the relief, precautions must therefore be taken with respect to interpretation, since the texture of the skin is highly anisotropic. Thereby, the choice of the scanning direction is an important factor for the evaluation. Makki et al., realizing this difficulty, extended the method so that a three-dimensional representation of the relief is provided, but the time required in order to reproduce one square centimeter of skin makes it prohibitive for routine use [21].

An alternative method was firstly proposed in 1981 [4]. It consists of combining image analysis and the "surface shadowing" principle, a method that NASA investigated to study the topography of the moon during the first Apollo flights. Applied to the topography of negative impressions, it provides three-dimensional information from a one square centimeter field in less than 5 min.

Under "grazing" illumination, the shadows formed behind the crests (i.e. grooves of the skin) can be selected by thresholding and then analyzed (Fig. 4, 5). In this way the *principal orientations* of the furrows, their line *density*, and *average depth* for each direction can be defined. From a mathematical model, the true skin surface area vs the apparent one can be calculated. This is the coefficient of developed skin surface (CDSS) measuring either tissue reserve or amount of deformability in order to avoid cracking of the SC and epidermis under stretching. The stereological parameters thus defined depend on a concept of fractality [22]. Since the skin surface is very irregular, euclidian measurements vary with magnification and angle of lighting. The results will mainly depend on the angle of light, which acts as a spatial filter. At an angle of 26°, for instance, furrows less than 15 μm will not be recognized. At 38°, it will not be possible to measure both primary lines and wrinkles on the same sample. In spite of these limitations, a large amount of data can be obtained from a large area of skin in a very short time, so that routine studies on many samples can be made, with the consequence of statistical improved. Alternatives to this method of image analysis have been proposed [23–25], but they do not allow three-dimensional investigation of the relief. Other methods are, however currently under study: densitometry on negative photographs [26], and profilometry by laser beam and by focusing under the microscope [27].

Aspects of Cutaneous Relief Depending on the Site

As mentioned in the previous section, the features of the microrelief depend on the organization of the collagen bundles in the papillary dermis. The direction of these bundles depends on the strains which they most often experience. This explains why the organization of skin microrelief varies according to the site of the body. Over exerted muscles, the skin pattern presents a highly anisotropic structure. For instance, the lines are denser along an axis perpendicular to the strain axis (i.e., limbs). This anisotropy is gradually developed and is far more marked on the skin of elderly people than on that of children, where the distribution is almost isotropic (star-shaped

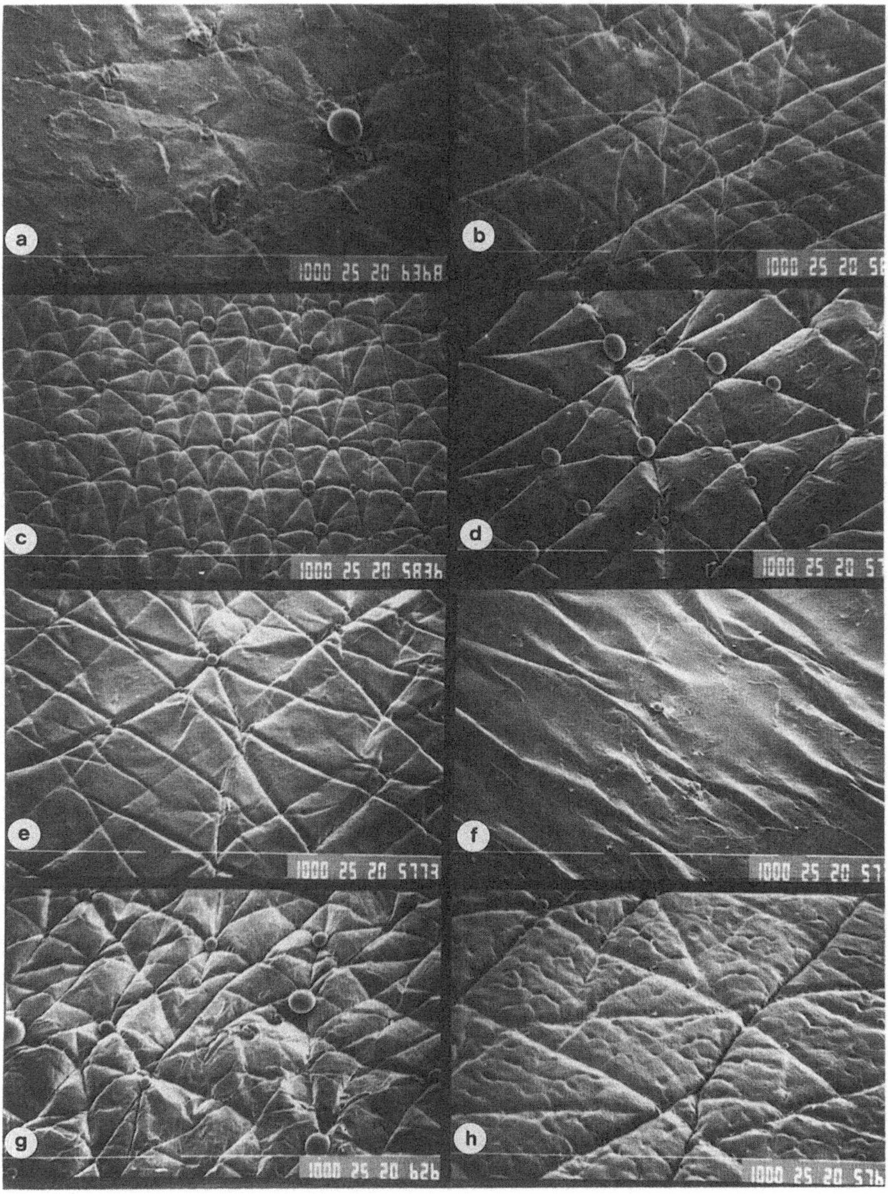

Fig. 6a–p. Scanning electron micrographs of skin from various body sites. **a**: Scalp: the surface appears stretched, resulting in a very flat pattern. The small mechanical movements on the cranial box might explain the absence of a reservoir of deformation for the skin. **b**: Forehead: this pattern is made up of wide parallelograms. The furrows are shallow and the "hills" are relatively flat. In contrast to the primary lines, the secondary lines are randomly distributed giving a weak periodicity to the image. **c**: Forearm: As found on the arm, this site has a typical pattern made up of isotropic features: a star-shaped plexus of furrows. The major feature is triangular leading to three primary ▷

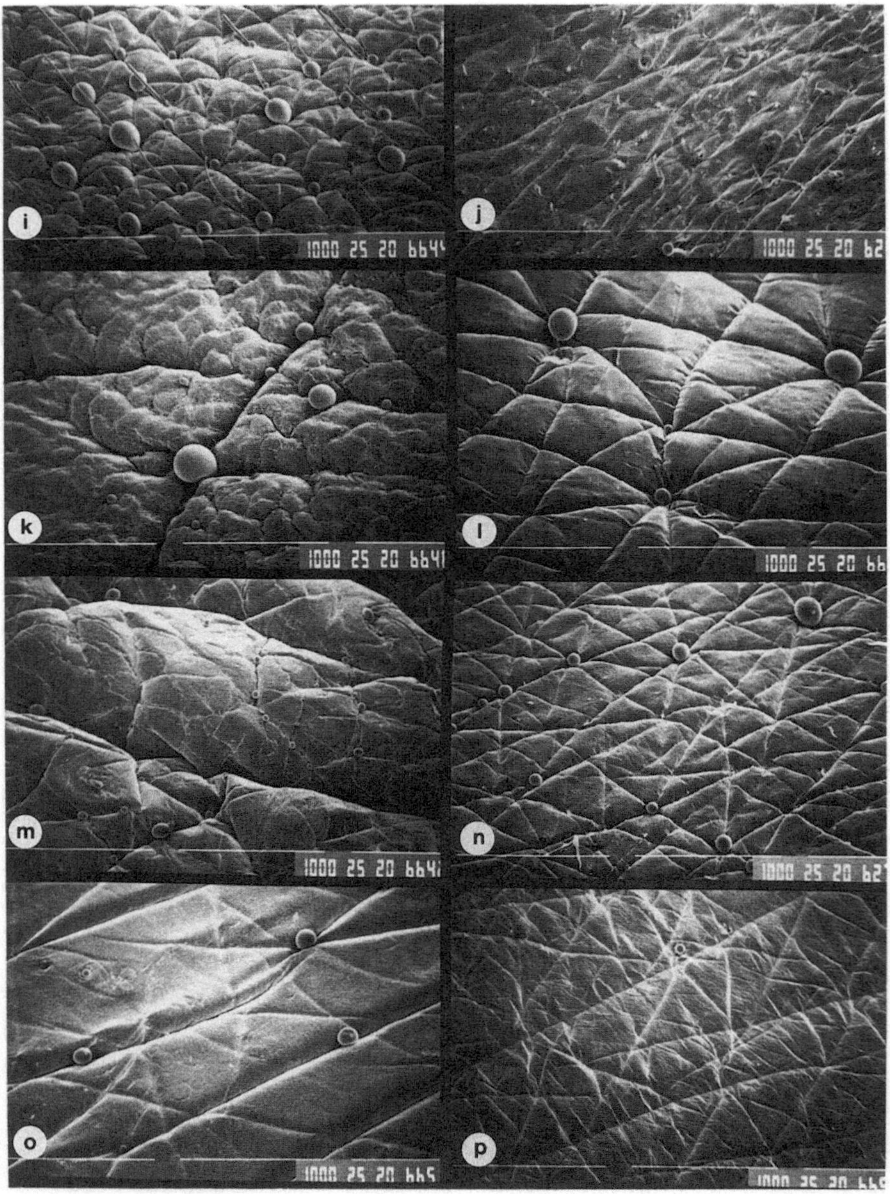

directions of lines whose periodicity is obvious. Sweat bubbles are at the intersections of the lines. **d**: Dorsal side of the hand: Very similar to the arm but with larger features. The hills are higher and consequently, the reservoir of deformation is increased to facilitate full mobility of this site in every direction. **e**: Calf: The network of primary lines is relatively anisotropic. Furrows criss-cross at an acute angle (about 30°), forming large trapezoid features; hills are flat and smooth and furrows are relatively shallow. **f**: Tibia: a completely unorganized pattern. The skin is tensed, with microplicated lines instead of furrows. A single orientation of lines does not allow any geometrical pattern ▷

images). These preliminary observations imply that a full description of the skin relief would be presumptive: any specialist in this field would agree that both individual features and genetic factors or geographical latitude, or race, or age, define, in fact, many different patterns.

In Fig. 6, scanning electron micrographs (SEMs) of the skin of a 30 year old woman and the bald scalp of a 35 year old man are shown as typical examples. The SEMs were performed at the same magnification and under the same incident angle.

The cranium and forehead relief are often marked by the presence of sebaceous lipids. Figure 7 shows how, starting from a clean scalp, the surface of the skin becomes overlaid with sebum. The skin is inhabited by a number of "guests" such as bacteria and fungi, which are very difficult to observe from impressions. This is because the density is relatively low (a few per about 100 μm^2) and because they may be concealed under corneocytes. However, examination of the forehead surface under high magnification frequently reveals *Demodex folliculorum* (Fig. 8) more or less buried in pilosebaceous outlets. This is an acarid which plays, in all likehood, a role in the pathogenesis of rosacea (P. Frosch., personal communication).

recognition. As seen for the head, underlaid skin is mostly by bone rather than muscle. **g**: Buttock: a dense star-shaped network made up of very deep primary furrows. The hills are very plump and the reservoir of deformation is high. Most previous publications classify this site as a nonexposed skin reference, normally protected since birth. The high tissue reserve implies that this site would receive constant mechanical assault (e.g., with respect to sitting). Thus, from a strictly mechanical point of view, this site would age faster than others. **h**: Upper foot: characterized by wide triangular features. Deep, abrupt, but spaced furrows frame large fields which are crossed by wide and flattened depressions. Hills look randomly riddled. **i**: Upper lip: typical pattern is made up of triangular features. The dense network is star-shaped and numerous hairs and bubbles emerge from criss-cross points. The great mobility of this site needs a pronounced relief. **j**: Nose: the presence of bone and cartilage tenses the skin, as in the scalp and tibia. A flat pattern without evident periodicity is characteristic of these sites. Discontinuous and rare primary lines can hardly be seen. Numerous sebaceous follicles show emerging vellus hair. **k**: Upper phalanx: this is a region closely associated with flexion and external rubbing. Next to the sites of articulation, there is a pattern of deep and abrupt furrows; the hills show enlarged features. Hyperkeratosis gives a deep appearance. **l**: Space between first and second metacarpus: made up of smooth hills. The star-shaped network defines large triangles resembling a "linen parachute;" this site is well fitted to buffer the wide variety of movements (prehensile motion). **m**: Elbow: parallel wrinkles are largely spaced and the image is almost anisotropic. The fish-scale appearance is characteristic of a hyperkeratotic region. Tertiary lines are pronounced. This region is perfectly well fitted for absorbing flexion-extension of the joint and constant rubbing. **n**: Breast: all of the geometrical features are found in this area: triangles, lozenges, trapeziums, etc. Hills are relatively flat and primary furrows are fairly deep, probably due to tension exerted by the underlying mammary gland. **o**: Kneecap: another example of an area in which bone is closely underlaid by skin. Anisotropy is as pronounced as seen in the elbow in order to absorb flexion of the joint. The primary lines are rectilinear, showing deep furrows, and the secondary ones are sparse. **p**: Popliteal area: highly protected against actinic damage and mechanical movements. Thus, the pattern is flattened, with randomly organized secondary lines defining triangular features of different sizes. *White bar* = 1 mm

a

b

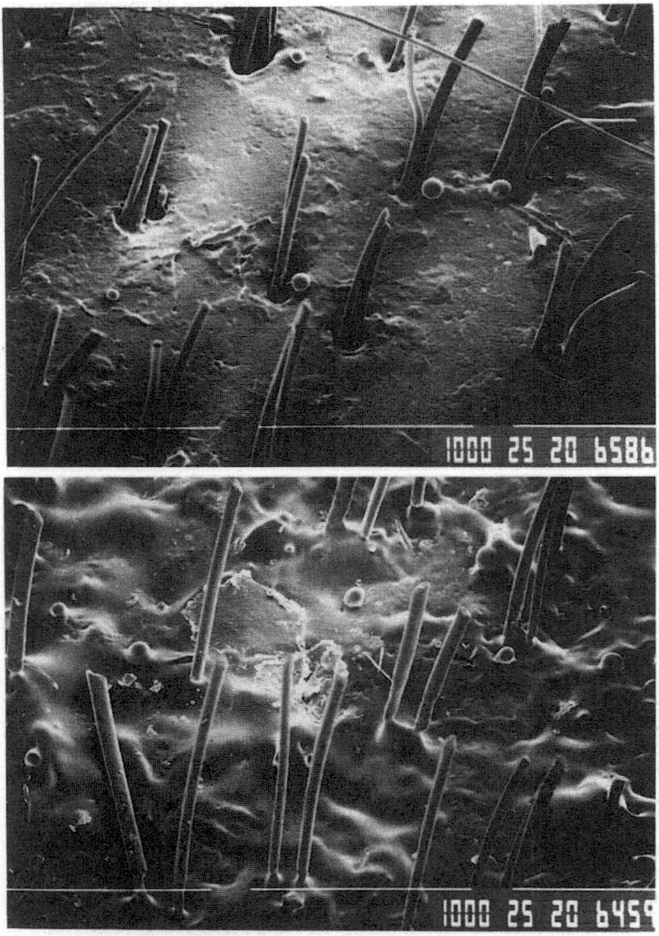

Fig. 7 a, b. Scanning electron micrographs of a hairy scalp **a** just after shampooing and **b** 48 h later. Sebum has filled the ducts and covered the whole surface.

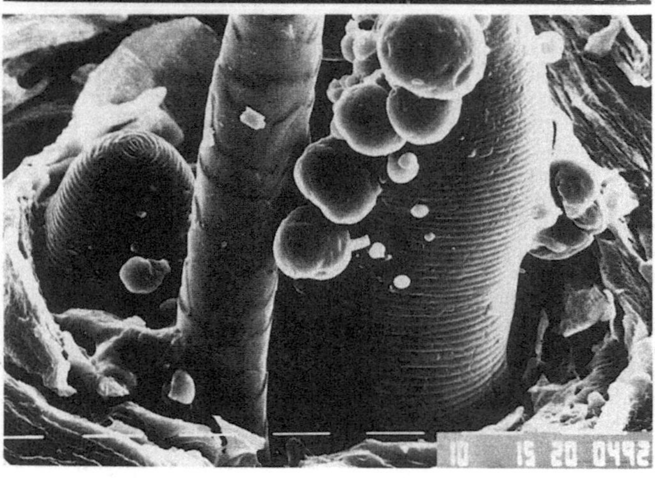

Fig. 8. *Demodex folliculorum* emerging from pilosebaceous duct. SEM white bar = 10 μm

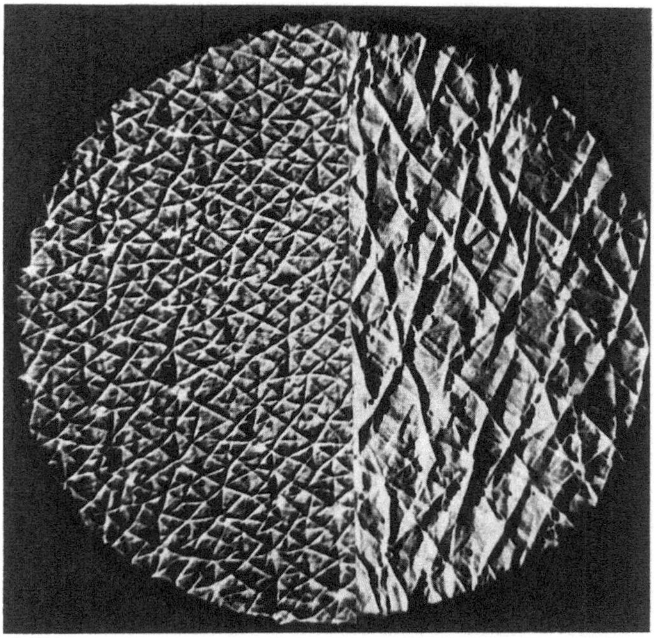

Fig. 9. Photographic montage showing evolution of the skin microrelief (forearm) between a young (*left*) and an old (*right*) subject.

Age and Cutaneous Relief

Figure 9 shows the forearm pattern of a 7 year old child and of a 79 year old woman. Over the years, the fine, star-shaped, isotropic network characteristic of childhood is replaced by a texture which reveals the underlying disorganization of the subpapillary dermis and of its junction with epidermis. At the different sites of the body, the skin adapts itself and undergoes deformations according to local stresses which, repeated throughout a lifetime, cause a certain remodeling of skin texture.

The sites at which most of the experimental investigations have been performed are: the ventral surface of the forearm [7, 28], the abdomen [21], and the face [29]. The volar forearm can be considered as an area which is relatively seldom exposed to the sun. It is therefore a useful site for describing the phenomenon of chronological aging. At this site, studies show a progressive decrease in line density after age 50 following a sharp increase in their depth. The situation is, in fact, more complex, as a fairly similar organization in all directions is gradually replaced by a certain anisotropy. For example, the density of the lines decreases along one axis but is compensated by a depth increase along another axis [7]. This emphasizes how important it is to consider every direction of the plane of the skin in these studies.

These changes in skin texture probably originate in the structural changes which take place throughout life in the dermis [30]. A gradual disappearance of oxytalan fibers and poor recovery of the conjunctive fibers after extension could explain this less homogeneous line distribution on the skin surface of elderly people. In some peculiar sites, such as the buttocks Fig. 10., the skin becomes exaggeratedly folded under the additional influence of gravity.

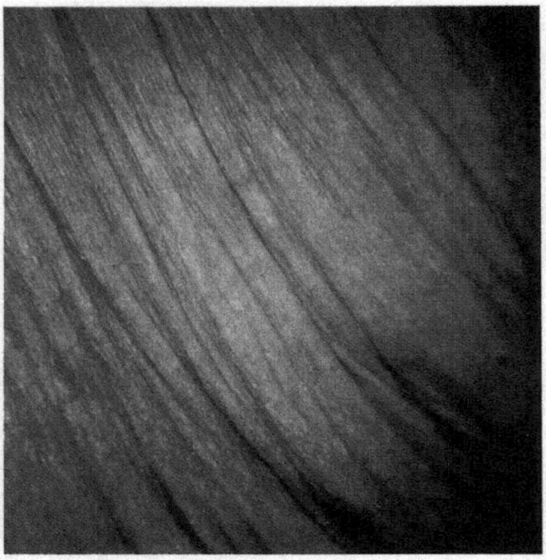

Fig. 10. Macrophotograph of the flabby skin of the buttock of an elderly woman. (Courtesy of Dr. O. de Lacharriere)

With respect to the problem of aging, it is instructive to compare how the microrelief changes on exposed and unexposed areas.

Figure 11 shows changes in the average depth of lines with age on the volar forearm and on the periorbital "crow's foot" area. The face suffers and stores the "attacks" of life which may be extrinsic, such as environmental factors (cold, sun, wind, etc.), or intrinsic such as genetic features. These factors contribute to the aging process as does lifestyle hygiene habits, and the personal characteristics which make up a personality. All these aspects explain the wide variations found in measurements made on the face.

Cutaneous Relief and the Environment

Among environmental factors, most research has focused on the effects of ultraviolet rays. Standard procedures exist for such a study, using solar simulators to expose the skin surface to well known doses of ultraviolet rays at different wavelengths.

These experimental procedures have shown that the application of single doses above the minimum erythematous dose causes a substantial change in the cutaneous relief a few days later (Fig. 12). Objective studies of these changes have produced a description of this phenomenon which, to a certain extent, mimics the aging process. These studies have shown that the lines become more widely spaced and that the average depth increases. Unlike what happens in aging, however, the CDSS does not seem to increase [6]. These changes reach a maximum between the fifth and seventh day after exposure and are probably the consequence of earlier microedema (48 h post-exposure), which progressively stretches the skin surface. This phenomenon vanishes on and after the 12th day when excessive SC desquamation occurs.

Fewer experiments have been done on the effect of prolonged and repeated exposure to the sun, but a recent study also concludes that lines become deeper and, to a certain extent, denser. Under particular test conditions, the CDSS dramatically increased [31].

a

b

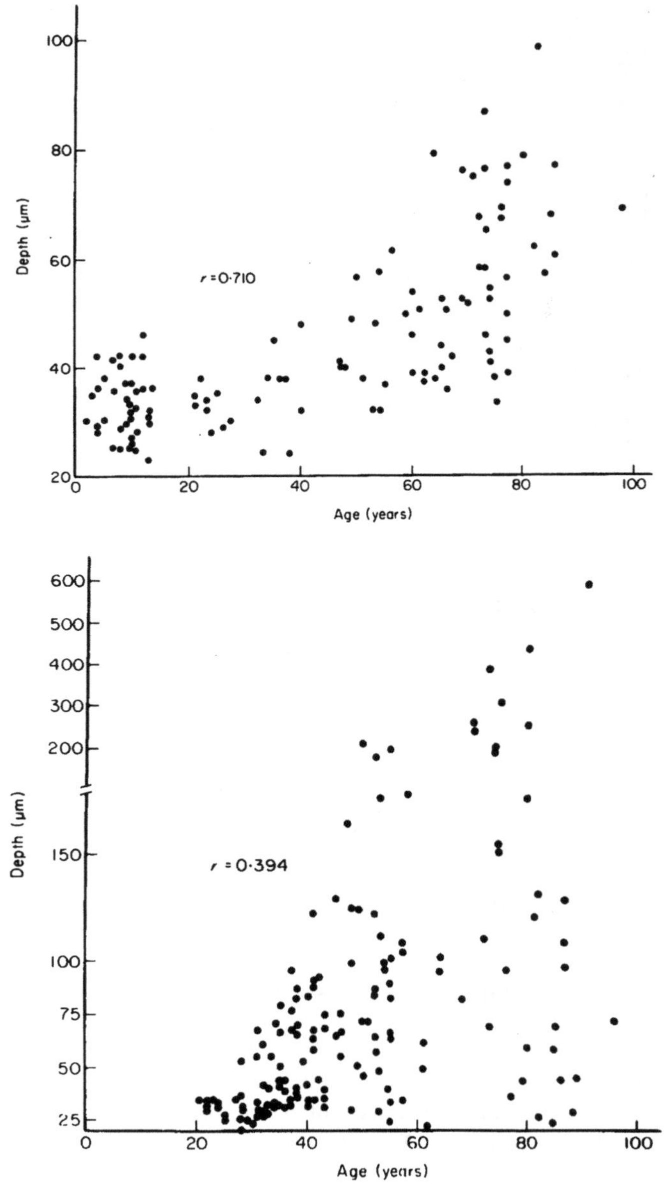

Fig. 11 a, b. Individual plots of the mean depth of skin furrows vs age; **a** volar forearm and **b** crow's feet wrinkles of the periorbital region.

The explanation for these changes can probably be found in the conclusions of histological research on animals after repeated exposure to radiation. Kligman et al., for instance, showed that elastolysis of oxytalan fibers occurred and that large quantities of amorphous elastotic material [32] were deposited in the subpapillary dermis. These changes are, however, reported to be reversible [33].

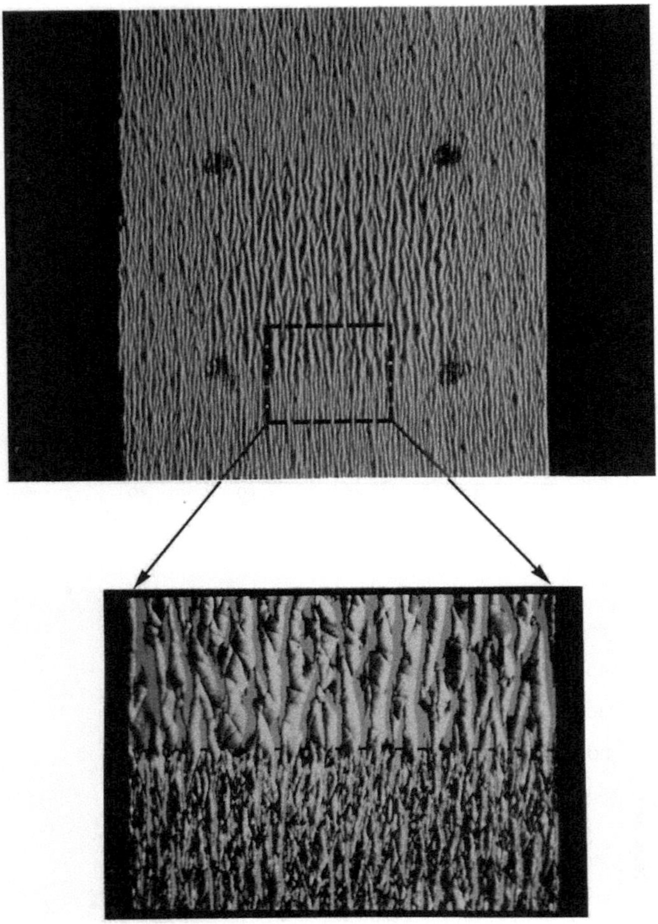

Fig. 12. Silflo replica of a UV exposed skin square (3 Minimal Erythema Doses) surrounded by protected skin. The image of the border between irradiated and protected zones is displayed on the TV monitor. The upper (*blue*) features correspond to the UV irradiated skin, showing enlarged and deep furrows compared to the lower (*orange*) nonexposed skin.

Pathology and Cosmetic Disorders – Topical Treatments

As noted in the Introduction, the skin microrelief actively contributes to the appearance of the individual. Appearance is the emphasis of the cosmetics market, which for many years now has taken into account various demands, chiefly regarding the "softness" of the skin and wrinkles. Dry skin, with which cosmetic products are concerned, are above all rough skins, with four main causes: (1) senile xerosis; (2) excessive desquamation after exposure to the sun, soaps or detergents; (3) common dry skin, principally on the face and legs, which is more marked in winter, and (4) dry skin in atopic dermatitis [34].

To control these conditions, which in fact can cause serious problems over a long-term period, various types of cosmetics are available whose efficacy can nowadays be easily and objectively measured. The methods used to illustrate the effect of these products on skin softness include in vivo measurement of the coefficient of friction and profilometric technique (see above).

a

b

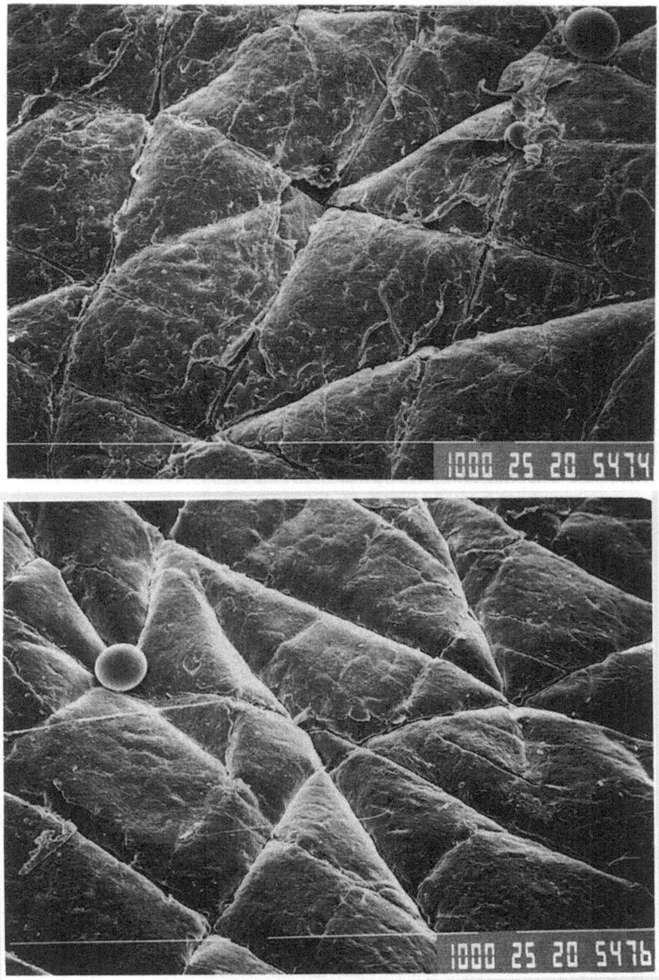

Fig. 13 a, b. Scanning electron micrograph of the surface of dry skin **a** before treatment and **b** after hydration with a cosmetic moisturizer.

Dry skin is characterized by groups of raised corneocytes and flakes, which give the skin a rough, cracked, gray appearance (Fig. 13a). After treatment, the skin surface becomes once again smooth (Fig. 13b). Profilometric studies of positive impression of the skin surface readily reveal these properties (Fig. 14).

The treatment of wrinkles is more recent, although the need is very old. Figure 15 illustrates changes in crows feet with age at the corners of the eyes. By the age of 25, these expression marks are constantly present. They become more pronounced and deeper with age, but to an extent which varies greatly from one individual to another, as shown in Fig. 11. The specific products supplied by leading cosmetic firms for the treatment of wrinkles seem to be increasingly active in attenuating, at least temporarily, these unattractive formations. Some studies have been published [35, 36] and

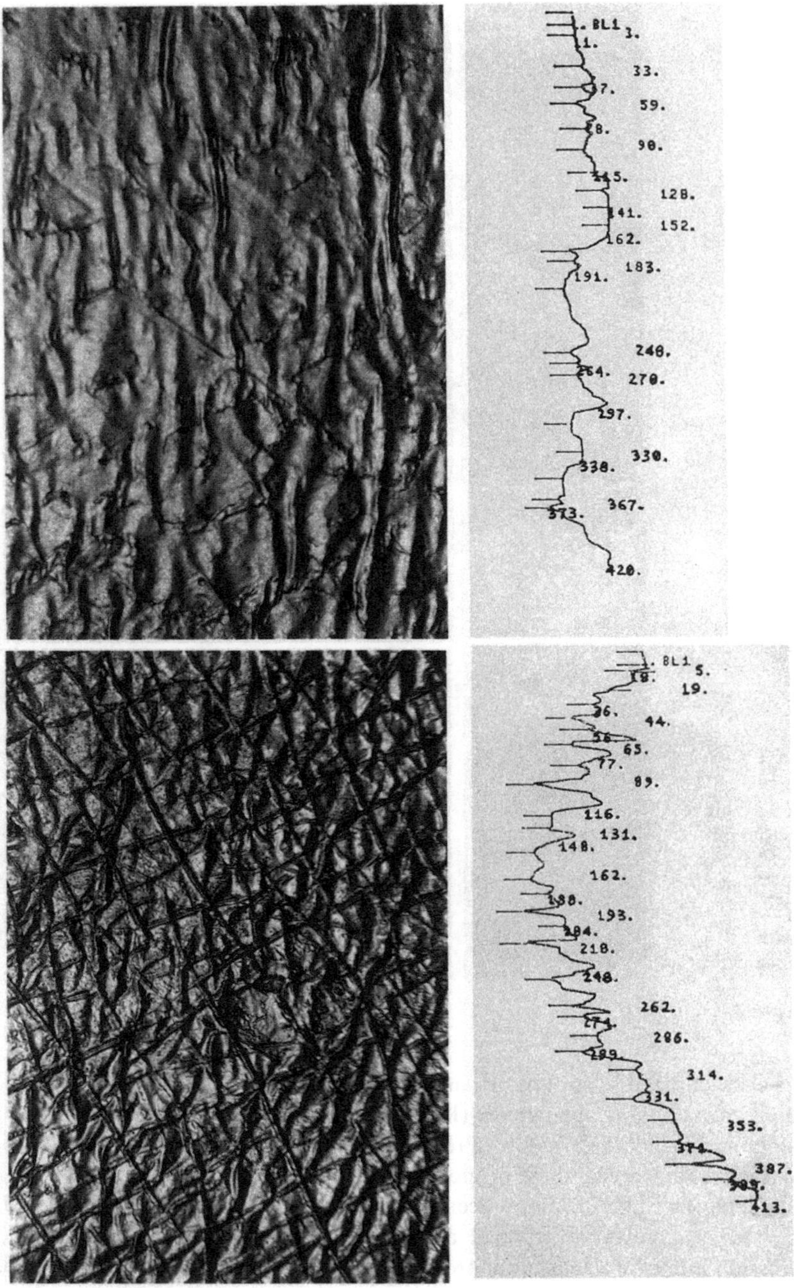

a

b

Fig. 14. Alcalmite positive casts of dry skin before and after cosmetic treatment. The *curves* represent surface profiles drawn by profilometry. *a*, Dry skin leads to a flat line profile due to the typical lack of the microrelief. *b*, After treatment, the microrelief has been restored; periodic furrows are recorded on the line profile. (Courtesy of Dr. T. Cook)

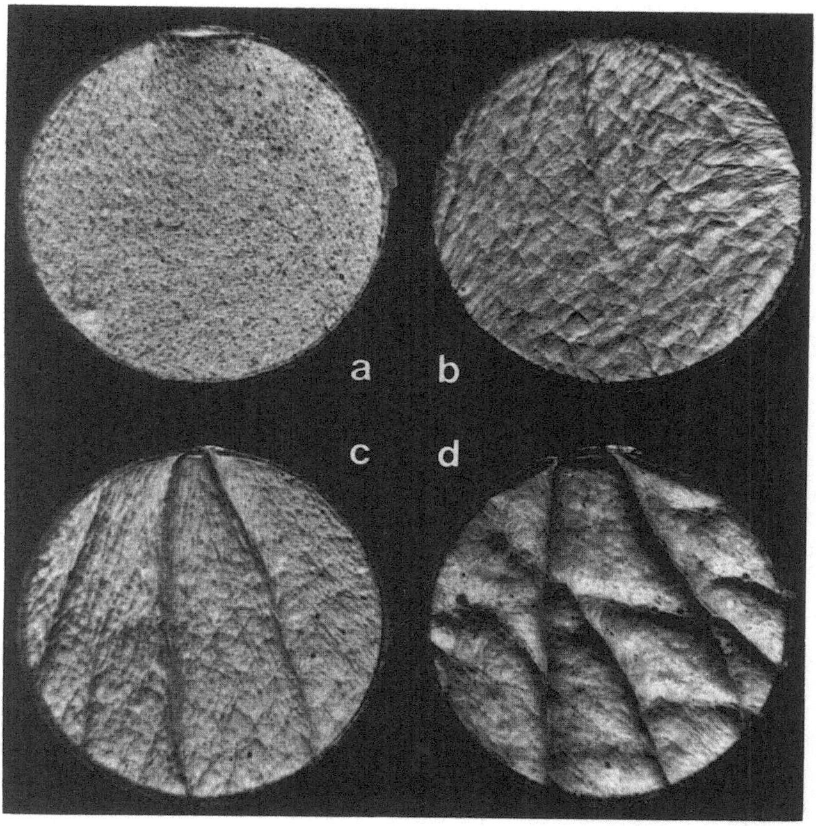

Figs. 15 a–d. Macrophotographs of crow's foot site at different ages: **a** 10 years old; **b** 25 years old; **c** 65 years old; **d** 65 years old with extensive sun exposure

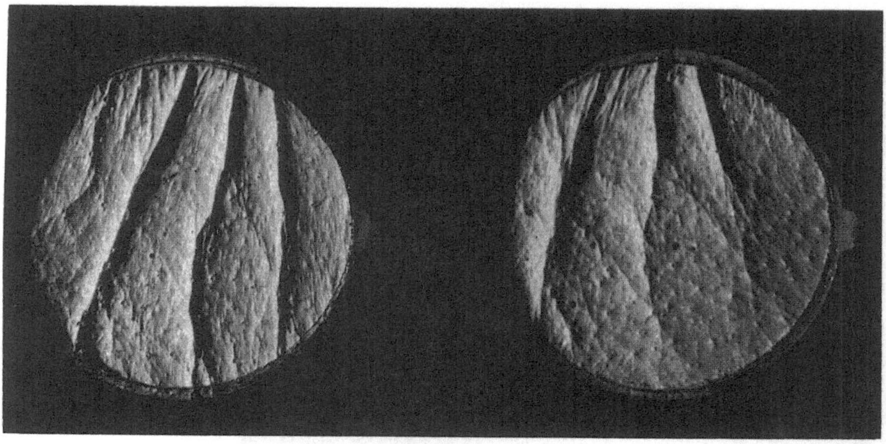

Fig. 16. Crow's foot wrinkles as displayed by the image analyzer before (*left*) and after (*right*) a 3 month therapy with 0,05% retinoic acid ointment.

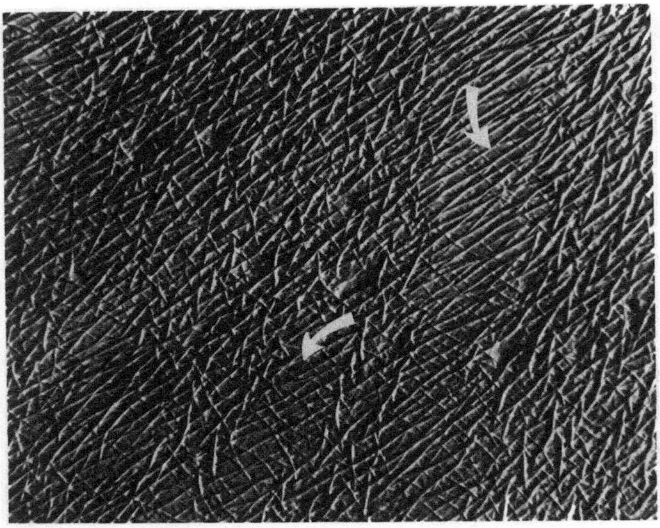

Fig. 17. Macrophotograph of striae distensae (*arrows*) characterized by the lack of one line orientation.

the authors have even reported what, according to them, might be either the most convenient age group or the most receptive one for such treatment (30–40 years old). Retinoic acid and derivatives, as a treatment of photodamaged skin, is currently being studied by many teams [37, 38]. Reduction of facial wrinkles seems to be one of the most visible result obtained with this treatment (Fig. 16)

Dermatological disorders lead to obvious changes in the skin microrelief. As mentioned earlier, the cutaneous relief mainly depends on the spatial organization of collagen bundles. This relief can be observed at the dermoepidermal junction. Among

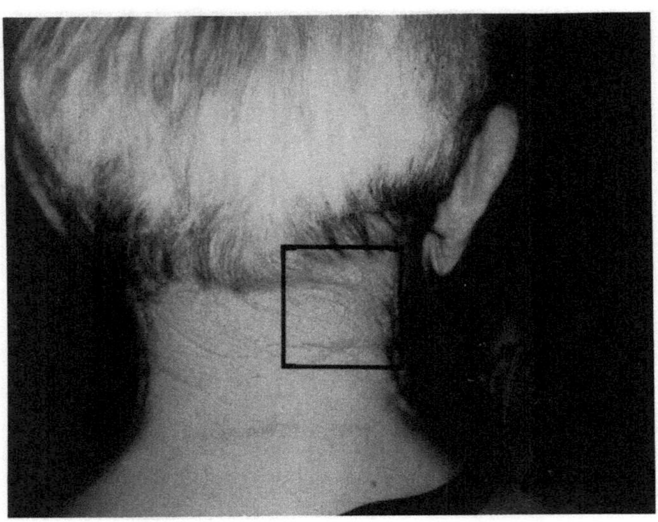

Fig. 18. Cutis rhomboidalis nucchae, **a** Overview; **b** Detail of the square area in **a**; **c** SEM of the rectangle in **b** *Arrow* indicates a normal star-shaped skin surrounded by elastotic-like patterns. (Courtesy of Dr O. de Lacharriere)

Fig. 18b

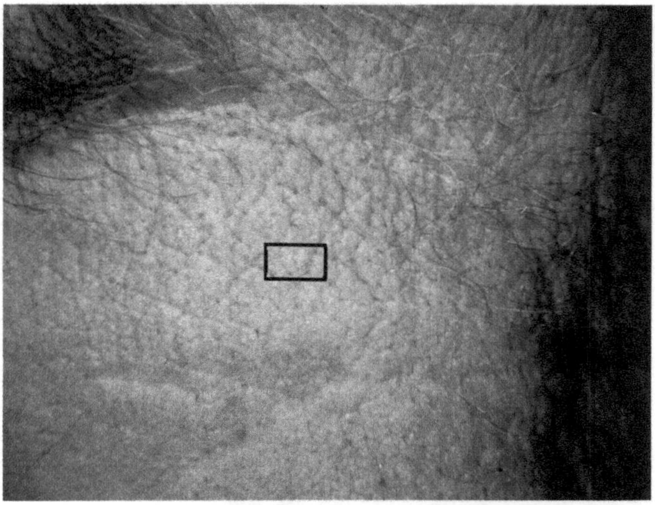

c

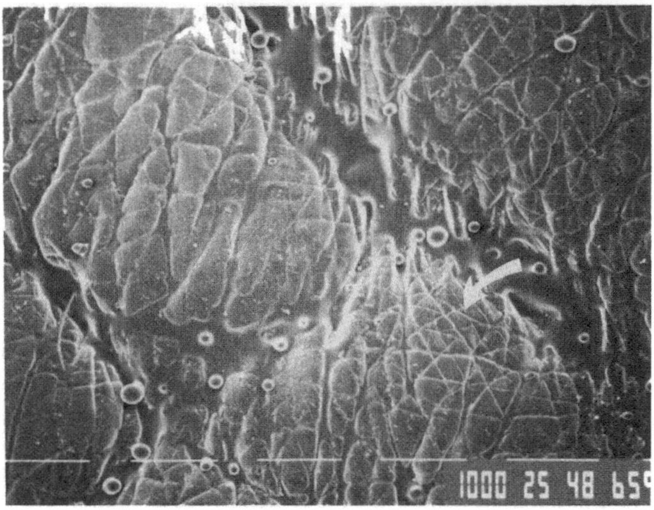

the different pathologies those originating from the dermis should be focused on. The best illustration is the "striae distensae" which are the consequence of fast and local skin stretching due to obesity, fast growth, or pregnancy. Their preferential localization is on the abdomen, hips, buttock, thigh, and breast. They are characterized by a shift of collagen bundles in the direction of the strain. On the surface (Fig. 17), independent of color modification, the microrelief is characterized by the lack of line orientation through a tubular area the boundaries of which are sharp and rectilinear.

Solar elastosis is a typical example of the destruction of the skin microrelief, as readily illustrated by the rhomboidalis nucchae (Fig. 18). It involves both dermis and epidermis. Dermal changes are expressed on the skin surface by large wrinkles. Epi-

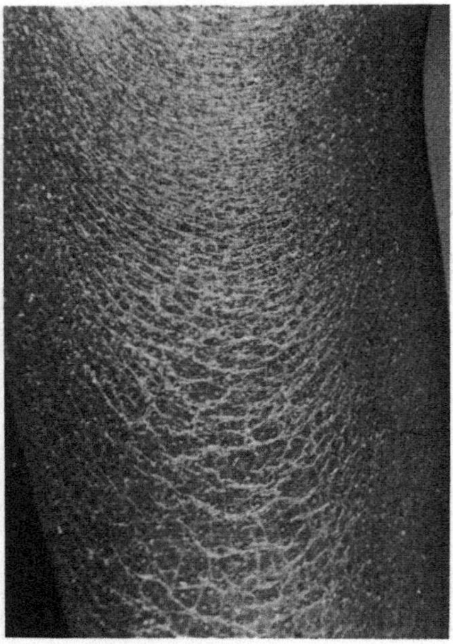

Fig. 19. Ichthyosis vulgaris (leg); scaly pigmented features are apparent. (Courtesy of Dr Y. de Prost)

dermal hyperplasia is expressed by the lack of the typically star-shaped image of crossing furrows.

Pathological disorders resulting from epidermal dysplasia and hyperplasia cover a large field. Psoriasis leads to a exaggerated thickening of epidermis and a disorganized stratum corneum from which the abnormal desquamative process leads to the formation of scales and clumps of cells.

In dealing with dry skin, we have shown that local modification of the microrelief is possible. In more severe situations, ichtyosis for example, excessive desquamative or thickening of the stratum corneum considerably changes the cutaneous relief (Fig. 19).

Conclusion

The skin surface represents the ultimate frontier of the human body, through which psychology and behavior may be transmitted, allowing the perception of an individual's personality by others. Physically, this surface is neither flat nor uniform. Its temperature and color may vary according to skin site and environment.

The major function of the skin is to act as a barrier which affords both protection and exchange between the organism and the outside world. It therefore plays a crucial role in maintaining the vital functions of the organism.

Despite its important implication in skin physiology, the skin surface has been scarcely studied in the past. As a matter of fact, investigations are just beginning; thus one can expect a better understanding through the new methods and techniques recently conceived by dermatologists and cosmetologists, to shortly follow. These new approaches allow description of the skin relief at various sites of the body and to follow its evolution with aging, sun exposure, and in response to pathological disorders.

In cosmetology, the effect of products on wrinkles or on dry skin can be described and quantified. These studies are, however, the first steps and constitute the initial data of a new field of research. They should shed light on our understanding of cutaneous physiology and in the role that the skin surface may play in the establishment of social relations. Regarding this duality, both dermatology and cosmetology will benefit from these new fields of research.

Acknowledgements. This article is dedicated to the late Dr. T. Cook, a pioneer in this field of research. Most of the figures presented in this chapter are taken from documents belonging to the Laboratoires de Recherche de l'OREAL, Département de Biophysique.

The authors are thus indebted to Ms A. M. Gracia and M. Huart who obtained and supplied the SEM documents. Dr. T. COOK (Elisabeth Arden, Indianapolis), Dr. O. de Lacharriere (Hospital Corentin Celton, Paris), Dr. G.E. Pierard (Hospital de Bavière, Liege), and Dr. Y. de Prost (Hospital Necker, Paris), are gratefully acknowledged for supplying some of the illustrations.

References

1. Graham JA, Kligman AM (1985) Physical attractiveness, cosmetic use and self perception in the elderly. Int J Cosmet Sci 7/2: 85–98
2. Hashimoto K (1974) New methods for surface ultrastructure: comparative studies or scanning electron microscopy, transmission electron microscopy and replica method. Int J Dermatol 13: 357–381
3. Feder M, Burggren W (1986) Comment respire la peau des vertébrés. Science Jan: 68–77
4. Corcuff P, de Rigal J., Leveque JL (1982) Image analysis of the cutaneous microrelief. International conference on bioengineering and the skin, Philadelphia, 1981. Bioeng Skin 4 1: 16–31
5. Langer K (1978) On the anatomy and physiology of the skin Br J Plast Surg 31: 3–8, 96–106, 185–199
6. Corcuff P (1985) Stereology of the skin surface: a comparison between aging and U. V. induced damages. In: Morganti P. Montagna W (eds) International symposium: a new look at old skin Rome 1985. International Ediemme Rome, pp 157–163
7. Corcuff P, de Rigal J, Leveque JL, Makki S, Agache P (1983) Skin relief and aging. J Soc Cosmet Chem 34: 177–190
8. Makki S, Agache P, Masouy P (1981) Quantitative assessment of skin aging through surface microtopography measurements. J Invest Dermatol 76: 428–433
9. Piérard GE, Franchimont C, Lapiere CM (1980) Aging as shown by the microanatomy and the physical properties of the skin. Int. J. Cosmet. Sci. 2 4: 209–214
10. Piérard GE, Hermanns JF, Lapiere CH (1974) Stéréologie de l'interface dermoépidermique. Dermatologica 149: 266–273
11. Schellander F, Headington J (1974) The stratum corneum – some structural and functional correlates. Br J Dermatol 91: 507–515
12. Ferguson J, Barbenel JC (1981) Skin surface patterns and the directional mechanical properties of the dermis. Marks R, Payne PA (eds) Bioengineering and the skin MTP, Lancaster, pp. 83–92
13. Takahashi M, Marks R (1986) Conformational and functional changes in the stratum corneum after forced extension. Bioeng Skin 2: 39–48
14. Corcuff P, Gracia AM, de Lacharriere O, Leveque JL (1989) Image analysis of the skin microrelief as a noninvasive method to approach the dermal architecture. In: Piérard G,

Piérard-Franchimont C (eds) The Dermis – from biology to diseases – monographies dermato pathologiques liégeoises. Franchimont, pp. 102–113
15. Ishida T, Kashibuchi M, Morita K, Yuasa S (1979) Measurements of skin roughness by computerized surface tracing and applications in cosmetics efficacy substantiation. Cosmet Toil 94: 39–47
16. Marks R, Pearse AD (1975) Surformetry: a method of evaluating the internal structure of the stratum corneum. Br J. Dermatol 92: 651–657
17. Makki S, Barbenel JC, Agache P (1979) A quantitative method for the assessment of the microtopography of human skin. Acta Derm Venereol (Stockh) 59: 285–291
18. Aubert L, Brun A, Grollier JF, Leveque JL (1982) A method to show the influence of cosmetic products on the cutaneous microrelief. Cosmet. Technol. Sci. 3: 265–270
19. Kadner H, Biesold C (1971) Zur Technik der Rauhigkeitsmessung der Hautoberfläche mit dem Perth-O-Meter. Dermatol Monatsschr. 157: 758–759
20. Cook TH (1980) Profilometry of skin – a useful tool for the substantation of cosmetic efficacy. J Soc Cosmet Chem 31: 339–359
21. Agache P, Mignot J, Makki S (1988) Microtopography of the skin and aging. Cutaneous aging 1: 475–499
22. Mandelbrot B (1975) Les objets fractals – forme, hasard et dimension. Flammarion, Paris
23. Nakayama Y (1985) Applications of image analysis to the microtopography of aging skin surface J Appl Cosmet 3: 106 (abstr)
24. Tankosic P, Burlet C (1986) Morphometric analysis of anisotropic and multioriented structures by use of an electronic image analyser (Quantimet 720): application to the study of the human cutaneous microrelief. Acta Stereolog 5/1: 87–92
25. Hoppe U, Sauermann G (1985) Quantitative analysis of the skin's surface by means of digital image processing J Soc Cosmet Chem 36: 105–123
26. Barton SP, Marshall RJ, Marks R (1989) A novel method for assessing skin surface topography. Bioeng Skin 3: 93–107
27. Gormley DE (1985) Automated optical profilometry. Bioengineering and the skin – San Francisco meeting, Sept. 1985
28. Hoppe U (1979) Topologie der Hautoberfläche. J Soc Cosmet Chem 30: 213–239
29. Corcuff P, Chatenay F, Leveque JL (1984) A fully automated system to study skin surface patterns. Int. J. Cosmet Sci 6: 167–176
30. Imayama S, Braverman IM (1989) A hypothetical explanation for the aging of skin. Am J Pathol 134/5: 1019–1025
31. Corcuff P, Francois AM, Leveque JL, Porte G (1988) Microrelief changes in chronically sun-exposed human skin. Photodermatology 5: 92–95
32. Kligman LH, Kligman AM (1985) Cutaneous photoaging by ultraviolet radiation. In: Maibach H, Lowe NJ (eds) Models in dermatology, vol 1. Karger, Basel, pp 59–68
33. Kligman LH (1986) Prevention and repair of actinic damage to skin. J. Soc. Cosmet. Chem. 37: 44
34. Linde YW, Bengtsson A, Loden M (1989) Dry skin in atopic dermatitis. Acta Derm Venereol 69: 311–319
35. Chanteloube F, Poulain E, Meybeck A (1982) Efficacy evaluation of anti-wrinkle products Cosmet Technol Sci 3: 277–281
36. Corcuff P, Chatenay F, Brun A (1985) Evaluation of anti-wrinkle effects on humans, Int J Cosmet Sci 7: 117–126
37. Bryce GF, Bogdan NJ, Brown CC (1988) Retinoic acids promote the repair of the dermal damage and the effacement of wrinkles in the UVB irradiated hairless mouse. J Invest Dermatol 91: 175–180
38. Grove GL, Grove MJ (1989) Optical profilometry: an objective method for quantification of facial wrinkles. J Am Acad. Dermatol. 3/2: 631–737

Quantitative Analysis of the Skin's Surface by Digital Signal Processing

U. Hoppe[1], R. Lunderstädt[2] and G. Sauermann[1]

Introduction

If you look at the nose
of your darling sweetheart
Magnified through a glass
It'll give you a start
For you'll find her complexion
Neither smooth nor clear
But pocked and pimpled
Like a wart hog's ear.
Michael Miller

The human skin's three dimensional surface is subjected to continuous structural changes. These result from the influences of the seasons, climate, diurnal rhythms, pathological conditions, age, psychic reactions, and cosmetics [1–6].

It is possible to quantitatively express the (normally slight) influences cosmetic preparations have on living human skin if one succeeds in thoroughly collecting all of the relevant data about the characteristics of the skin's structure. These characteristics are generally global in nature (based upon the mean values of a number of subjects), as the skin's surface has revealed itself to be a stochastic process which only conditionally permits individual descriptions.

Our work relies on a measurement technique which we first described in 1976. Its reproduction by other authors has demonstrated its great reliability [7–11].

Some modifications of the previously described methods were necessary in order to obtain a more exact analysis of the reactive capabilities of the human skin. These will be discussed in more detail later. The actual analyses were carried out by a digital computer. This required the development of the appropriate programs. The results thus obtained may be divided into three types concerned with (1) the geometry (topology) of the skin's surface, (2) the distributions, and (3) the spectral representations.

The last of these were determined with the aid of the Fast Fourier Transformation (FFT). In the concluding section of this paper, we shall present some elaborations having to do with not only the measuring apparatus, but also with multidimensional representations of the skin and the skin's "dynamics."

[1] Paul Gerson, Unna, Forschungszentrum Beiersdorf AG, 2000 Hamburg and
[2] Universität der Bundeswehr, Holstenhofstr. 35, 2000 Hamburg

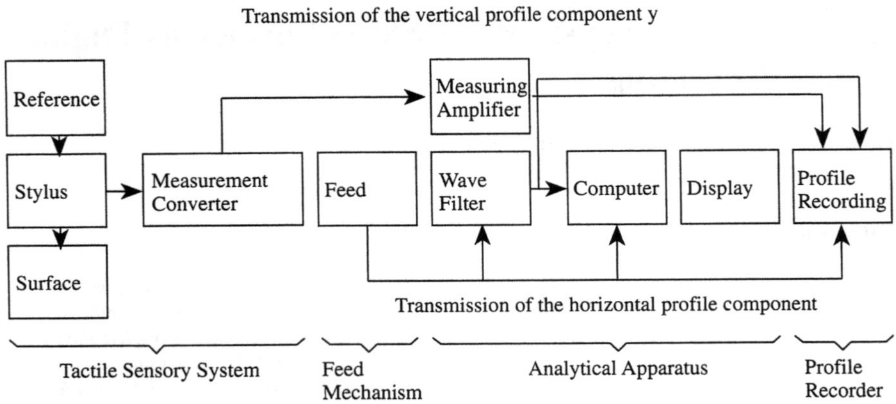

Fig. 1. Electromechanical sensing apparatus, according to DIN 4772

Data Collection

The methods used to obtain data on surface structures have been described in detail elsewhere [3, 4, 12]; the following schematic diagram illustrates the procedures used in attaining roughness profiles (Fig. 1)

By itself, this sensing apparatus is not sufficient for a state-of-the-art manipulation of the data it provides. For this reason, an analog magnetic tape is connected to a measuring amplifier. The collected data are recorded in situ on this tape. Next, this record is fed into a powerful digital computer, which then reads and digitalizes the data before providing an off-line analysis. The following illustration provides a schematic view of this process.

The end results are graphic, two-dimensional representations of skin samples which provide momentary records of the overall kinetics of the skin's topology (Fig. 2)

An unusually large number of measured points are required in order to comprehensively measure a skin sample. In our study, we thus restricted ourselves to dealing with just six profile segments per sample, each 4 cm in length, and all sharing a common midpoint. To be sure, these data are not enough to compute a geometric reconstruction of the skin sample it was obtained from; they do, however, permit one to recognize any anisotropies which may be present. The geometry used for obtaining these profile segments is shown in Fig. 3. The samples studied are skin impressions taken from the inner side of the forearm. The direction $\varphi = 0°$ is oriented towards the hand (north south), the direction $\varphi = 90°$ towards the body (ventrally/east west). In the corresponding fashion, the segments 1, 2, 3, 4, 5 and 6 are defined by intervals in which $\Delta\varphi = 30°$.

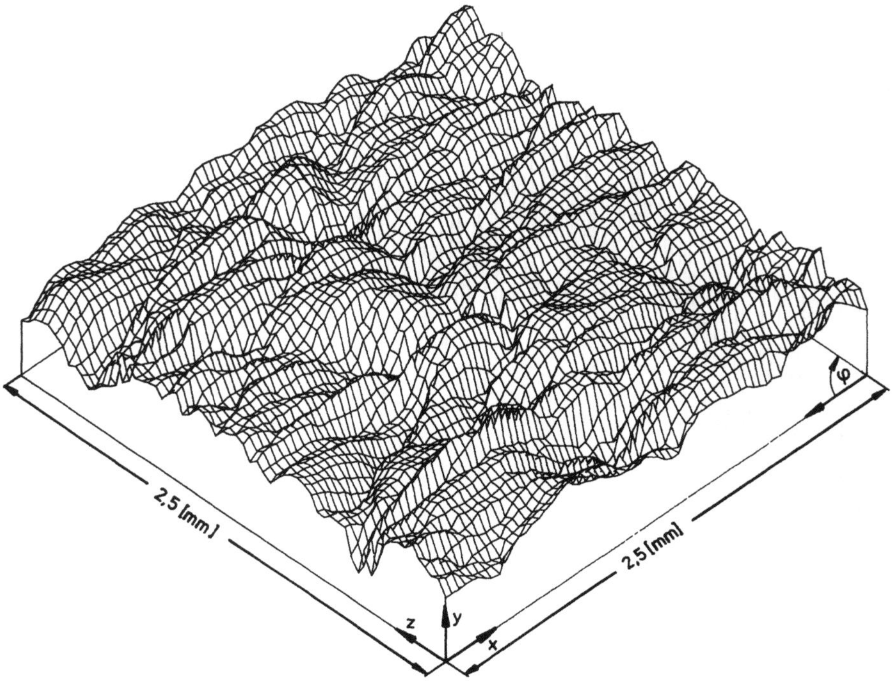

Fig. 2. Two-dimensional representation of a skin sample

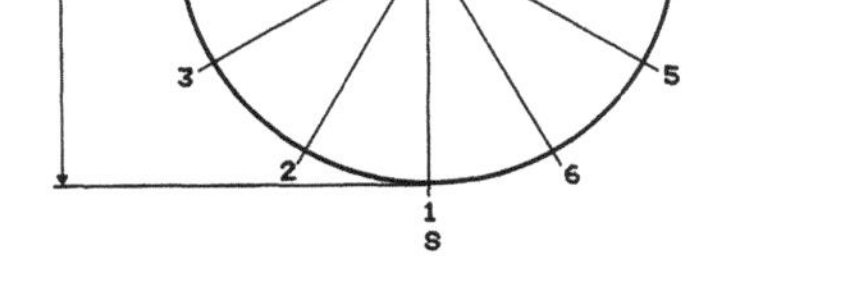

Fig. 3. Geometry of scanning

Preprocessing of Data

The data obtained through these procedures is stored in the computer. It is not yet available for immediate analysis. The signals possess both means deviating from "O" and fundamental waves which need to be eliminated. Normally, a wave filter suitable for this purpose would be used [12], but this method was not used in the present study. Instead, filtering occurred directly at the signal source through application of the appropriate computer algorithms [13]. Figure 4a presents a view of an uncorrected

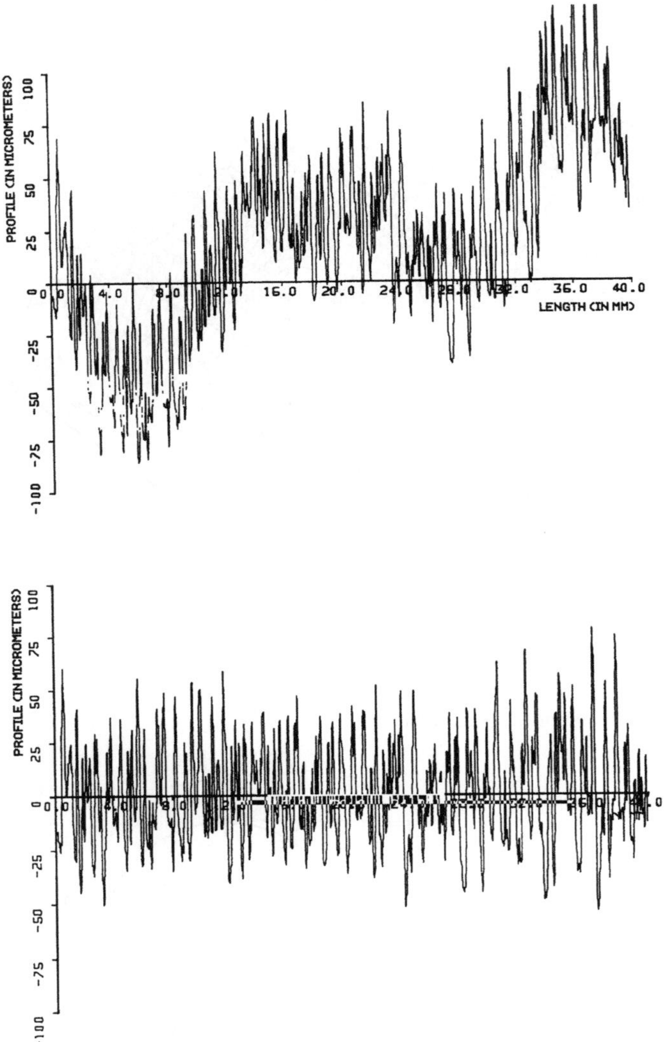

a

b

Fig. 4a, b. Uncorrected (**a**) and corrected (**b**) longitudinal section

profile section; the various natural oscillations in the data signal may be clearly seen. These problems are eliminated quickly and efficiently by means of an extremely elegant mathematical procedure, the so-called "migrating parabolae" (Fig. 4b).

The "migrating parabolae" is a very powerful principle, yet it is interesting that, up until now, it has rarely been used in practice.

The data corrected in this way are then "mirrored" by the computer, as they were taken from a negative impression of the skin sample under investigation. This step helps to avoid errors in measurement which could result from the production of a second (positive) impression (since a different type of material would have to be used

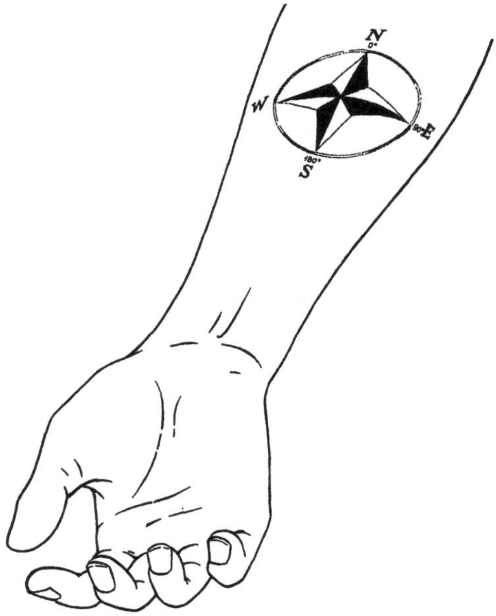

Fig. 5. Geometry for obtaining a longitudinal section

in order to avoid the possibility that the two impressions adhere together). Thus, all of the findings of this study are based upon a positive profile, even though only a single negative impression was made in each of the experimental stages.

Execution and Analysis

Prior to the beginning of the experiment, we determined the skin roughness of 19 female volunteers (aged between 24 and 58 years, $\bar{x} = 41$ years) using the replication technique just described [1–6]. Samples were taken of the skin on the inner side of both forearms. It had been previously determined that there were no significant differences in the skin roughness (untreated condition) of the individual subjects' left and right forearms (test conducted in January and February i.e., winter). Following this, the subjects treated twice a day (in the morning and in the evening) a selected area of one forearm with a standard water-in-oil-cream. The left/right positions of the skin areas to be tested had been previously randomized within the collective sample. Five weeks after the beginning of the study, both the treated areas and the contralateral untreated skin areas were marked with nail polish. This was done 12 h after the last application of the "W/O" cream.

Skin impressions were then obtained from both the treated and the untreated areas; for this, the arm was held out, with the palm facing upwards (Fig. 5). As nail polish had been used to mark the directions "north," "south," "east," and "west," it was possible to precisely position the impression while measurements were being taken.

One method of determining the effects of a cosmetic treatment is to analyze the roughness of the skin [1–6]. This provides information about the topology of the epidermal surface. Following this step, (statistical) distributions are determined. These are, first of all, important for hte topology; in addition, they provide an indication of the extent to which the skin's surface is statistical and by which (known) distribution it can be mathematically described. The third part of our study deals with spectral analyses. These go beyond the more global findings provided by the roughness and distributions and permit more individually oriented conclusions.

Each of the measured profile segments offered 4.096 points of measurement. As a total of six segments per impression were evaluated, this project (with its 19 volunteer subjects) evaluated a total of 466.944 points of measurement.

Roughness

The determination and analysis of roughness was carried out following guidelines set in the German Industrial Standards (*Deutsche Industrie Norm* = DIN) [12]; the appropriate definitions have been given in detail elsewhere. We determined the following roughness measures: the individual roughness depth (R_{ti}), the mean roughness depth (R_z), the smoothness depth (R_p), the arithmetic mean roughness value (R_a), and the square root mean roughness value (R_g). These measures of roughness vary in quality. The smoothness depth (R_p), the arithmetic mean roughness value (R_a), and the square root mean roughness value (R_g) are especially useful as they represent integral means, i.e., genuine means. These three measures are important because only genuine means may be used to describe stochastic and partially stochastic processes. Of these, the square root mean roughness value (R_g) is the most significant. This value, by definition, is identical with the standard deviation (s_o) of the surface structure. As a principle, the following important relation holds for Gaussian processes [14]:

$$R_v \equiv \frac{R_a}{R_q} = \sqrt{\frac{2}{\pi}} \cong 0.7978$$

R_z, R_p, R_q, R_a, and R_a/R_q–were determined for all 19 subjects, for both the untreated and treated conditions. This was done using the profile segments in the 6 directions in which $\varphi = 0°, 30°, 60°, 90°, 120°, 150°$. The resultant values are given in the following tables 1 and 2.

Table 1. Mean roughness values for all subjects (n = 19) (untreated condition)

$\bar{R}$[μm]	0°	30°	60°	90°	120°	150°	$\bar{R}_\varphi$
$\bar{R}_z$	191.92	183.86	183.40	177.22	176.04	187.24	183.28
$\bar{R}_p$	143.85	147.16	139.38	129.43	138.67	145.22	140.61
$\bar{R}_q$	34.73	34.62	32.65	31.78	33.54	34.13	33.57
$\bar{R}_a$	27.30	27.24	25.67	24.98	26.35	26.80	26.39
$\bar{R}_a \bar{R}_q$	0.7860	0.7868	0.7862	0.7860	0.7856	0.7852	0.7861

Table 2. Mean roughness values for all subjects ($n = 19$) (treated condition)

$\bar{R}[\mu m]$	0°	30°	60°	90°	120°	150°	$\bar{R}_\varphi$
$\bar{R}_z$	180.36	166.94	161.85	147.62	138.66	176.79	162.04
$\bar{R}_p$	129.12	117.34	114.68	117.27	114.07	120.24	118.78
$\bar{R}_q$	32.32	31.36	29.33	29.35	28.64	31.51	30.42
$\bar{R}_a$	25.20	24.83	23.26	23.03	22.52	24.82	23.95
$\bar{R}_a\ \bar{R}_q$	0.7797	0.7933	0.7930	0.7846	0.7863	0.7876	0.7873

Table 3. Changes in roughness values (measurements taken before to and after treatment) ($n = 19$)

$\Delta\bar{R}[\mu m]$	0°	30°	60°	90°	120°	150°	$\Delta\bar{R}$
$\Delta\bar{R}_z$	− 11.56	− 16.92	− 21.55	− 29.60	− 37.38	− 10.45	− 21.24
$\bar{r}_z$	− 6.02	− 9.20	− 11.75	− 16.70	− 21.23	− 5.58	− 11.58
$\Delta\bar{R}_p$	− 14.73	− 29.82	− 24.70	− 12.16	− 24.60	− 24.98	− 21.83
$\bar{r}_p$	− 10.23	− 20.26	− 17.72	− 9.39	− 17.73	− 17.20	− 15.52
$\Delta\bar{R}_q$	− 2.41	− 3.26	− 3.32	− 2.43	− 4.90	− 2.62	− 3.15
$\bar{r}_q$	− 6.93	− 9.41	− 10.16	− 7.64	− 14.60	− 7.67	− 9.38
$\Delta\bar{R}_a$	− 2.10	− 2.36	− 2.41	− 1.95	− 3.83	− 1.98	− 2.44
$\bar{r}_a$	− 7.69	− 8.66	− 9.38	− 7.80	− 14.53	− 7.38	− 9.24

Table 3 shows that roughness values fell as a result of treatment, an effect that was both expected and desired. Expressed quantitatively, the mean decreases were:

1. Mean roughness depth $\bar{r}_z = -11.58$ (%)
2. Smoothness depth $\bar{r}_p = -15.52$ (%)
3. Square root mean roughness value $\bar{r}_q = -9.38$ (%)
4. Arithmetic mean roughness value $\bar{r}_a = -9.24$ (%)

Another interesting finding shown in Table 3 is that the numerical values differ widely over the various directions. This indicates the presence of epidermal anisotropies. For this reason, Fig. 6 and Fig. 7 give the values for R_z, R_p, R_q, and R_a, for both the treated and the untreated conditions, again as a function of φ.

It can be plainly seen that all of the measures of roughness exhibit their smallest values in the direction of $\varphi = 90°$. This is especially true on R_z in the treated condition.

The anisotropies demonstrated in this way were subjected to further investigation. This involved the determination of all the standard deviations for all of the directions.

The skin's anisotropy can be seen in both the untreated and the treated conditions (Table 4). The finding that $\bar{R}_q$ and s_q exhibit more variability after treatment than before is evidently due to the fact that a treatment's effects vary from individual to individual. Summing up, we can say that both the roughness values and their standard deviations are minimal in the neighborhood fo $\varphi = 90°$. This is obviously a naturally advantageous direction in which the most pronounced results may be expected!

When these findings are correlated with the ages of the subjects and with seasonal factors, then the effects of treatment again become plain [1–6].

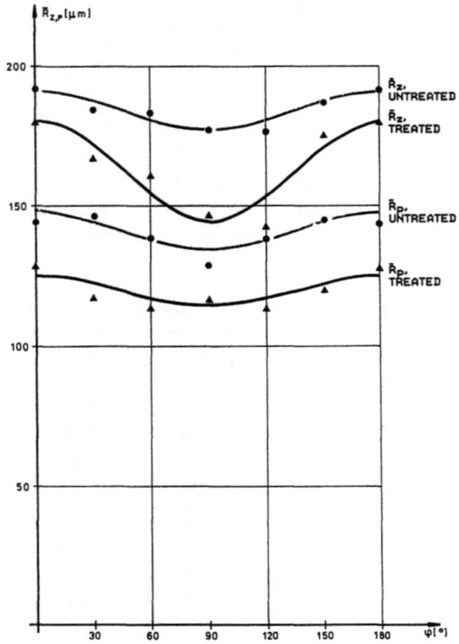

Fig. 6. Roughness R_z and R_p before and after treatment

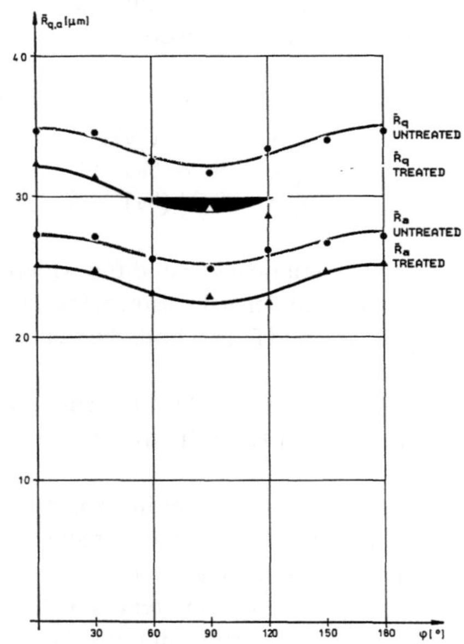

Fig. 7. Roughness R_q and R_a before and after treatment

These age correlations shall not be considered further at the present time, yet they are directly contained in the findings we have already discussed. For the relatively large standard deviations s_z and s_q are ultimately the result of age factors. The upshot is that the topology of the skin's surface is composed of both deterministic (periodic) and stochastic components, a crucial finding which will be considered in more detail in a moment. For now, however, we can point out that the computed values indicate that the distributions which can be expected to exhibit an almost Gaussian behavior [14].

$$\begin{array}{lll}\bar{\bar{R}}_v \text{ untreated} & = (\bar{\bar{R}}_a/\bar{\bar{R}}_q) \text{ untreated} & = 0.7861\\ \bar{\bar{R}}_v \text{ treated} & = (\bar{R}_a/\bar{R}_q) \text{ treated} & = 0.7873\\ (R_v \text{ theoretical} & & = 0.7978)\end{array}$$

Table 4. Standard deviations for $\bar{R}_z$ and $\bar{R}_q$ in untreated and treated conditions

$s_{z,q}$[μm]	0°	30°	60°	90°	120°	150°	$\bar{s}_{z,q}$
s_z	65.74	43.20	33.15	44.56	47.91	58.88	48.90
$s_z/\bar{R}_z$[%]	34.25	23.49	18.07	25.14	27.21	31.44	26.68
s_q	7.08	5.92	4.56	4.98	6.35	6.50	5.96
$s_q\bar{R}_q$[%]	20.30	17.12	13.91	15.63	18.91	19.10	17.71
treated							
s_z	63.75	42.95	36.62	31.61	28.17	39.96	40.51
$s_z/\bar{R}_z$[%]	35.34	25.73	22.63	21.41	20.31	22.60	25.00
s_q	9.11	8.06	5.61	4.89	4.66	7.61	6.86
$s_q/\bar{R}_q$[%]	28.11	25.73	19.10	16.63	16.25	24.14	22.51

Distributions

In order to obtain and investigate the distributions of the profile segments, one must first compute the corresponding histograms. An exact examination of these histograms indicates that the factors skewness and kurtosis must also be included in any analysis attempting to thoroughly describe all of the values of the Gaussian normal distribution.

From Fig. 8 it can be seen that the effects of treatment are primarily reflected in the amplitudes; the statistics of the distribution are, with respect to a treatment, generally invariant. The changes which do occur are in the direction of a normal distribution. A precise analysis of the histograms reveals that the surface of the human epidermis can be best characterized as a disturbed normal distribution. The "disturbances" result from the presence of both skewness and kurtosis. Thus, four statistical parameters are necessary to mathematically describe the distribution functions: mode and/or mean, standard deviation, skewness, and kurtosis see [15–17] for methods of computing these factors).

Physically, this means that we have a surface structure which generally features "shallow valleys" and "high-peaked mountains." This finding is important in that it means that the distributions can be computed analytically using known parameters. The troublesome task of preparing histograms is thereby eliminated.

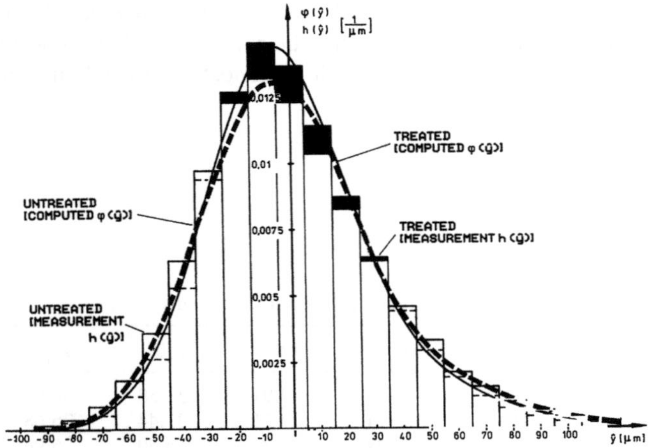

Fig. 8. Complete histogram as computed and as measured

Spectral Analysis

Up to now, this discussion of the various roughness values and distribution functions has been more global. We shall now refine our considerations through the use of spectral analyses. To this end we drew upon spectra, correlation functions, and the quantities derived therefrom.

Fourier Series and Fourier Integrals

A deterministic and continuous date sequence may be approximated with the aid of the Fourier series development [12]. The breaking down of such a sequence into its separate periodic and stochastic components, i.e., working out a Fourier series, is also known as Fourier analysis and spectral analysis. The sequence is called an amplitude curve and, also, a Fourier amplitude spectrum. The square of the amplitude spectrum is the auto spectrum (power spectrum). In our explanatory example (Fig. 9).

The amplitude spectrum is composed of just two discrete lines. As this discussion proceeds on the assumption that the data sequence is both periodic and continuous, and as these preconditions are not fulfilled in the present case, it is necessary to turn to the discrete Fourier transformation (DFT). Here, the underlying assumptions are that the data sequences are only present in a discrete form and that these, moreover, are finite. These conditions are normally met by scanning systems and are basic to the Fourier series. First, all of the surveyed skin structures are detected and analyzed using the FFT [18]. Of course, this method does not provide us with discrete amplitude spectra and autospectra; instead we obtain envelopes for these spectra. All of the topological information about the subject group's skin structures reappear in these spectra. To a certain extent, these spectra present the mathematical picture of the "normal" skin.

As Figs. 10–13 show, the autospectra consist of periodic components together with statistical background noise. One striking finding contained in these spectra is that we find an especially great accumulation of square amplitudes in the areas in which

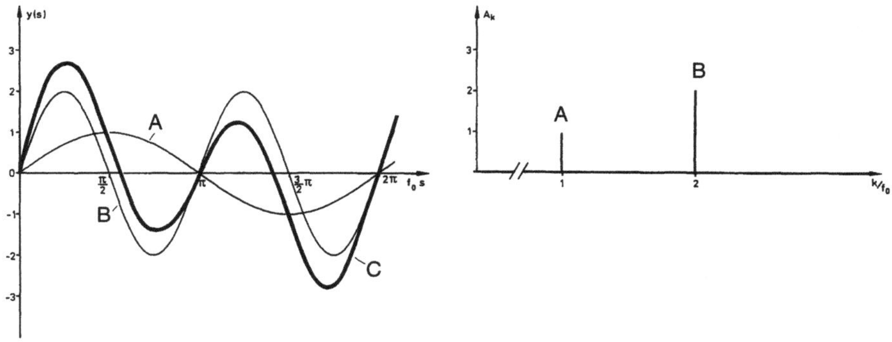

Fig. 9a.b. **a** Principle of the Fourier development. **b** Spectrum of amplitudes K = s/fo; A_k, amplitude (relative units). Oscillation C is defined as C = A + B

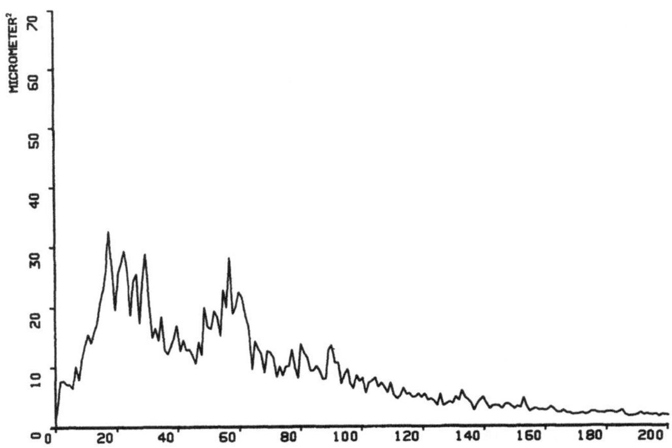

Fig. 10. Auto-spectrum over all directions; untreated condition

K = 20, 60, and 90. The frequencies F = 0.5, 1.5 and 2.25 (1/mm) are obviously quite prominent. The figures show that a cosmetic treatment with a W/O cream significantly lowers the square amplitude and, therewith, the amplitudes of the skin surfaces (the measured values also indicate that such changes take place) (see Tables 5 and 6). The drop occurs along the entire frequency range, a finding which is not revealed by the roughness values and distributions alone. A treatment with a W/O cream results in a homogenizing of the spectra; this effect is particularly pronounced in the realm of K = 60. Only traces of the periodic components remain in the mean spectra. This lends further support to the previously made claim that the periodic processes seen in the individual spectra are the realization of a stochastic process.

The effects of a cosmetic treatment are quite easily seen when the mean autospectra (i.e. φ 90°) for all directions are compared. This reflects the differences between the treated and untreated condition (Fig. 14).

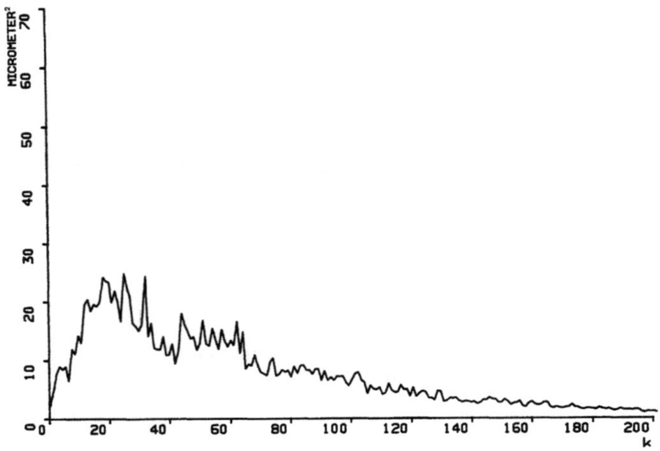

Fig. 11. Auto-spectrum over all directions; treated with a W/O cream

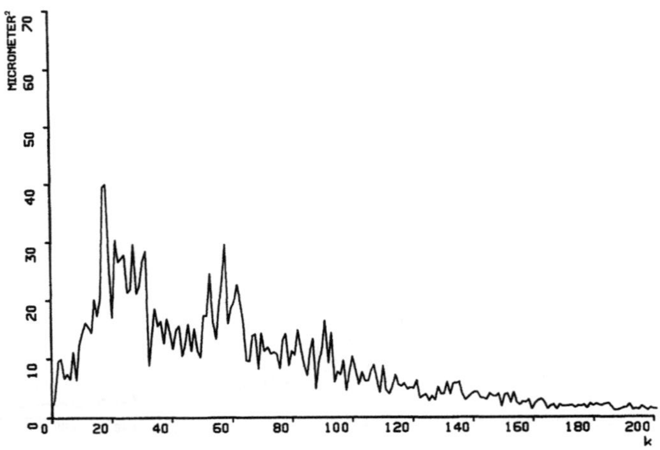

Fig. 12. Auto-spectrum means for the direction 90°, untreated condition

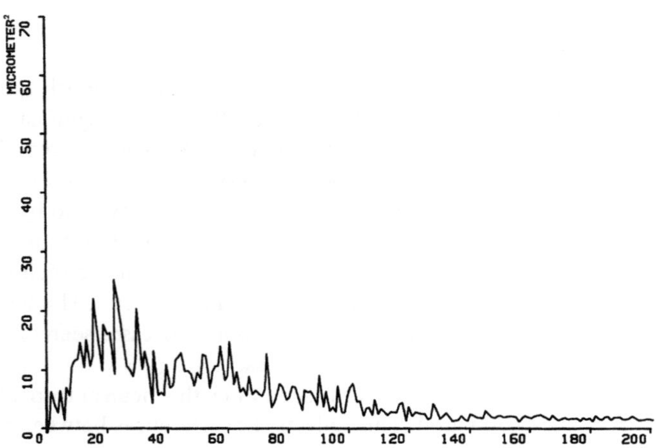

Fig. 13. Auto-spectrum means for the direction 90°, treated with W/O cream

Table 5. Means of the autospectrum for all subjects (untreated)

Parameter	0°	30°	60°	90°	120°	150°	Mean
$\bar{E}[\mu m^2]$	1970	1966	1931	1966	1984	1968	1964*
$s_{\bar{E}}[\mu m^2]$	377	338	324	333	373	352	349
$\frac{s_{\bar{E}}}{\bar{E}}$ [–]	0.191	0.171	0.168	0.169	0.188	0.178	0.177
$\frac{s_{\bar{E}}}{\bar{E}} \cdot 100\%$	19.1	17.1	16.8	16.9	18.8	17.8	17.7
$\bar{f}_m \frac{1}{mm}$	1.59	1.59	1.59	1.60	1.62	1.60	1.60
$\frac{1}{\bar{v}}$ [mm]	0.201	0.199	0.199	0.200	0.201	0.200	0.200

* Calculated up to K * 1024.

Table 6. Means of the autospectrum for all subjects (treated)

Parameter	0°	30°	60°	90°	120°	150°	Mean
$\bar{E}[\mu m^2]$	1519	1470	1420	1437	1485	1577	1484*
$s_{\bar{E}}[\mu m^2]$	555	457	378	399	494	534	470
$\frac{s_{\bar{E}}}{\bar{E}}$ [–]	0.365	0.310	0.266	0.277	0.332	0.338	0.316
$\frac{s_{\bar{E}}}{\bar{E}} \cdot 100\%$	36.5	31.0	26.6	27.7	33.2	33.8	31.6
$\frac{\bar{E}_{treated}}{\bar{E}_{untreated}}$	0.771	0.747	0.735	0.730	0.748	0.801	0.755
$\bar{f}_m \frac{1}{mm}$	1.60	1.60	1.59	1.60	1.58	1.57	1.59
$\frac{\bar{f}_{m\ treated}}{\bar{f}_{m\ untreated}}$	1.00	1.00	1.00	1.00	0.97	0.98	1.00
$\frac{1}{\bar{v}}$ [mm]	0.207	0.202	0.201	0.203	0.204	0.206	0.203
$\frac{v_{untreated}}{v_{treated}}$	1.029	1.105	1.010	1.015	1.014	1.030	1.015

* Calculated up to K * 1024.

Correlation Functions

The capabilities of the Fourier transformations are not exhausted with the computation and analysis of spectra. They find additional application within the framework of correlation theory, where they help to extract added data from the signals. The autocorrelation function (ACF) is a measurement of the "internal relationship" of a signal for various arguments s and s+r. The important advantage of the ACF is that, by following its development, it becomes possible to make statements about the signal itself. In

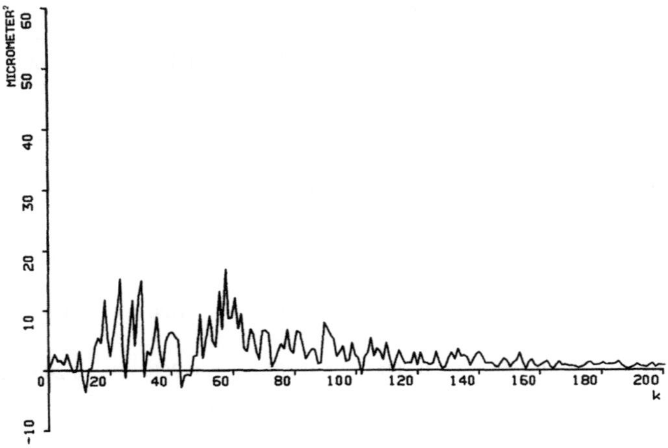

Fig. 14. Autospectrum over all directions; difference between treated and untreated condition

particular, the ACF can be used to separate the deterministic (especially periodic!) components of a signal from the stochastic components. The autocorrelation functions were then calculated for all subjects and all profile segments. Here, again, we find that both the periodic component of the ACF and the stochastic component are easily recognized and differentiated from one another. This provides us with decisive evidence in support of the claim that the periodic components of the epidermal surface are the realization of a stochastic process.

Spectral Analysis of the correlation functions

By means of a spectral analysis of the correlation functions of those regions in which the estochastic signal components have abated, it was possible to quantitatively separate the periodic components of a signal from its stochastic components. This is a very arduous procedure which will not be detailed here, although one interesting finding should be mentioned. While we found that the overall energy exhibits an almost completely isotropic behavior in the untreated condition (a fact which has already been pointed out), an anisotropy is present in the treated condition (an analogous situation was found with the roughnesses). For $\varphi = 90°$, $\bar{E}_{tr}$ is minimal. The energy $\bar{E}_p$ of the periodic component displays a different behavior: *it is anisotropic both before and after treatment*. These findings are depicted graphically in Fig. 15 in the untreated condition, $\bar{E}_p$ is maximal at $\varphi = 90°$. In contrast, $\bar{E}_p$ is minimal following treatment. The energy of the stochastic component ($\bar{E}_s$) behaves anisotropically in the untreated condition (with a minimum at $\varphi = 90°$; in the treated condition, $\bar{E}_p$ is practically isotropic. This means that the periodic component of the skin's surface is more strongly affected by a treatment than is the stochastic component. With $\bar{E}_p$, the effects of treatment are maximal at $\varphi = 90°$ and minimal at $\varphi = 0°$. The opposite relationships hold true for $\bar{E}_s$.

In other words, we find that a treatment leads to a reduction of the periodic structures. The skin becomes more lawless, i.e., "more uniform."

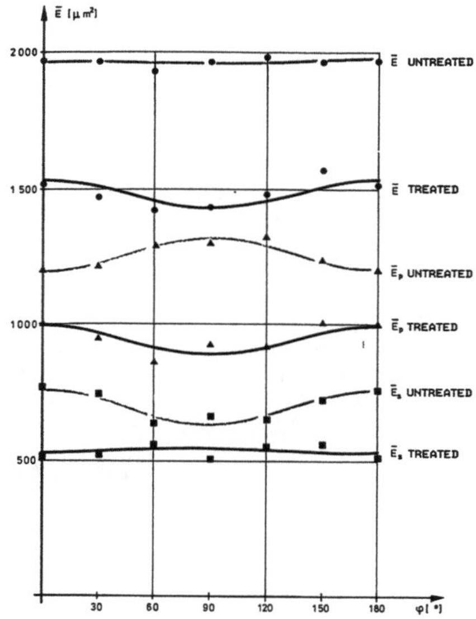

Fig. 15. Amounts of energy, before and after treatment

Future Prospects

The experiments described herein concentrated on investigating the roughness, distributions, and spectra of the untreated and treated human skin. While some of the findings pertaining to roughness and distributions have been previously published [1–6], the discussion of the spectra is new. The experimental work made use of preexisting apparatus. This apparatus is powerful (in the classical sense), yet it still does not entirely fulfill the needs of state-of-the-art signal processing. One method for improving both resolving power and processing speed is that of Bitz [19], in which characteristic roughness values are obtained by means of diffused light.

This entire discussion is based solely on the investigation of profile segments, in other words, our modes of procedure were onedimensional. In the final analysis, such methods are unsatisfactory, as an adequate description of the topology of the skin's surface is only possible when two dimensions are used. While computer programs suitable for the purpose have been developed, the lack of appropriate data has prevented their extensive use. In an attempt to test the power of such a program, we measured an untreasted skin sample from a single volunteer. The total surface area of this sample was 10 mm x 10 mm = 100 mm^2. Each direction (profile segment) was broken down into 256 points, corresponding to a scanning distance between points = 0.04 mm. The skin surface was reconstructed using the 65 536 points thus measured (Fig. 3).

The two-dimensional Fourier transformation is an indispensable aid for state-of-the-art procedures of picture processing. Its use, however, presupposes the availability of an extremely powerful computer (powerful in terms of both data processing capabilities and processing speed). The two-dimensional autospectrum shown in Fig. 16 and the two-dimensional representation of the ACF (Fig. 17) contain all of the topological

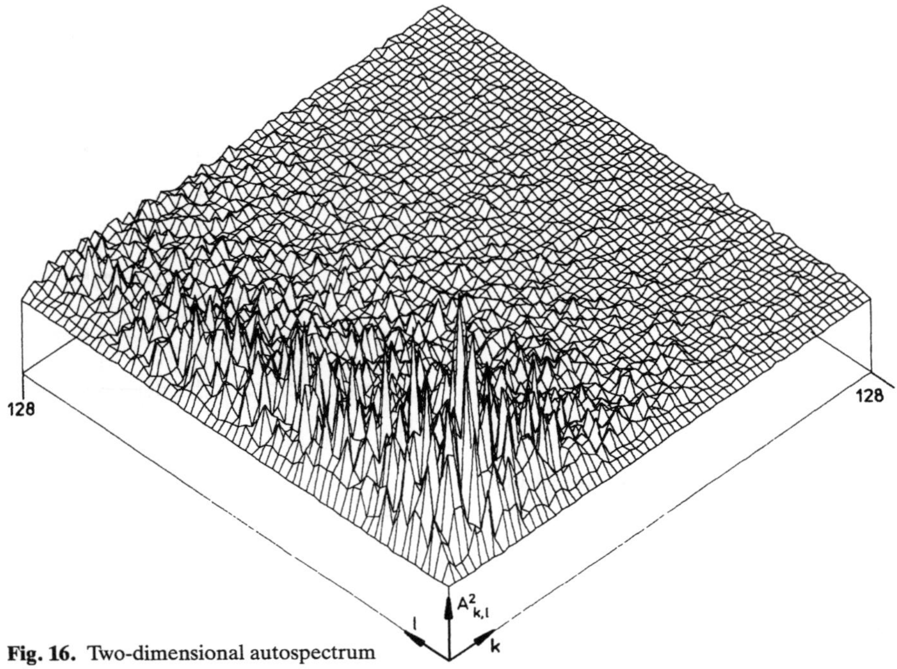

Fig. 16. Two-dimensional autospectrum

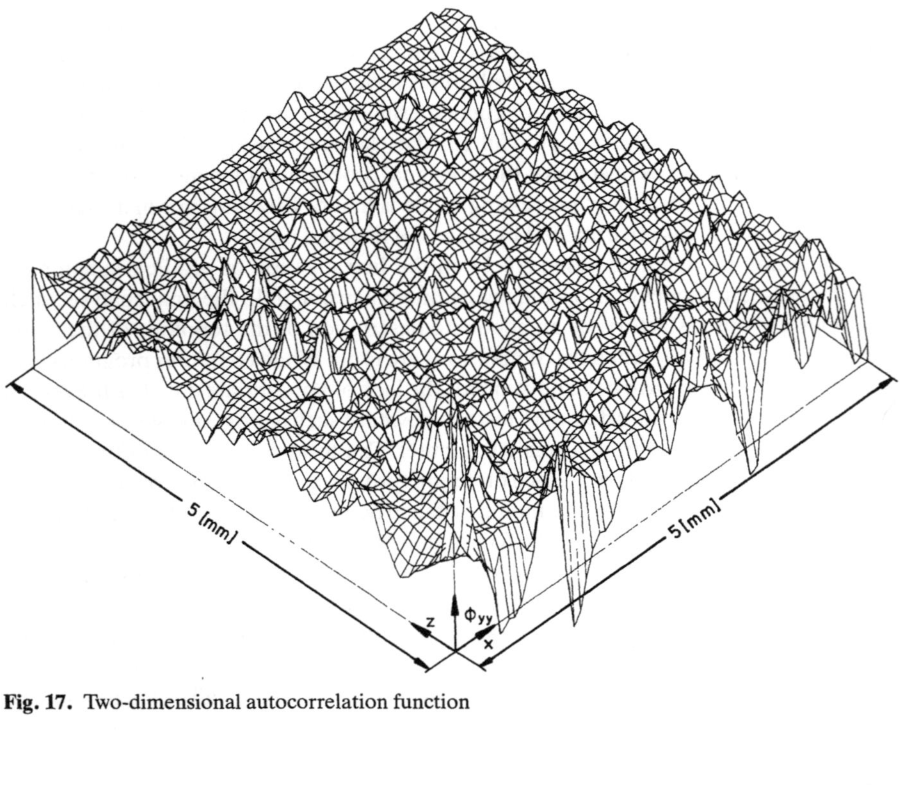

Fig. 17. Two-dimensional autocorrelation function

information about the skin's surface structure. Both the stochastic components and the occurrences of periodicities are quite graphically presented.

Finally, we should like to make a few comments about the "dynamics" of the skin. All of the investigations conducted for this study are of a purely static nature, i.e., they represent "snapshots" of equilibrium states. Of future importance is a method which would consider the behaviour of the skin over time (some preliminary thoughts on this subject can be found in [1–6]. In order to be able to precisely describe the effects of a given treatment, it would be necessary to know when such effects begin, how they develop, and how long they continue. Only then would we fully know what the effects of any particular cosmetic preparation are. Arranging findings sequentially provides an indication of the temporal behavior (kinetics). For example, roughnesses, distributions, spectra, and the values derived from them can be expressed as a function of time. This is another area for future research, one which would require genuine innovation.

References

1. Hoppe U (1976) Topologie der Hautoberfläche. Symposium "Stratum corneum" Berlin, 3–4 December 1976
2. Hoppe U Müller L (1977) Verfahren zur Bestimmung der Rauhigkeit der Oberfläche der menschlichen Haut. DBP 2719341; 30 April 1977
3. Hoppe U (1979) Topologie der Hautoberfläche. J Soc Cosmet Chem 30: 213–239
4. Hoppe U (1981) "Stratum corneum" Struktur und Function. Klaschka F (ed) 1981 In: Cosmetic technology. Grosse, Berlin, pp 141–158
5. Hoppe U (1981) The topology of the skin, part I. Cosmet Technol Febr. 1981 XX: 54–59
6. Hoppe U (1981) The topology of the skin part II. Cosmet Technol March 1981 XX: 32–38
7. Cook TH (1980) Profilometry of skin – a useful tool for the substantiation of cosmetic efficacy. J Soc Cosmet Chem 31: 339–359
8. Cook TH, Craft TJ, Brunelle RL, Norris F, Griffin WA (1982) Quantification of the skin's topography by skin profilometry. Int J Cosmet Sci 4: 195–205
9. Barbenel JC, Makki S, Agache P (1980) The variability of skin surface contours. Annals of Biomedical Engineering 8 (2) 175–182
10. Marks R, Nicholls SC (1981) Drugs which influence the stratum corneum and techniques for their evaluation. Clin Exp Dermatol 6: 419–427
11. Makki S, Mignot J, Nadvornik IM, Agache P (1982) Statistical analysis of human skin microtopographical profiles. Proceedings of the 12th IFSCC congress, Paris 13–17 September 1982, E 2, pp 257–269
12. Deutsche Norm DIN 4760 bis 4766, 4768 und 4769, 4771 bis 4775. Beuth, Berlin.
13. Bendat JS, Piersol AG, Random data: analysis and measurement procedures. Wiley, (1980) New York
14. Mesch F (1980) Beschreibung rauher Oberflächen durch zweidimensionale Korrelationsfunktionen und Spektren. V. Oberflächenkolloquium, Dresden
15. Lunderstädt R, (1980) Rechnerorientierte Verfahren der Regelungstechnik, Teil III: Stochastische Systeme. Lecture, Hochschule der Bundeswehr Hamburg (HSBwH), Hamburg
16. Papoulis A (1965) Probability, random variables and stochastic processes Mc-Graw Hill, New York
17. Korn GA, Korn TM (1961) Mathematical handbook for scientists and engineers. Mc-Graw Hill, New York
18. Oppenheim AV, Schafer RW (1975) Digital signal processing. Prentice Hall, Englewood Cliffs
19. Bitz G (1982) Verfahren zur Bestimmung von Rauhigkeitskenngrößen durch Specklekorrelation. VDI Fortschrittsbericht, part 8, no. 47, Düsseldorf

Noninvasive Methods for the Determination of Skin Hydration

A. Triebskorn and M. Gloor*

Introduction

In 1953, Blank [1] showed that water makes up 10%–20% of the stratum corneum. As soon as the amount of water decreases below 10%, the skin develops a rough and dry looking appearance. Kligman [17], in 1963, maintained that the lipids of the skin surface were of no essential significance for the appearance of the horny layer, rather that the appearance of the skin is mainly due to the water content of the horny layer. Based on the postulated affiliation between stratum corneum hydration and the macroscopic aspect of the skin, diverse methods for assessing horny layer hydration have been developed (for details see Gloor's outline in chapter 3 of [7].

The aim of our own investigations was to answer the following questions: (1) To what extent do the results achieved by some of the frequently used hydration assessment methods correlate with one another. (2) The water content of which layer of the stratum corneum is determined by the various methods? (3) Do changes in the water content of the horny layer which are within the physiological range impact the appearance of the skin, as may be supposed on the basis of Blank's [1] work? Before addressing these questions, some of the more frequently used in vivo techniques will be outlined.

Methods

Capacitance Measurement with the Corneometer-technique

The fundamentals of this method were developed by Bingmer and Tronnier. The method is based on the dielectric constant of water ($\varepsilon_r \approx 81$), which is very high in comparison with that of other substances. The probe is designed as a scatter-field capacitor (Fig. 1). By a polymer foil of defined thickness, it is separated from the horny layer, which forms the major part of the dielectric measured. Due to the above mentioned high ε_r of water, the dielectric characteristics of the stratum corneum depend on its water content, to a large extent, so that a range of determinations is possible. State of the art equipment which is available on the market includes the Corneometer CM 820 (Courage and Khazaka, Cologne, FRG). Possible sources of error or potential sources of variation in the method are, according to the location of the measurement site, sweat production, filling of the sweat gland ducts, the number of hair follicles, the electrolyte content of the stratum corneum, and artefacts from applied topical agents.

* Hautklinik des Städtischen Klinikums Karlsruhe, Moltkestrasse 18, 7500 Karlsruhe, Germany

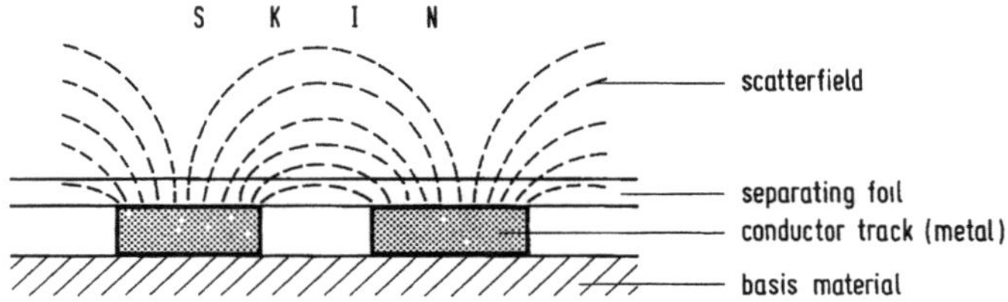

Fig. 1. Principle of the corneometer probe. Metallic conductor tracks are separated from the skin by a polymer foil covering the probe. During the measurement, an electric scatterfield penetrates the skin. The dielectric measured is highly dependent on the water content of the stratum corneum, due to the high dielectric constant of water

Resonance Frequency Measurement

This method was first described by Tronnier and Wagener [33]. The principle is based on the fact that changes in the water content of the stratum corneum also induce changes in the mechanical properties of the horny layer. A stylus conducts the oscillations produced by a frequency generator onto the skin. At a certain distance, these oscillations are registered by a receptor stylus. The oscillation generating and receiving functions may also be taken over by a single stylus. While measuring, the frequency of the magnetic system is gradually raised, and the intensity of the oscillation of the skin can be registered as a function of the frequencies used. Thus, determination of the resonance frequency of the skin is possible. The more the stratum corneum hydration increases, the lower the resonance frequency of the skin.

The thickness of the horny layer, the thickness and tension of the skin, and the nature of underlying tissues (e.g., bone, muscle) are to be considered as sources of error. By using the same sites for measuring before and after an experimental application of topical agents, some sources of error may be eliminated.

A further method using the mechanical properties of the skin for the determination of stratum corneum hydration was described by Potts et al. [24], a few years ago. These authors made use of an instrument which evaluates, at frequencies between 8 and 1016 Hz, the dynamic mechanical properties of the skin by measuring the propagation and impairment of shear waves.

Electric Conductance / Resistance Measurements

Diverse electric signals may be attained from human skin, for example, the galvanic skin response and the skin potential level (for detailed explanations see [34]). To gain insight in to skin hydration in vivo, we are interested in changes of the skin resistance level. In normal skin, this is a tonic value which shows little change during the course of the day.

Variations in the method include the option of AC/DC current or voltage, and the electrode design (form, surface, contact pressure, material, humid/dry, polarizable/ nonpolarizable, unipolar/bipolar, etc.). For AC measurement techniques, additional options include current intensities, voltages, and frequencies used. The distinct procedures only permit statements on certain aspects of the correlation between the electric properties of the skin and its structure or physiological state. This is due to the complicated architecture of the skin, with its heterogenous laminar structures but also, e.g., variously filled sweat glands and sebaceous gland ducts. As all morphological elements are taken into account, electric measurements on the skin are often difficult to interpret.

Special Aspects of DC Resistance/Conductance Techniques

According to Edelberg [5], the resistance of the skin accounts for at least 90% of the resistance value measured between two arbitrary sites of the surface of the body. According to Keller [16], the skin resistance measured when using DC is mostly to be interpreted as a polarization resistance, more precisely "as a combination of several kinds of polarizable capacitors and diverse unpolarizable resistors ..., which are partly switched in a parallel, partly in a serial way to capacitors." Rothman [28], too, considers skin resistance to be a "pseudoresistance" because of the polarization phenomena. These phenomena may be responsible for the fact that resistance values up to the range of 10^{10} Ω, i.e., up to the giga-ohm range, are found, thus demanding high standards for the accuracy to the measurement equipment. Similar maximal values were also reported by Wienert et al. [36] and Campbell et al. [3]. Keller states that two basic types of capacities contribute to the origin of polarization: double layer capacities and diffusion capacities.

Sources of error may be the hair follicles and the filling state of the sweat gland ducts as electric paths with low resistance; therefore, an appropriate temperature of the room (22°C), a constant relative humidity (50%–55%), and possibly the suppression of sweat gland activity by drugs (scopolamine methylbromide) may be advised for measurements of stratum corneum hydration.

In DC resistance measurement with dry electrodes on the nonsweating subject, the high resistance value of the horny layer lies in series with the much lower resistance of the layers below. Therefore, the resistance of the horny layer determines the resistance value measured and reflects essentially the relative dryness of the stratum corneum and also its electrolyte content, to a certain degree.

When applying an electrolyte solution as an electrode medium, the humidification of the horny layer causes a reduction of the electric resistance to a minimum. In that case, the resistance measured does not indicate the hydration but, more likely, the thickness and density of the stratum corneum and the permeability of the underlying layers. Therefore, dry electrodes should be used for measurements of stratum corneum hydration.

Special aspects of AC Impedance/Conductance Techniques

According to Lawler et al. [20], no inductive properties can be attributed to the skin. Therefore, only the capacitive properties of the skin and its real ohmic resistance determine its impedance when using AC techniques. With rising frequency, the capacitance diminishes. Thus, the impedance diminishes, too. There is little doubt, according to Edelberg [5], that the impedance equals the ohmic resistance of the skin when using frequencies above 10 kHz. Thus, when the intensity of the polarization is diminished with rising frequencies, it is completely eliminated from the resistance value measured.

For details of the diverse resistance/impedance/conductance techniques described in the literature, see Clar [4], Campbell et al. [3], Wienert et al. [36], and Tagami et al. [30]. For our own investigations, we used a specially constructed AC conductance instrument with dry electrodes made of stainless steel, which permits measurements at 1.5 and 15 kHz [32]. For DC resistance measurements, we used another specially designed instrument with a total measurement range up to 20 giga-ohms, for which we also used dry electrodes made of stainless steel.

Infrared Spectroscopy Using the Attenuated Total Reflectance Method

This method was first employed in dermatologic research in the 1970s by Putnam [26] and Osberghaus et al. [22]. For years, infrared spectroscopy has been an established method for physics, chemistry and for technical analysis in industry.

Basic Physical Principles

First, a short summary of the most important physical principles. The use of infrared spectroscopy is based primarily on the principle of the weakening of infrared radiation by absorption in a different medium (besides the weakening of a ray via scattering by small solid particles). Absorption of infrared light is possible only when the molecules stimulated have a dipolar electric structure. Such molecules are called infrared-active. Tissue proteins and water as well are infrared-active substances. The absorption of infrared light occurs inside these molecules or parts of these molecules via two mechanisms:

(1) by way of oscillation, when the infrared light frequency is the same as the innate frequency of the molecules, and
(2) by way of rotation. The priming of rotation states by absorption of photons is possible at various frequencies. Pure priming of rotation states alone, however, occurs only at radiation frequencies in the far infrared spectrum and is of no importance in photometry.

Often, both mechanisms mentioned occur simultaneously as "combined excitation." As a result of the frequency dependency of oscillation or rotational energy, every substance or functional unit of a substance has its own typical absorption maxima or transmission minima at certain frequencies. These maxima or minima are specific for the substance or for a functional unit. When absorption maxima of a test substance are shown graphically in the infrared spectrum, one obtains a diagram that, because of the specificity of certain absorption maxima for certain chemical groups, can directly give clues as to the molecular constitution of the substance.

Support for the Usefulness of Infrared Spectroscopy in Dermatologic Research

Why can infrared spectroscopy be used in dermatology or cosmetic research? As mentioned before, Osberghaus et al. [22] used infrared spectroscopy for dermatologic research in the manner to be described here. In the same manner, Gloor and various coworkers [8, 9] used this method to examine other research aspects.

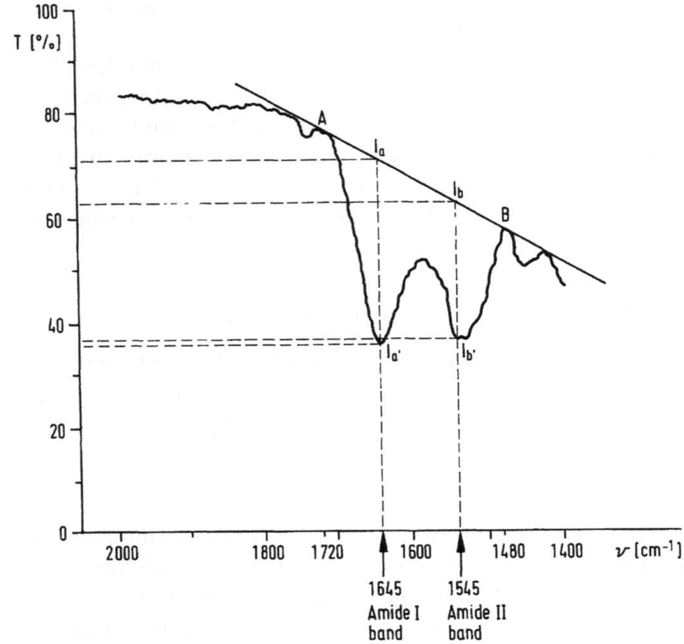

Fig. 2. Infrared spectrogram of human stratum corneum (part). The amide I band at 1645 cm^{-1} is sensitive to the presence of water in the stratum corneum, whereas the amide II band at 1545 cm^{-1} is independent of the water content. By a graphing procedure, the baseline method (see text), the moisture factor as measure of stratum corneum hydration is evaluated

Amide groups of tissue proteins have a total of six absorption bands in the infrared spectrum. Two of these lie at the wave numbers (reciprocal value of the wavelength) 1545 cm^{-1} and 1645 cm^{-1} (Fig. 2). The absorption at the so-called amide I band at 1645 cm^{-1} follows stimulation of a C=O (carbonyl group) stretch oscillation; absorption at the so-called amide II band at 1545 cm^{-1} after stimulation of a C-N stretch oscillation and a C-N-H deformation oscillation. Very close to the amide I band, i.e., at 1640 cm^{-1}, we find a strong disturbance band for water, which arises by OH-deformation-oscillation and overlaps onto the amide I band at 1640 cm^{-1}. Thus, the amide I band reacts sensitively to an increase in water content in stratum corneum protein. Contrarily, amide II band behavior is not influenced by the presence of water. The different relationship in intensity between the two bands can thus be used as a relative dimension for measurement of stratum corneum hydration. For a quantitative evaluation of stratum corneum hydration, one takes the quotient of the maximal extinction values of both amide bands using the so-called baseline method. This quotient is also called the hydration factor.

Further infrared absorption bands that react sensitively to the presence of water lie at 3400 cm^{-1} (stimulation of OH-stretch oscillation) and at 2100 cm^{-1}. Potts et al [25] consider the latter absorption band to be of particular importance because, despite its weak delineation, it lies in a spectral range where the skin and the majority of topical agents show no absorption. In another baseline method, these authors use the absorption band at 2100 cm^{-1} as a dimension for measuring water concentration in the stratum corneum.

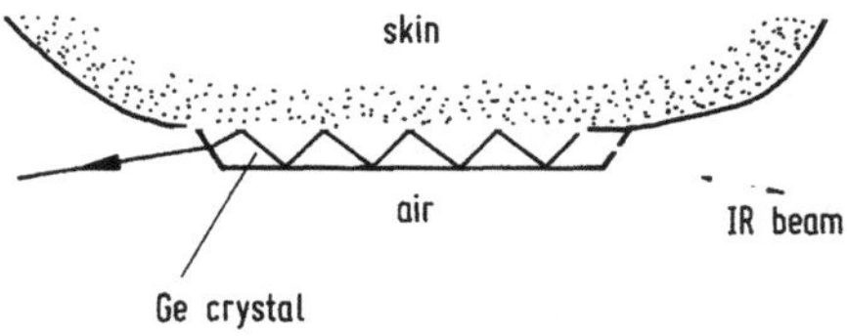

Fig. 3. Principle of the FMIR (frustrated multiple internal reflection) method. Infrared radiation enters one side of a germanium crystal. Due to the high reflecting potential of germanium, as a medium with high optical density, the greatest part of infrared radiation is repeatedly reflected inside the crystal, at the borders of the optically lower dense media in contact with the crystal (here: skin and air), before it leaves the crystal at the opposite small edge. Only a minimal amount of the infrared radiation penetrates into the skin, where it is nearly completely absorbed.

Apparatus

The apparatus for carrying out dermatologic research consists of an infrared spectral photometer (for example, model 297, Perkin Elmer and Co., FRG) with an additional unit for measurement according to the attenuated total reflectance method (ATR). For this purpose, an FMIR (frustrated multiple internal reflection) accessory is adequate. The measurement principle is based on the ATR of an IR ray at the surface between an optically denser medium (here, a germanium crystal) and an optically thinner medium (here, air or skin). The method has established itself in industry for the inspection of surfaces of materials, e.g., textiles, and is employed as follows:

The FMIR accessory (Fig. 3) is installed in the sample compartment of the photometer. The flexor side of the forearm is placed upon the horizontally situated germanium crystal so that the stratum corneum has direct contact with the surface of the crystal. Due to the crystal's high reflection capacity, the ray is reflected in numerous directions on the surfaces between the crystal and the skin or between crystal and air. On the other end of the compartment, the ray leaves the crystal. However, only a portion of the infrared radiation is reflected inside the crystal: A small part of it enters the optically thinner medium, that is the stratum corneum of the skin, when the reflection angle of the ray at the surface of the crystal reaches and overcomes a so-called critical angle. The light that exits here is then almost completely absorbed.

The reduction of the total inner reflection, and with it the decrement in infrared intensity, is used as a dimension for measuring absorption. The penetration depth of the infrared light perpendicular to the specimen lies in the magnitude of a few microns [10]. In comparison, the stratum corneum thickness in the skin of the flexor forearm is approximately 15 μm. Method variability arises when a zinc-sulfide crystal instead of a germanium crystal is employed or when a Fourier transformation infrared spectrophotometer (for example, Analect FX- 6 200, Laser Precision, Irvine, CA) which delivers a wide range of measurement data is used. Both variations have been employed by Potts et al. [25].

Infrared Spectroscopy – Applications in Cosmetic Research

In questions pertaining to cosmetics, it is of greater interest to know to what extent various topical agents influence the moisture level of the stratum corneum. Problems can arise here because the water content of topical agents influences the amide I band, while other topical agent components can change the water-independent amide II band. As an example, we cite a comparison of the infrared spectrum analysis of untreated skin and the infrared spectrum of soft soap (Sapo kalinus) treated skin from an experiment by Gloor et al. [8]. The amide I band of soft soap treated skin derives from the water content of the soap being used, the amide II band derives from the asymmetric oscillation stimulation of the carboxylate group of the fatty acid component of the same soap. The soap shows an absorption maximum of the symmetric carboxyl group at 1400 cm^{-1}.

Presuming that the absorption maximum at 1545 cm^{-1} from the carboxylate group and the other maximum at 1400 cm^{-1} from the carboxyl group are proportional to each other, a correction factor can be calculated by comparing them with the infrared absorption of untreated skin at 1400 cm^{-1}, thus eliminating the error introduced by the topical agent. Osberghaus et al. [22], in their test of a moisturizer, were also able to compute a correction factor to eliminate the error caused by the topical agent. Potts et al. [25] attempted to eliminate the error caused by topical agents by using the water-dependent infrared absorption at 2100 cm^{-1} as a reference point for moisture. In this spectral range, it is said that absorption is influenced neither by the skin nor by topical agents frequently used. The authors mentioned were the first who were able to prove in in vitro tests with stratum corneum preparations that a quantitative relationship between infrared absorption and water concentration in the stratum corneum (in g/cm^3) exists. Due to these findings, it may be possible in the future to establish a direct relationship between hydration elevations in the stratum corneum with the help of dermatologic or cosmetic topicals and the water concentration at the site treated.

Photoacoustic Spectroscopy

According to Kölmel et al. [18], in this method the periodic heating of a sample by the absorption of chopped light is detected by a sensitive microphone which measures the pressure oscillations in an adjacent sealed gas volume. The photoacoustic signal depends on both the optical and the thermal properties of the sample, since signal generation is determined by the diffusion of heat from the sample interior to the sample-gas interface. For the investigation of the hydration properties of the horny layer, this seems to be one of the most depth-sensitive methods. For further details, see also Rosencwaig [27].

Scanning Electron Microscopy

For a description and evaluation of this technique, see the chapter by Leveque in this volume.

Profilometry

For the registration of the skin surface profile and for the calculation of diverse measures of surface roughness, it is suitable to use electromechanical surface measurement equipment similar to tap-cut instruments (*Tastschnittgeräte*), used for many years in the metal and technical industries to monitor product surfaces.

These instruments have a tapping diamond, which is located on a movable fixed magnetic stylus and which is conducted horizontally at constant speed over a pre-

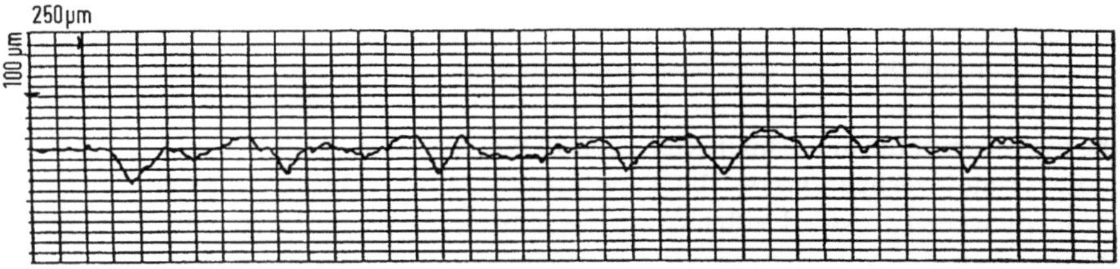

Fig. 4. Profilogram of a positive cast of the stratum corneum

conceived distance of the profile. The resulting vertical deviations of the stylus change the surrounding magnetic field by electric induction. This signal is amplified and is passed on to a profile diagram plotter or is used for the calculation of the preprogrammed roughness parameters in the computation portion of the instrument. At last, the profile of the sample on graph paper (Fig. 4) including an exact value for roughness is obtained. The scrub of the positive cast is negligibly low. The quantitative evaluation of the surface roughness is made with the aid of standardized roughness parameters (DIN 4760–4768) R^a, R^p, R^t, R^z, R^m. Out of those, R^a, R^p and R^t have proven to be especially appropriate for describing the roughness of the skin surface.

Profilometry can be used either directly on negative casts, as described, e.g., by Hoppe [12], or on polymer positive casts, which have been printed from highly precise, skin surface reflecting, negative casts. For details of the procedure, see Post [23] and Leveque (this volume).

In our own investigations, checking of the polymer positives was always performed in three directions with 45° angle differences.

Clinical Applications

Capacitance measurement with the corneometer, as used in the past e.g., by Thune [31] and Werner [35] for hydration measurements with patients suffering from atopic dermatitis, is both easy to handle and reliable. It must be kept in mind, however, that the layer of the stratum corneum which is taken into account principally depends on the thickness of the separating foil and the frequency used. Among the above mentioned methods, the corneometer might be regarded as one of the least expensive ones.

According to Tronnier [33] the resonance frequency measurement is a method which has proved to be efficient in practical tests of cosmetics and topical agents, with the great advantage of giving clues to the plasticity of the horny layer, i.e., to the property itself which one intends to affect by the application of moisturizing topical agents. However, the results gained with this measurement device await further confirmation by other investigators.

For the time being, electric impedance/conductance techniques are probably mainly employed not for dermatologic or cosmetic investigations, but for psychophysiologic experiments (e.g., determination of the galvanic skin response) or biofeedback techniques. The DC resistance measurement instrument described by Wienert et al. [35] was used by Keilhauer et al. [14, 15] at the North Sea and in the alpine climate for hydration measurements with patients suffering from atopic dermatitis. The equipment described by Tagami et al. [30] and by Blichmann and Serup [2] for measurements on eczematous skin works at a high frequency AC of 3.5 MHz. It functions with dry electrodes and has the asset that both impedance and capacitance measurements are possible. In earlier investigations, Tagami et al. [30] described that with this apparatus the hydration of the most superficial layers of the stratum corneum is determined. The more recent investigations of Obata and Tagami [21] with this instrument – which has meanwhile been provided with a new more sensitive probe – on a simulation model of stratum corneum have shown that skin conductance did not only correlate very well with the water content in the superficial layer of the simulation model, but also with the water content of the stratum corneum model as a whole. The authors report a penetration depth of the current of approximately 5 mm in this experimental constellation. Assuming that the measurement of the water content of the stratum corneum after instantaneous water absorption is mainly affiliated with the amount of rapidly absorbed and lost "bound water," Tagami et al. [29] described a water sorption/desorption test which provides, within a few minutes, information on the hygroscopic properties and the water binding capacity of the stratum corneum.

Although infrared spectroscopy using the ATR method is a complicated and costly method, the advantage is that the penetration depth of infrared radiation lies in the range of a few microns. Thus, the part of the horny layer in which the water content is determined can be well defined. Recent research by Potts et al. [25] indicates that, under certain circumstances, an exact quantitative relationship between infrared absorption and water concentration in the stratum corneum may be detected. If this should prove to be reliable, there would be far more domains in which it could be used.

As remains to be shown, changes of the relief and profile of the skin surface, as a function of changes in the moisture content of the horny layer, seem to be detectable only with technically and mathematically complicated procedures. For the moment, the most concise procedure might be that described by Hoppe et al. [13]

Investigations in Our Own Laboratory

Experimental Series 1

The goal of these experiments was to examine to what degree diverse methods of measurement provide results comparable to one another and to find out what parts of the horny layer are affected by moisture content. To do this, we performed measurements under standardized conditions in two series consisting of 17 healthy volunteers each.

We measured the water content of the stratum corneum of the flexor forearm using following methods:

1. Direct current resistance measurement with the aforementioned specially constructed instrument
2. Alternating current conductance measurement at 15 KHz with the aforementioned specially constructed instrument
3. Electric capacity measurement using a prototype of the Corneometer CM 420 (Schwarzhaupt Medizintechnik, Köln, FRG; more recent types, e.g. CM 820, now produced by Courage and Khazaka, Cologne, FRC)

4. Measurement of transepidermal water loss (TEWL) using the Evaporimeter EP 1 (Servo Med, Vällingby, Sweden)
5. Infrared spectroscopy using the aforementioned ATR method

With all of these methods, measurements were made on unmanipulated skin. With infrared spectroscopy, additional measurements were performed on the same skin area after five and ten adhesive tape strippings. Our examinations showed (Table 1, 2), that, except for the transepidermal water loss measurement method, all of the above mentioned examination methods yielded results that correlated with the infrared spectroscopy method. Since the penetration depth of infrared light into the stratum corneum is extremely small, as noted above, the following statements can be made: *While direct current resistance measurement takes in the moisture content of the most superficial layer of the stratum corneum, the capacity measurement method yields results from deep layers of the stratum corneum. If the alternating current conductance method is employed, both superficial and deep aspects of the stratum corneum can be reached. Due to the correlation of the infrared spectroscopic test results with those of several other in vivo methods, its competence and usefulness in dermatologic research has been underscored.*

Table 1. Measurement of the hydration of the stratum corneum of the flexor forearm

Series (n= 17)	Mean value	SD
DC resistance (ohm)	6.02×10^8	8.25×10^8
TEWL (g/m^2xh)	9.39	2.46
IR spectroscopy on skin surface (MF)	1.208	0.079
IR spectroscopy after 5 adhesive tape strippings (MF)	1.270	0.060
IR spectroscopy after 10 adhesive tape strippings (MF)	1.314	0.059
Series 2 (n= 17)		
AC conductance, 15 KHz (scale units)	30.38	25.95
Capacity (Locale units)	48.16	1.54
IR spectroscopy on skin surface (MF)	1.305	0.076
IR spectroscopy after 5 adhesive tape strippings (MF)	1.388	0.060
IR spectroscopy after 10 adhesive tape strippings (MF)	1.416	0.064

TEWL, transepidermal water loss; IR, infrared; MF, moisture factor.

Table 2. Correlations between several methods used to assess hydration of the stratum corneum

	IR spectroscopy (surface)	IR spectroscopy adhesive tape (5 strapping)	IR spectroscopy (10 adhesive tape strippings)
DC resistance	−0.5371[a]	−0.5116[a]	−0.1477[b]
TEWL	0.0474[b]	0.0289[b]	−0.0789[b]
Capacity	0.3285[b]	0.2653[b]	0.6076[a]
AC conductance, 15 kHz	0.4904[a]	−0.3483[b]	−0.5089[a]

IR, infrared; TEWL, transepidermal water loss
[a] Significant for a $\leq$ 0,05
[b] Not significant (Spearman's rank correlation test)

Thus, a conclusion based on empirical data could be drawn about those layers of the stratum corneum which are preferentially evaluated by the diverse methods.

Experimental Series 2

The goal of these experiments was to find out if hydration of the horny layer – by an occlusion lasting several hours – which could be detected with certainty by several methods of measurement would also have significant effects on the skin surface relief. Therefore, we performed measurements under standardized conditions in a series of 17 healthy male volunteers, age 19–29 years, before and after a 4 h occlusion of the volar aspect of the forearm. The following methods were applied:

1. Measurement of the TEWL with the Evaporimeter EP 1
2. DC resistance measurement with the above mentioned specially constructed instrument
3. Infrared spectroscopy with the above described ATR technique
4. Profilometry with a tap-cut instrument used in industry (Perth-o-meter, Typ Universal S 4 PD and Perth-o-graph) on positive casts made of an acrylate polymer (Palavit G), which had been taken from negative casts of the skin made of a highly precise, skin surface reflecting, silicon plastic (Silasoft). We considered, as Post [23] and Hoppe [12] did, R_t, R_p, and R_a to be characteristic measures of roughness.
5. Scanning electron microscopy on positive casts made of a polyvinylacetate polymer (Mowital B), which were prepared in the usual way for evaluation at a magnification of 100x and an aspect angle of 45°

The results of the objective methods used are shown in Table 3. Infrared spectroscopy DC resistance measurement and determination of the TEWL indicated the highly significant expected differences in the stratum corneum hydration following occlusion treatment ($a \leq 0.0001$, Wilcoxon test for matched pairs), whereas this was not the case for the profilometric measurements of roughness (not significant for $a \leq 0.05$, Wilcoxon test for matched pairs). Visual evaluation (by several persons) of matched SEMs before and after occlusion showed no significant changes in the skin surface relief, in particular no swelling of the surface of the stratum corneum or formation of numerous wrinkles, as might have been expected according to Harris [11].

Thus, our results show that short-term occlusion (4h) leads to an enhancement of stratum corneum hydration which could clearly be shown with the aid of infrared spectroscopy, DC resistance measurement, and determination of TEWL. By contrast, our investigations using profilometry and scanning electron microscopy imply that the relief of the skin surface was not significantly changed.

Our findings are contradictory to those of Harris, who found significant changes of the relief and roughness of the skin surface based on scanning electron microscopic investigation of skin biopsies after a 72 h occlusion at a magnification of 500x. Due to differences in the study design, however, those investigations cannot be compared to ours without reservation. Harris chose an occlusion time of 72 h for his experiments, i.e., 18 times longer than in our study. A 72 h occlusion may lead to secondary effects by growth of bacteria of the skin flora with destruction of corneocytes by bacterial proteinases. Furthermore, the magnification scales used for the SEM investigations were different (Harris, 500x; in our study, 100x). Our findings do correspond with those of several authors: Post [23], too, could not find a definite relation between the water content of the horny layer and the relief of the skin surface using infrared spectroscopy, profilometry, and scanning electron microscopy for her investigations. Garber [6] also could not detect any significant changes of the surface of the stratum corneum by the use of scanning electron microscopy after a 1 h water soak. After applying topical agents, Hoppe [12], at first, found only very rare significant differences in the skin surface relief when five roughness parameters were determined on several skin casts. Only after the development of technically as well as mathematically more complicated procedures [12,13] did this author and coworkers detect significant differences in the skin surface after application of topicals. In contrast to our investigations, however, Hoppe did not directly correlate profilometry to the determination of stratum corneum hydration using other methods. The smoothing effect of topicals shown by him might have been caused by the lipid components of the topicals applied. Giving due consideration to the investigations mentioned, we draw the subsequent conclusion to experimental series 2: *Restricting oneself to the physiological range of variation of the stratum corneum hydration, the impact of the water content of the horny layer alone on the relief of the skin surface has mostly been overestimated.*

Table 3. Results of various methods to measure hydration of the stratum corneum following a 4 h occlusion of the volar aspect of the forearm.

	before occlusion (mean/sp)	after occlusion (mean/sp)	T value[a]
IR spectroscopy (moisture factor)	1.209/ 0.062	1.541/ 0.120	153*
DC resistance (Ohm)	5.14×10^8/ 8.33×10^8	1.12×10^7/ 8.15×10^6	1*
TEWL ($g/m^2 \times h$)	8.29/ 2.64	45.02/ 14.42	153*
Profilometry			
R_p	23.16/ 4.75	20.85/ 4.10	35 n.s.
R_a	13.49/ 2.04	12.70/ 1.94	46 n.s.
R_t	106.10/ 14.13	109.02/ 15.19	96.5 n.s.

IR, infrared; TEWL, transepidermal water loss.
* significant for $\alpha \leq 0.0001$; other T values not significant: $\alpha \geq 0.05$.
[a] Wilcoxon test for matched pairs.

When profilometry or scanning electron microscopy procedures are to be used for dermatologic or cosmetologic studies, only more advanced procedures, for example, the profilometry method described by Hoppe et al. [13] or the scanning electron microscopy technique described by Leveque (this volume), should be considered as suitable.

As can be seen from the aforementioned studies, the noninvasive methods characterized above have been developed to such an extent that they permit reliable statements concerning stratum corneum hydration by topical agents. Nevertheless, methods which permit a differentiation of the water content of the horny layer into "free" and more or less "bound" water, i.e., into extra- and intracellulary located water, and which, as a goal, are practicable in a non-invasive manner remain to be developed.

References

1. Blank IH (1953) Further observations on factors which influence the water content of stratum corneum. J Invest Dermatol 21: 259–271
2. Blichmann C, Serup J (1987) Hydration studies on scaly hand eczema. Contact Dermatitis 16: 155–159
3. Campbell SD, Kraning KK, Schibli E, Momil ST (1977) Hydration characteristics and electrical resistivity of stratum corneum using a noninvasive four-point microelectrode method. J Invest Dermatol 69: 290–295
4. Clar, EJ (1981): Skin impedance measurement: a means to study stratum corneum barrier properties and hydration state. In: Klaschka, F (ed) Stratum corneum – Struktur und Funktion. Berliner Dermatologisches Symposium. Grosse, Berlin
5. Edelberg, R (1971): Electric properties of skin. In: Elden, HR (ed) Biophysical properties of the skin. Wiley, New York
6. Garber, CA (1978): Characterizing "moistured skin" by scanning electron microscopy. Cosmet Toil. 93: 74–83
7. Gloor, M (1982): Pharmakologie dermatologischer Externa. Springer, Berlin Heidelberg New York
8. Gloor, M, Hirsch, G, Willebrandt, U (1981): On the use of infrared spectroscopy for the in vivo measurement of the water content of the horny layer after application of dermatologic ointments Arch Dermatol Res 271: 305–313
9. Gloor M, Willebrandt, U, Thomer, G, Kupferschmid, W (1980): Water content of the horny layer and skin surface lipids. Arch. Dermatol. Res. 268: 221–223
10. Günzler H, Böck H, (1975): IR-Spektroskopie. Eine Einführung. Verlag Chemie, Weinheim
11. Harris DR, Papa, CM Stanton, R. (1974): Percutaneous absorption and the surface area of occluded skin – a scanning electron microscopic study. Br J Dermatal 91: 27–32
12. Hoppe U (1979): Topologie der Hautoberfläche. J Soc Cosmet Chem 30: 213–239
13. Hoppe U, Lunderstädt R, Sauermann, G (1986): Quantitative Analyse der Hautoberfläche mit Hilfe der digitalen Signalverarbeitung Ärztl Kosmetol 7: 13–37
14. Keilhauer A, Wienert V, Borelli S (1982): Die Hautfeuchtigkeit bei Neurodermitikern in alpiner Klimazone. Akt. Dermatol. 8: 146–149
15. Keilhauer A, Wienert V, Pürschel W (1982): Die Hautfeuchtigkeit bei Neurodermitikern in maritimer Klimazone. Z. Hautkr 57: 1477–1486
16. Keller P (1963): Elektrophysiologie der Haut. In: Marchionini A, Spier HW (eds) Normale und pathologische Physiologie (Handbuch der Haut- und Geschlechtskrankheiten. [Suppl], vol I, part 3) Springer, Berlin Göttingen Heidelberg der Haut I.
17. Kligman AM, (1963): The uses of sebum. Br J Dermatol 75: 307–319
18. Kölmel K, Nicolaus A, Giese K, (1985): Photoacoustic determination of the water uptake by the upper horny layer of non-eczematous skin in atopic dermatitis. Bioeng. Skin 1: 125–131
19. Kronzucker H, Zehner B, (1980): Prinzipien der Prozess-Meßtechnik: 2. Analysengeräte. Schnäckerl, Karlsruhe
20. Lawler JC, Davis MJ, Griffith EC, (1960): Electrical characteristics of the skin. J. Invest Dermatol 34: 301–308
21. Obata M, Tagami H, (1989): Electrical determination of water content and concentration profile in a simulation model of in vivo stratum corneum. J Invest Dermatol 92: 854–859

22. Osberghaus R, Gloxhuber C, van Raay HG, Braig S, (1978): Hydagen F, ein neuer Hautfeuchtigkeitsregulator – Methoden und Ergebnisse des Wirkungsnachweises. J Soc Cosmet Chem. 29: 133–146
23. Post, H. (1983): Hautoberflächenprofil und Hornschichtfeuchtigkeit. Inauguraldissertation, University of Heidelberg
24. Potts, RO, Christman, DA, Buras, EM (1983): The dynamic mechanical properties of human skin. J Biomech 16: 365–372
25. Potts, RO, Guzek, DB, Harris, RR, McKie, JE (1985): A noninvasive, in vivo technique to quantitatively measure water concentration of the stratum corneum using attenuated total-reflectance infrared spectroscopy Arch Dermatol Res 277: 489–495
26. Putnam NA, (1972): Attenuated total reflectance studies of the skin. J Soc Cosmet Chem 23: 209–226
27. Rosencwaig A, Pines E (1977): Stratum corneum studies with photoacoustic spectroscopy. J Invest Dermatol 69: 296–298
28. Rothman S (1954): Physiology and biochemistry of the skin, Chapter 2: Electrical behavior. University of Chicago Press, Chicago
29. Tagami H, Kanamaru Y, Inoue K, et al (1982): Water sorption-desorption test of the skin in vivo for functional assessment of the stratum corneum. J Invest Dermatol 78: 425–428
30. Tagami H, Ohi M, Iwatsuki K, et al. (1980): Evaluation of the skin surface hydration in vivo by electrical measurement. J Invest Dermatol 75: 500–507
31. Thune P (1989): Evaluation of the hydration and the water-holding capacity in atopic skin and so-called dry skin. Acta Derm Venereol (Stockh) Suppl 144: 133–135
32. Triebskorn, A (1983): Hornschichtfeuchtigkeit und Hautoberflächenrelief – Beitrag zur Frage der gegenseitigen Abhängigkeit und zur Methodologie. Inaugural dissertation, University of Heidelberg
33. Tronnier H, Wagener HH (1952): Über die Frequenzleitfähigkeit der menschlichen Haut. Dermatologica 104: 135–151
34. Walschburger P (1975): Zur Standardisierung und Interpretation elektrodermaler Meßwerte in psychologischen Experimenten. Exp Angew Psychol 22: 514–533
35. Werner Y (1986): The water content of the stratum corneum in patients with atopic dermatitis; measurements with the corneometer 420. Acta Derm Venereol (Stockh) 66: 281–284
36. Wienert V, Hegner G, Sick H, (1981): Ein Verfahren zur Bestimmung des relativen Wassergehaltes des Stratum corneum der menschlichen Haut. Arch Dermatol Res 270: 67–75

Transepidermal Water Loss Measurement by Means of an Evaporimeter

R. A. Tupker, J. Pinnagoda, P.-J. Coenraads, and J. P. Nater*

Introduction

The skin is the interface of an organism with its environment, and therefore the basic role of the skin is protection, e.g., against water loss and entrance of external factors, such as irritants. The location of the permeation barrier depends on the physicochemical characteristics of the substance concerned. Blank has noticed that the water diffusion rate was dependent on the number of stratum corneum layers stripped [5]. Based on this observation, the stratum corneum is considered to provide a uniformly impermeable layer which constitutes the main barrier against diffusional water loss [6]. The epidermal layers underneath the stratum corneum (i.e., viable epidermis) have a predominantly hydrophilic nature; water-soluble substances can be transported easily via the intercellular fluids. Lipophilic substances tend to accumulate and/or bind in the stratum corneum layers [25]. For the majority of compounds, therefore, the stratum corneum is the main penetration barrier [34].

The total amount of water vapor passing the skin can be divided into water vapor passing the stratum corneum by passive diffusion and water vapor loss as a result of sweating [31]. Originally, the term "transepidermal water loss" (TEWL) indicated the amount of water vapor passing the stratum corneum by passive diffusion [31]. Nowadays, TEWL refers to the total amount of the water loss through the skin. The term "insensible perspiration" [31] would better denote total water loss, since, in this way, a clear distinction can be made between the two processes (passive diffusion and sweating) on the basis of terminology. To conform with the more recent publications, however, we adhere to the term "TEWL" in the broader definition (total water vapor loss). Therefore, it must be kept in mind that TEWL is a reflection of stratum corneum barrier function for water only when there is no sweat gland activity.

The first primitive attempts to evaluate water loss from human skin were already made in the seventeenth and eighteenth centuries by determining the weight reduction of the whole body on a weighing scale. In the twentieth century, the following methods have been developed in order to measure water loss through limited areas of the skin:

1. Methods based on unventilated chambers. Water loss is determined gravimetrically; the increase in weight of a hygroscopic material is a measure of water loss of the skin per unit time and skin surface [40].

* Occupational Dermatology Unit, State University Hospital, PO Box 30.001, 9700 RB Groningen, The Netherlands.

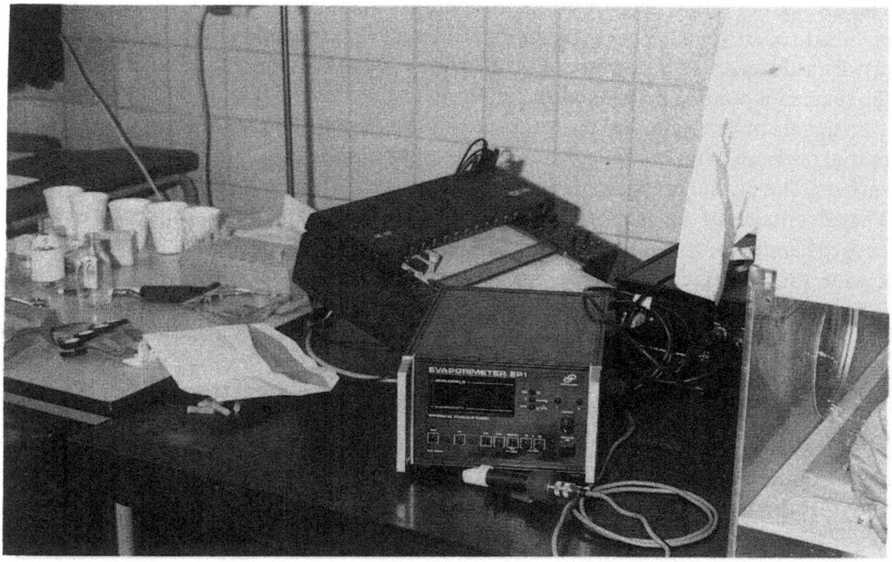

Fig. 1. The ServoMed evaporimeter

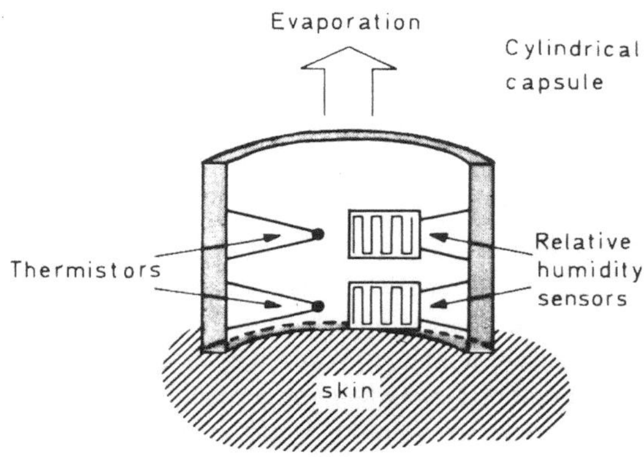

Fig. 2. Arrangement of sensors in the probe of the ServoMed evaporimeter (Adapted from Nilsson 1977 [26])

2. Methods based on ventilated chambers. A carrier gas with a known water content and at a known gas flow rate is passed through a chamber placed with its open end on the skin. The water loss of the tested skin area is proportional to the gas flow rate and the increase in water content of the carrier gas. The water content of the gas can be analyzed gravimetrically [3] or electrohygrometrically [1, 40, 42].
3. More recently, a method based on gradient estimation has been developed [26]. Gradient estimation depends upon determination of the vapor pressure gradient in the air layer adjacent to the skin. This gradient can be considered as proportional to the exchange of water vapor from the skin.

The operating principle of the ServoMed evaporimeter (ServoMed AB Stockholm, Sweden) (see Fig. 1) is based on the method of gradient estimation [26].

The measuring probe head of this instrument contains two sensor units, placed in the enclosure of an open cylinder (diameter of 12 mm). Each sensor unit consists of a humidity transducer and a thermistor (Fig. 2). The probe head is applied parallel to the skin, the sensor units being positioned at a different distance to the skin surface (3 and 9 mm). The signals of the humidity transducers and thermistors can be used to compute the partial pressure of the water vapor and the temperature at these positions above the skin surface. The partial pressure gradient and water vapor loss rate can thus be calculated. The advantages of the evaporimeter compared with other methods are, that it is rather easy to handle, it is portable, and has a fast display and a high reproducibility. However, a wide range of factors may decrease the reproducibility of this instrument. These include individual-related, environment-related, and instrument-related factors [29].

Control of the majority of the above mentioned influencing factors was achieved by methods described elsewhere [29]. The aims of the studies presented in this chapter were to investigate the following phenomena using the evaporimeter:

(1) individual variation in susceptibility to repeated exposure to the anionic detergent sodium lauryl sulfate (SLS) and its relationship to preexposure barrier function (experiment 1) [43];
(2) individual differences in time course of TEWL after a single 24 h SLS exposure (experiment 2) [44]; and
(3) to study which personal characteristics determine the individual susceptibility to irritants (experiment 3) [45].

Method

Evaluation

In all three experiments, TEWL measurements were performed with the ServoMed evaporimeter EP1C. The measurements were performed in an air-conditioned room at a constant temperature of 20° C and a relative humidity of 45% ± 5%. To avoid measurement errors caused by air currents, the experiment was performed in a transparent box into which the subject had placed the forearm. The top side of the box was left open to avoid build-up of heat and/or water vapor from the arms. The instrument was zeroed only once daily using its own offset button prior to the first measurement. The probes were clamped in order to avoid transfer of heat from the operator's hand [29]. After an acclimatization period of 15 min, the probe was applied parallel to the skin surface. These measures were intended to minimize interference by sweating. The electronic filters (10 and 20 s) available for damping fluctuations [39] were used after the display values had stabilized (30–45 s). TEWL was recorded, after the stabilization period, on a chart strip recorder (BBC SE 120, Austria). Only in case a straight horizontal line was obtained for at least 30 s, was the height of this line taken as the value measured. After each measurement, the instrument was allowed to return to zero on its own, with its own probe cover in place.

Clinical changes at the exposed sites were graded according to Frosch and Kligman [12]: (a) erythema: slight redness, spotty or diffuse (1+); moderate redness (2+); intense redness (3+); fiery red with edema (4+); (b) scaling: fine (1+); moderate

(2+); severe with large flakes (3+); (c) fissures: fine cracks (1+); single or multiple broader fissures (2+); wide cracks with hemorrhage or exudation (3+). After evaluation, fresh solutions were applied.

Exposure

In each experiment 0.3 ml of a solution was applied to a disc of absorbent Whatman paper of a diameter of 20 mm and 1.0 mm in thickness (number 2589C, Schleicher & Schuell, The Netherlands). Each disc fitted into a round, flat, plastic chamber (Agfa Bayer, Leverkusen, Germany) with an inside diameter of 22 mm. These chambers were attached to a metal strip which was fixed to the skin of the volar side of each forearm with nonadhesive bandages.

In the different experiments, the relationship between time of exposure to the irritants and TEWL measurement was as follows:

Experiment 1
This involved a repeated exposure to 0.5% (g/100 ml) SLS (Merck, USA). Two applications, lasting 45 min each, were made on 4 consecutive days on this site (eight applications in total). The minimal time interval between these two applications was 3 h. After removal of the test material, the skin was cleaned with running water and dried with a paper towel. TEWL was measured on day 1 (baseline TEWL, BASE) and day 5 (REPET). A total of 37 healthy volunteers (20 females and 17 males, ages 20–48 years) (who were free from skin diseases collaborated in the study, which was performed from the end of March until the beginning of June and in September, 1987.

Experiment 2
A single 24 h exposure to 0.5% SLS was administered. After removal of the material on day 2, the skin was cleaned and dried as mentioned above. TEWL was measured before exposure to SLS, on day 1 (BASE) and on days 2 (2 h after removal of the patch), 3, 4, 5, 8, and 10. A total of 35 healthy individuals without any skin ailment (17 females and 18 males, age 19–61 years) cooperated in the study, which was performed from April to June, 1988.

Experiment 3
This involved a 3 week repeated exposure to various irritants. Two daily applications, lasting 45 min each, were made 5 days a week for 3 consecutive weeks (a total of 28 applications). A 0.1% SLS solution was applied at a site 110 mm proximal to the right wrist; 2.3% disodium lauryl 3-ethoxysulfosuccinate (SUC, anionic detergent) (Rewopol 30, 40, Rewo Benelux, Doodewaard, The Netherlands) 110 mm proximal to the left wrist; 2.0% Shellsol K (SOL, aliphatic solvent) (Shell, Amsterdam, The Netherlands) 190 mm proximal to the left wrist. On the right forearm, a more distal site, positioned 70 mm from the wrist joint, was occluded using the same chamber but without any solution and thus served as a control site. TEWL measurements of these sites were carried out on every first and fifth day of each week, before the solutions were applied.

On day 1, the forearm skin was scored for dryness by means of a visual scoring system (positive score when the skin looked and felt dry or rough). There were three groups of subjects:

1. Group AD: 20 persons with healed atopic dermatitis (AD). Selection criteria were the diagnostic criteria for AD according to Hanifin and Rajka [19] and a minimal symptom-free period of 2 weeks. Only persons with a past AD were tested, since the presence of (some type of) dermatitis itself may enhance susceptibility [4]. This group consisted of four men and 16 women, ranging in age from 17 to 33 years (mean, 25 years).
2. Group CD: 18 persons with healed allergic contact dermatitis (CD). Selection criteria were past dermatitis which could be explained by relevant contact allergens, no evidence of (past) AD or (past) dyshidrotic dermatitis, and minimal symptom-free period of 2 weeks. Subjects having a past CD were included to investigate whether AD is unique with respect to altered susceptibility. This group consisted of eight men and ten women, age 20–49 years (mean, 31 years).
3. Group C: 18 control subjects without any past or present skin ailment. This group consisted of 10 men and 8 women, age 20–35 years (mean, 28 years).

The experiment was conducted from February to April, 1989.

Statistical Analysis

Experiment 1
The least squares method was used to obtain the linear regression equation of REPET on BASE [22] using the GLM statistical package described by SAS.

Experiment 2 and 3
Analysis of variance was used for comparison of mean TEWL and mean age between the groups. Differences were considered to be significant for a p value < 0.05. The chisquare test was used to calculate the difference between the three groups with respect to sex and skin dryness.

Multiple linear regression models were calculated for the TEWL values after exposure to the irritants as dependent variables and evaluated by the p value of the partial F tests [22]. In each regression model, various combinations of personal characteristics (baseline TEWL, skin dryness, etc.) as independent variables were evaluated.

Results

Our Own Observations

Experiment 1
Large interindividual differences in both preexposure baseline TEWL (BASE) were observed and in TEWL, following 4 days of repeated SLS exposure, on day 5 (REPET) (Fig. 3). A strong correlation was found between BASE and REPET (R = ap).

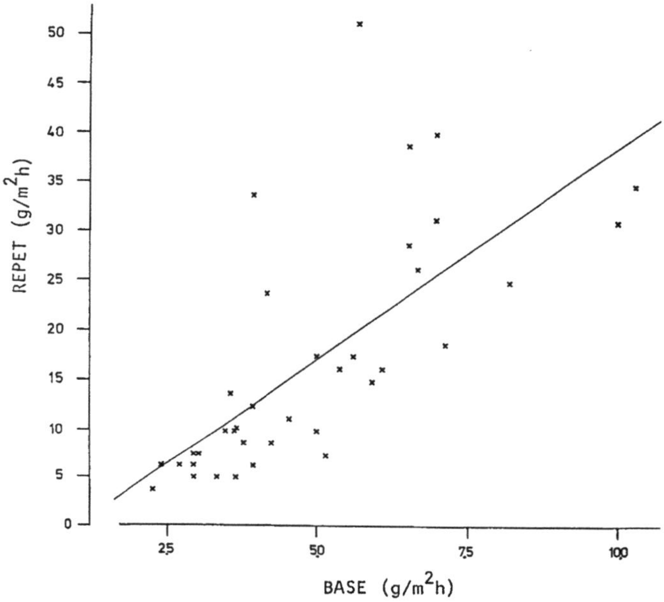

Fig. 3 Relationship between REPET and BASE. Plots and fitted linear regression line of transepidermal water loss (TEWL) on the 5th day of exposure to SLS (*REPET, y-axis*) and TEWL before exposure (*BASE, x-axis*) in 37 volunteers. Regression equation: REPET = −4.7 + 4.4 x BASE, with $SE_{\beta} = 0.73$ and $R = 0.71$

The clinical findings on day 5 showed only nine persons with a high total visual score: four had a total score of 2+; three had a total score of 3+; one had 4+; and one had 5+.

All volunteers with a high visual score ($n = 9$) had a high REPET value (≥20.0). All individuals except one ($n = 10$) with a high REPET value had a high visual score.

Experiment 2

A striking interindividual difference in TEWL time course after the single exposure was noticed; some individuals had their highest TEWL value on the day of removal of the patch (day 2), whereas in others, TEWL continued rising during the subsequent days after patch removal. Thus, the subjects could be divided into four subgroups (groups 1–4), according to the day of their maximum TEWL value after the 24 h SLS exposure (days 2–5, respectively). Figure 4 depicts the time course of TEWL at site 1, before and after the 24 h single application, for the total group and for the various subgroups. The mean total scores of the clinical manifestations followed a time pattern similar to that of the mean TEWL values for the different subgroups.

Interindividual variation in TEWL value was highest during the first days after the single exposure and became smaller in the second week. This was also true for the variation in TEWL time course after removal of the SLS patch. The latter was expressed as the difference in TEWL level between day 2 and day 3, 4, 5, etc. (DIFF 2–3, DIFF 2–4, DIFF 2–5, etc.) and was also highest in the first days after exposure.

Experiment 3

Each agent caused a significant increase in mean TEWL value during the exposure period. On day 19, a high total visual score (≥ 2) at the sites exposed to SLS, SUC, and

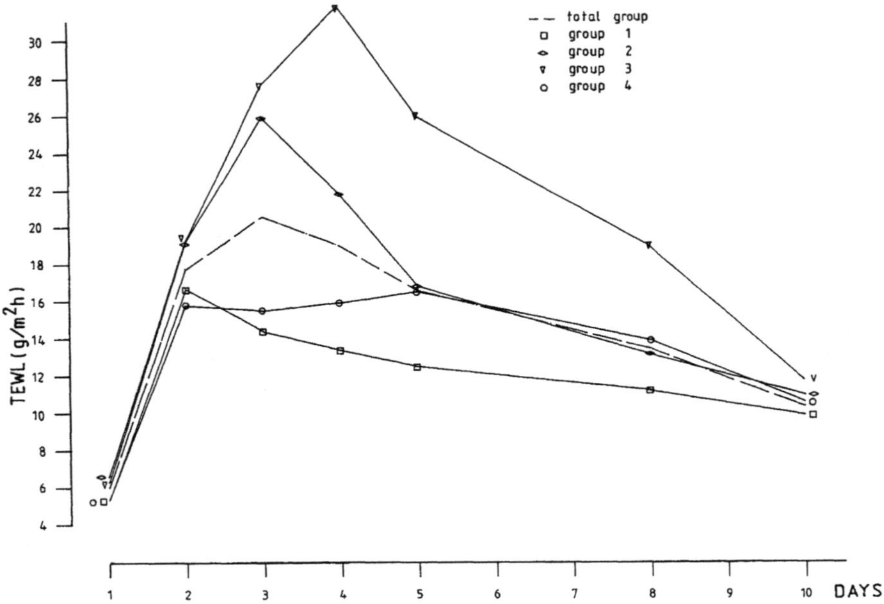

Fig. 4. Time course of transepidermal water loss (TEWL) (g/m^2h) before and after a single sodium lauryl sulphate (SLS) exposure. Values are means for the total group ($n = 35$) and for the different subgroups: *group 1* (maximal TEWL level on day 2; $n = 14$); *group 2* (maximal TEWL level on day 3; $n=16$); *group 3* (maximal TEWL level on day 4; $n = 4$); *group 4* (maximal TEWL level on day 5; $n = 1$)

SOL, was observed in 2, 2, and 0 individuals, respectively. In each case, the clinical signs were accompanied by a clear TEWL increase ($\geq 5g/m^2$ h).

Group AD consisted of more persons with clinically dry skin ($n = 7$) than group CD ($n = 3$) (not significant) and group C ($n = 1$) (significant).

Figure 5 shows that the mean preexposure baseline TEWL value (BASE) of group AD was significantly higher than that of the other two groups. Group AD had higher TEWL values than groups CD and C throughout the entire period at the exposed sites.

For the total group, higher postexposure TEWL values were observed in clinically dry skin than in nondry skin. Within each group also, dry skin had a (in several cases significantly) higher susceptibility than nondry skin.

There was a significant correlation between TEWL values on day 19 of the sites exposed to SLS, SUC, and SOL ($R = 0.6–0.85$). By means of multiple linear regression analysis one is able to estimate the importance of a given factor (independent variable) for the phenomenon (dependent variable) which is influenced by this factor. By taking more than one independent variable in the model it is possible to compare the significance of each of these variables for the dependent variable. In our case, when we take, for example, the TEWL value an day 19 at the site exposed to SLS as the dependent variable, it was found that the independent variable BASE had a more significant contribution ($p = 0.03$) to this dependent variable than DRY ($p = 0.2$) (Table 1). When all three independent variables were present in the model, the contribution of AD was not significant. In the absence of BASE, however, AD had a significant contribution in most models.

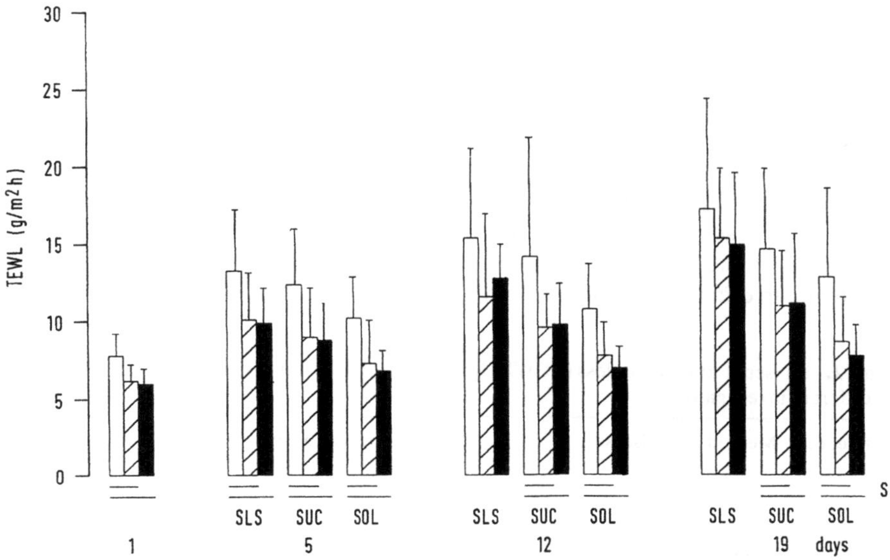

Fig. 5 Differences between groups AD (history of atopic dermatitis), CD (history of contact dermatitis), and C (controls) in mean transepidermal water loss value (g/m^{2}h) before and after exposure at different sites on various days. (*Black bar*, Group AD; *hatched bar, group CD*; *blank bar*, group C; *s* denotes significant difference ($p < 0.05$) between the groups

Table 1. Multiple regression analysis with transepidermal water loss (TEWL) on the 19th day of exposure at different sites as dependent variables and four combinations of baseline TEWL (BASE), dry skin (DRY), and history of atopic dermatitis (AD) as independent variables

Combination of independent variables		Site	
	SLS	SUC	SOL
BASE	0.03[a]	0.003	0.001
DRY	0.2	0.007	0.004
BASE	0.06	0.03	0.03
AD	0.8	0.2	0.3
AD	0.4	0.04	0.01
DRY	0.2	0.02	0.005
BASE	0.06	0.03	0.04
DRY	0.2	0.01	0.006
AD	0.8	0.5	0.5

SLS, sodium lauryl sulfate; SUC, disodium lauryl 3-ethoxysulfosuccinate; SOL, Shellsol K.
[a]*p* value denotes the significance of that variable's contribution to the model; all dependent variables and BASE are continuous; AD and dry are dichotomous.

Clinical Applications

The TEWL rate can be determined by two factors (see introduction): (1) barrier function of the epidermis and (2) sweat gland activity. Clinical application of TEWL measurement is based on these two parameters.

Barrier Function of the Epidermis

A higher TEWL has been noticed on involved skin in various types of dermatitis than on uninvolved sites [2, 7, 41] (Table 2). Shahidullah et al. have observed an increased TEWL on the involved and uninvolved skin in dermatitis related to the severity of the disease [41]. TEWL on uninvolved skin of patients with dermatitis showed larger variations in time than TEWL measured on a similar site in subjects without dermatitis [41]. Uninvolved skin of patients with manifest AD was demonstrated to have a higher TEWL than the same skin region of subjects without dermatitis [9, 48] (Table 2). Serup and Staberg studied the time course of TEWL after a single irritant (SLS) exposure in an attempt to differentiate allergic from irritant skin reactions [37].

Table 2. Transepidermal water loss (TEWL) (g/m^2h) on involved and uninvolved skin as reported by different investigators

Reference	Method	Disease	Number of subjects	Mean TEWL of involved skin	Number of subject	Mean TEWL of uninvolved skin
Baker [2]	Ventilated chamber	Psoriasis	12	23.4		
		Pityriasis rubra pilaris	10	14.5		
		Ichthyosis vulgaris	3	3.3		
		Psoriasis			16	2.5
		Atopic dermatitis			22	2.9
		Controls			132	2.8
Finlay et al. [9]	Evapori-meter	Atopic dermatitis			3	11.6
		Controls			11	2.9
Frost et al. [15]	Ventilated chamber	Psoriasis	3	4.8		
		Epidermolytic hyperkeratosis	7	3.4		
		X-linked ichthyosis	5	2.6		
		Ichthyosis vulgaris	5	2.1		
		Lamellar ichthyosis	4	2.3		
		Controls	11	1.8		
Grice and Bettley [16]	Ventilated chamber	Psoriasis	27	31.0		
		Dermatitis	8	27.0		
		Erythroderma	10	26.0		
		Ichthyosis	18	10.0		
		Controls	58	3.0		
Lamke et al. [24]	Evapori-meter	First degree burn	12	11.6		
		Second degree burn	30	178.1		
		Third degree burn	20	143.2		
		Granulating wound	21	214.1		
		Controls	60	8.5		
Van der Valk et al. [48]	Evapori-meter	Atopic dermatitis			10	8.7
		Irritant contact dermatitis			17	6.4
		Controls			19	6.5
Frosch and Czarnetzki [14]	Evapori-meter	Wounds treated				
		with acitretin	8	16		
		with isotretinoin	5	19		
		Controls	6	8		

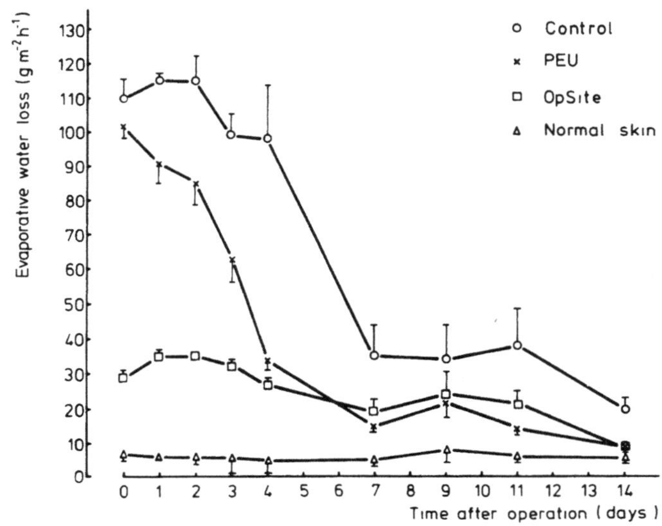

Fig. 6. Evaporative water loss from partial thickness wounds in guinea pigs covered with a permeable membrane or with the relatively impermeable OpSite membrane, or left air-exposed as control during the first 2 weeks after excision. (Adapted from Jonkman et al. [20])

In psoriasis, TEWL is elevated on the plaques [11,16,30] and is not dependent on the degree of scaling [38] (Table 2). The clinical course showed a strict parallel with the TEWL values [16, 30], and TEWL has been used successfully in monitoring the healing effect of antipsoriatic therapy [11, 30] Furthermore, TEWL was shown to be more sensitive in detecting early skin changes, since TEWL deteriorated in 12 out of 14 patients before clinical exacerbation became obvious [30].

TEWL was found to be significantly increased in four forms of ichthyosis compared with control subjects without a skin condition [15] (Table 2). Also in patients with ichthyosis, the magnitude of increase in TEWL paralleled the severity of the scaling [15].

TEWL measurement has been used frequently to monitor the epidermal repair process in (burn) wounds. Soon after the burning, TEWL was extremely elevated, dependent on the degree of burn [24] (Table 2). The permeability of different grafts and artificial membranes can be assessed in vitro and in vivo [20, 24]. Evaporative water loss has been shown to be preeminently suited for the evaluation of epidermal regeneration of partial thickness wounds in guinea pigs which were covered with different artificial membranes or left uncovered [20] (Fig. 6). A triphasic water loss behavior was observed, being related to the phases of epidermal wound healing as determined histologically: epidermal closure, parakeratosis, and maturation of the stratum corneum [20].

TEWL measurement was the most differentiating parameter in regard to the demonstration of delay in wound healing by retinoids in diabetic rats [14].

Hammarlund et al. have found a linear relationship between TEWL and ambient percent relative humidity (RH) in 19 neonates [18]. At high RH (60%) TEWL was 40% lower than at low RH (20%). By determining TEWL from different parts of the body and calculating the areas of the corresponding surfaces, the total cutaneous water loss could be obtained (8.1 g/m^{2}h) [18].

Premature neonates have an increased TEWL compared with term infants [35]. Most preterm infants lose up to 13% of their body weight as TEWL during the first days after birth, gradually diminishing with age. This high TEWL is accompanied by a large heat loss [35]. Semipermeable polyurethane membrane produced a significant TEWL reduction in 18 premature infants: 21.1 ± 2.0 g/m^{2}h before application vs 10.5 ± 1.4 g/m^{2}h with membrane in place [23]. After 4 days of continuous dressing, TEWL returned to 22.8 ± 3.0 g/m^{2}h [23].

Sweat Gland Activity

Serup and Rasmussen have observed a significantly lower TEWL on the flexor and extensor sites of hands and forearms in 68 patients with generalized scleroderma than in 66 control subjects [36]. The TEWL decrease in scleroderma was probably due to sweat gland atrophy [36].

A higher TEWL was noticed in patients with Parkinson's disease than in healthy subjects, before and after heating provocation, as a result of sweating [47]. This TEWL increase was significantly correlated with the severity of the disease and indicated an extensive autonomous nervous system dysfunction in Parkinson's disease [47]. In contrast, a decreased sweat response after sympathomimetic stimulation, as measured by TEWL, was noted on the forehead in 31 patients suffering from cluster headache [32].

During rapid eye movement (REM) sleep, significant lower TEWL values were noted on the forehead than during quiet wakefulness or non-REM sleep [21].

In a patient with cholinergic urticaria, we have demonstrated an increase of TEWL on gustatory provocations of increasing strength [46]. These provocations (lemon, sal ammoniac licorice, and doubly salted licorice) were accompanied by erythematous macules and a sensation of warmth and itching of increasing severity, finally evolving into weals typical for cholinergic urticaria. A threshold dependency in the development of cholinergic urticaria was therefore proposed [46].

Discussion

Our Own Observations

Our work has been focused on the use of TEWL measurement by means of the Servo Med evaporimeter in the evaluation of irritant skin reactions. Many investigators have noticed variations in TEWL on uninvolved or unexposed skin, due to intra- and interindividual differences in TEWL [7, 11, 48]. These variations may interfere with results from experimentally and clinically oriented work. Therefore, the intraindividual variation should be considerably smaller than the interindividual variation. This latter requirement is of particular importance for the characterization of individuals by their baseline TEWL (experiments 2 and 3). Recently, our group has demonstrated that the intraindividual variation by site was substantially lower (15.5%) than the interindividual variation (84.5%) [28]. This was also true for the variation by days, although less clearly (intraindividual, 20.6%; interindividual 79.4%) [28]. This temporal variation may be explained by day to day differences in skin surface temperature, skin hydration state, and ambient relative humidity.

In persons with a high preexposure TEWL (BASE), the barrier function of the stratum corneum is apparently impaired from the start. This allows SLS to penetrate and damage the skin more easily, resulting in a high TEWL value after exposure. It may be possible, therefore, to "predict" the skin's response to SLS by knowing its preexposure TEWL value.

After the 24 h single SLS exposure, we measured TEWL 2 h after the removal of the patch, since in a previous study it has been demonstrated that it took 2 h for TEWL on the water-patch site to return to a level only slightly elevated above its own baseline value [27]. Baker and Kligman advised waiting as long as 3 h after removal of a patch [1].

In the majority of the subjects, epidermal injury and clinical signs were most pronounced 24 h after removal of the patch. This late peak irritation reaction may be caused by the fact that the damaging influence of SLS continues after removal of the patch, since the major part, once absorbed, remains in the upper skin layers until it is eliminated. In this study, we have observed that the skin's response to a single 24 h SLS exposure may be different among individuals, particularly in the first days after removal of the patch. This heterogeneous reaction pattern may constitute a problem in deciding to choose the right moment for evaluation of patch results; one might consider taking two readings (on days 2 and 3, for example), as has been recommended for allergic patch testing [10].

We postulate that the difference in TEWL levels between day 2 and a subsequent day corresponds to the efficacy of epidermal repair, indicating the importance of skin adaptation capacity.

The TEWL value after 3 weeks of repeated exposure to SLS, SUC, and SOL was taken as a measure of susceptibility to these irritants. In this study, it was noticed that there is a significant correlation between BASE and the TEWL value after 3 weeks of repeated exposure to the above-mentioned irritants. Also, skin dryness was significantly associated with higher susceptibility towards SUC and SOL. The higher susceptibility of group AD (history of atopic dermatitis) than groups CD and C indicates that past AD is unique with regard to enhanced skin susceptibility, probably owing to an impaired preexposure barrier function and/or the presence of skin dryness. Susceptibility to irritants may be not only dependent on preexposure barrier function of the stratum corneum, but also on other factors, such as reactivity of cellular targets underneath the stratum corneum [13] and adaptation capacity (see experiment 2).

When scoring irritant reactions by means of an evaporimeter, the substances should be applied over an area which is sufficiently large (about 20 mm in diameter), since it involves extensive experience to position the measuring probe cylinder (diameter, 12 mm) exactly on the site concerned.

Clinical Applications

Measurement of TEWL is a rapid and relatively simple procedure which may render information concerning the most essential function of the skin, namely, being a barrier. From the foregoing examples of clinical applications, it is evident that TEWL measurement may be of practical value.

Patients with generalized erythroderma are at high risk due to excessive loss of water, heat, and proteins. Assessment of TEWL would establish the total amount of water loss through the damaged skin and thus give an indication of the heat loss due to the cooling effect of its evaporation. This holds true not only for erythroderma, but also for severe (burn) wounds, in preterm infants, etc.

Furthermore, TEWL measurement has been proven to be a good mirror of the clinical severity of various skin conditions. Higher TEWL values were noted in dermatitis, psoriasis, pityriasis rubra pilaris, and ichthyosis. This increase in TEWL can be explained by a loss of barrier function and probably also by the effect of higher skin temperature [16]. It is likely that TEWL is elevated in a host of other skin ailments in which the barrier function is impaired, such as those characterized by parakeratosis and epidermal atrophy.

Therefore, evaporimetry may be a useful tool in the investigation of the influence of external (season) or individual factors and the efficacy of different treatment regimes in a multitude of skin diseases.

Exact determination of the degree of sweating was useful in disorders in which sweat gland activity is altered such as scleroderma, Parkinsons's disease, and cluster headache. Possible other applications in this direction may be: genetic counseling in hereditary disorders such as congenital ectodermal aplasia, determination of the extent of autonomous dysfunction in Hansen's disease, etc. In this field, TEWL measurement is superior to older methods aimed at estimating the sweat gland function (starch/iodine test, visualization of individual sweat droplets, collection of sweat in bags or pads; [8]) with respect to reproducibility and accuracy. Furthermore, monitoring of sweating was useful in the investigation of cholinergic urticaria and physiological phenomena, such as during sleep.

References

1. Baker H, Kligman AM (1967) Measurement of transepidermal water loss by electrical hygrometry. Arch Dermatol 96: 441–452
2. Baker H (1971) Déperdition d'eau trans-épidermique. Ann Dermatol Syph 98: 289–296
3. Bettley FR, Grice KA (1965) A method for measuring the transepidermal water loss and a means of inactivating sweat glands. Br J Dermatol 77: 627–638
4. Björnberg A (1968) Skin reactions to primary irritants in patients with hand eczema. An investigation with matched controls. Thesis, Gotenburg
5. Blank IH (1953) Factors which influcence the water content of the stratum corneum. J Invest Dermatol 21: 259–269
6. Blank IH, (1965) Cutaneous barriers. J Invest Dermatol 45: 249–256
7. Blichman C, Serup J (1987) Hydration studies on scaly hand eczemas. Contact Dermatitis 16: 155–159.
8. Champion RH (1986) Disorders of sweat glands. In: Rook AA, Wilkinson DS, Ebling FJG et al. (eds) Textbook of dermatology. Blackwell, Oxford, pp 1884–1887.
9. Finlay AY, Nicholls S, King CS, Marks R (1980) The 'dry' noneczematous skin associated with atopic eczema. Br J Dermatol 102: 249–256.
10. Fregert S, Hjorth N, Magnusson B, Bandmann HJ, Calnan CD, Cronin E, Malten KE, Meneghini CL, Pirila V, Wilkinson DS (1969) Epidemiology of contact dermatitis. Trans St Johns Hosp Dermatol Soc 55: 17–35.
11. Frödin T, Skogh M, Molin L (1988) The importance of the coal tar bath in the Ingram treatment of psoriasis. Evaluation by evaporimetry and laser Doppler flowmetry. Br J Dermatol 118: 429–434.
12. Frosch PJ, Kligman AM (1979) The soap chamber test. A new method for assessing the irritancy of soaps. J Am Acad Dermatol 1: 35–41

13. Frosch PJ (1989) Irritant contact dermatitis. In: Frosch PJ, Dooms-Goossens A, Lachapelle JM, Rycroft RJG, Scheper RJ (eds) Current topics in contact dermatitis. Springer, Berlin Heidelberg New York, pp 385–398
14. Frosch PJ Czarnetzki BM (1989) Effect of retinoids on wound healing in diabetic rats. Arch Dermatol Res 281: 424–426
15. Frost P, Weinstein GD, Bothwell JW, Wildnauer R (1968) Ichthyosioform dermatosis: III. Studies on transepidermal water loss. Arch Dermatol 98: 230–233.
16. Grice K, Bettley F (1967) Skin water loss and accidental hypothermia in psoriasis, ichthyosis, and erythroderma. 4: 195–198.
17. Grice KA (1980) Measurement of transepidermal water loss. In: Jarret A (ed) Physiology and pathophysiology of the skin VI. Academic, London, pp 2116–2118.
18. Hammarlund K, Nilsson GE, Öberg PA, Sedin G (1977) Transepidermal water loss in newborn infants: I. Relation to ambient humidity and site of measurement, and estimation of total transepidermal water loss. In: Nilsson GE (ed) On the measurement of evaporative water loss. Thesis, Department of Medical Engineering, Linköping University, Sweden
19. Hanifin JM, Rajka G (1980) Diagnostic features of atopic dermatitis. Acta Derm Venereol (Stockh) 92: 44–47.
20. Jonkman MF, Molenaar I, Nieuwenhuis P, Klasen HJ (1989) Evaporative water loss and epidermis regeneration in partial-thickness wounds dressed with by a fluid-retaining versus a clot-inducing wound covering in guinea pigs. Scand J Plast Reconstr Surg 23: 29–34
21. Kahn A, Rebuffat E, Blum D, Sottiaux M, Van de Merckt C, Dramaix M, Montauk L (1987) Transepidermal water loss during sleep in infants. Sleep 10: 111–115.
22. Kleinbaum DG, Kupper LL (1978) Applied regression analysis and other multivariable methods. Duxbury, Scituate
23. Knauth A, Gordin M, McNelis W, Baumgart S (1989) Semipermeable polyurethane membrane as an artificial skin for the premature neonate. Pediatrics 83: 945–950
24. Lamke L-O, Nilsson GE, Reithner HL (1977) The evaporative water loss from burns and the water-vapour permeability of grafts and artificial membranes used in the treatment of burns. Burns 3: 159–165.
25. Menczel E, Bucks DAW, Wester RC, Maibach HI (1985) Skin binding during percutaneous penetration. In: Bronaugh RL, Maibach HI (eds) Percutaneous absorption. Mechanisms, methodology, drug delivery. Dekker, New York; pp 43–56.
26. Nilsson GE (1977) Measurement of water exchange through the skin. Med Biol Eng Comput 15: 209–218.
27. Pinnagoda J, Tupker RA, Coenraads PJ, Nater JP (1989) Prediction of susceptibility to an irritant response by transepidermal water loss. Contact Dermatitis 20: 341–346.
28. Pinnagoda J, Tupker RA, Smit JA, Coenraads PJ, Nater JP (1989) The intra- and inter-individual variability and reliability of transepidermal water loss measurements. Contact Dermatitis 21: 255–259.
29. Pinnagoda J, Tupker RA, Agner T, Serup J (1990) Guidelines for transepidermal water loss (TEWL) measurement. A report from the standardization group of the European Environmental and Contact Dermatitis Society. Contact Dermatitis 22: 164–178.
30. Rajka G, Thune P (1976) The relationship between the course of psoriasis and transepidermal water loss, photoelectric plethysmography and reflex photometry. Br J Dermatol 94: 253–261.
31. Rothman S (1954) Insensible water loss. In: Physiology and biochemistry of the skin. University of Chicago Press, Chicago, pp. 153–200, 233–243.
32. Salvesen R, de Souza-Carvalho D, Sand T, Sjaastad O (1988) Cluster headache: forehead sweating pattern during heating and pilocarpine tests. Variation as a function of time. Cephalalgia 8: 245–253.
33. Schaefer H, Zesch A, Stüttgen G (1982) Skin permeability. Springer, Berlin Heidelberg New York, pp 590–625
34. Scheuplein RJ, Blank IH (1971) Permeability of the skin. Physiol Rev 51: 702–747.
35. Sedin G, Hammerlund K, Nilsson GE, Stromberg B, Öberg PA (1985) Measurements of transepidermal water loss in newborn infants. Clin Perinatol 12: 79–99.
36. Serup J, Rasmussen I (1985) Dry hands in scleroderma. Including studies of sweat gland function in healthy individuals. Acta Derm Venerol (Stockh) 65: 419–423.

37. Serup J, Staberg B (1987) Differentiation of allergic and irritant reactions by transepidermal water loss. Contact Dermatitis 16: 129–132.
38. Serup J, Blichman C (1987) Epidermal hydration of psoriasis plaques and the relation to scaling. Measurement of electrical conductance and transepidermal water loss. Acta Derm Venereol (Stockh) 67: 357–359
39. ServoMed Evaporimeters (1981) Operation handbook. ServoMed, Stockholm
40. Shahidullah M, Raffle EJ, Frain-Bell W (1967) Insensible water loss in dermatitis. Br J Dermatol 79: 589–597.
41. Shahidullah M, Raffle EJ, Rimmer AR, Frain-Bell W (1969) Transepidermal water loss in patients with dermatitis. Br J Dermatol 81: 722–730.
42. Spruit D, Malten KE (1966) The regeneration rate of the water vapour loss of heavily damaged skin. Dermatologica 132: 115–123.
43. Tupker RA, Coenraads PJ, Pinnagoda J, Nater JP (1989) Baseline transepidermal water loss (TEWL) as a prediction of susceptibility to sodium lauryl sulphate. Contact Dermatitis 20: 265–269.
44. Tupker RA, Pinnagoda J, Nater JP (1990) The transient and cumulative effect of sodium lauryl sulphate on the epidermal barrier assessed by transepidermal water loss: interindividual variation. Acta Derm Venereol (Stockh) 70: 1–5.
45. Tupker RA, Pinnagoda J, Coenraads PJ, Nater PJ (1990) Susceptibility to irritants: role of barrier function, skin dryness and history of atopic dermatitis. Br J Dermatol 123: 199–205.
46. Tupker RA, Doeglas HMG (1990) Water vapour loss threshold and induction of cholinergic urticaria. Dermatologica 181: 23–25
47. Turkha JT, Myllyla VV (1987) Sweating dysfunction of Parkinson's disease. Eur Neurol 26: 1–7.
48. Van der Valk PGM, Nater JP, Bleumink E (1985) Vulnerability of the skin to surfactants in different groups of eczema patients and controls as measured by water vapour loss. Clin Exp Dermatol 10: 98–103
49. Vickers CFH (1963) Existence of reservoir in the stratum corneum. Arch Dermatol 88: 20–23.

Simultaneous Measurement of Thickness and Compressibility of a Skin Fold

D. Lubach, G. Neumann, and M. Kietzmann

Introduction

The thickness of a skin fold is usually measured with mechanical instruments such as a vernier caliper or a skin fold caliper [4].

A problem encountered when using such mechanical instruments is the fact that there actually is no definable skin fold thickness because skin can be compressed. Even the manipulation necessary to create a skin fold causes a deformation. The pressure needed for measuring skin fold thickness with a mechanical instrument also changes the fold. Application of constant pressure has been used to avoid this difficulty. However, it must be noted that compressibility of skin shows individual variation so that identical pressure can have a variable effect on skin fold thickness depending on skin plasticity.

Skin folds can best be formed on the volar aspect of the forearm and on the dorsum of the hand since there is only little subcutis and the epidermis is loosely attached to the underlying tissue.

The smaller the distance between opposing skin pushed together to form a skin fold, the smaller the amount of subcutaneous fat grasped in the process. Skin fold thickness measurements referring to physiologic and pathologic conditions of the dermis should include as little subcutaneous fat as possible. For this reason, application of the skin fold method is limited to certain areas of the body.

Method

It is clear from the above that exact measurement of a particular skin fold is impossible because the formation of such a fold is a dynamic process. It is, however, possible to calculate the diameter of a skin fold. We have developed a method that utilizes continuous compression of a skin fold over a defined time span [9–11]. The decrease of skin fold thickness caused by compression is measured at certain intervals, i.e., every 5 s in most cases. Compression of the skin fold is terminated after 25–30 s. Entering the measured points in a coordinate system (x-axis equals time) produces a typical asymptotic curve. The curve can be transformed into a straight line by using a logarithmic time axis. This straight line can be described by the equation $y = a-bx$. The intercept a with the y-axis is taken as a measure of the skin fold thickness in millimeters.

Hautklinik Linden, Medizinische Hochschule Hannover, Ricklinger Str. 5, 3000 Hannover 91

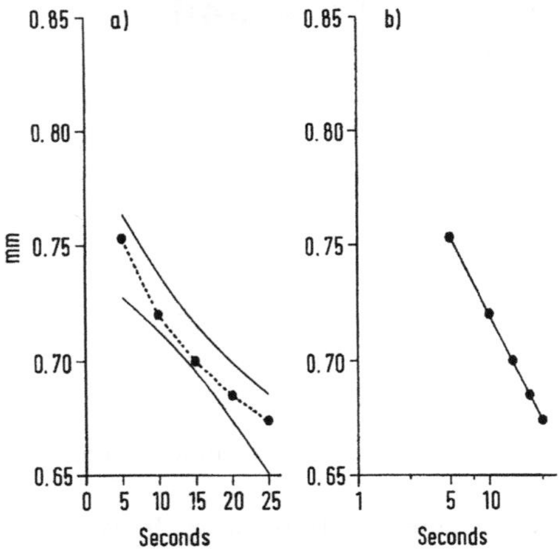

time	SFT (mm)
5	0.753
10	0.720
15	0.700
20	0.685
25	0.674
y = 0.833 − 0.049 x	

Fig. 1a, b. Example of a compressibility and skin fold thickness (CT) measuring procedure. Five individuals measurements at intervals of 5 s (**a**). Transformation of the curve into a straight line by use of a logarithmic time axis (**b**). *SFT*, skin fold thickness

Due to the logarithmic transformation of time axis or y-axis, a is defined at log 1 = 0, i.e., 1 s. The line is characterized by the slope $-b$. The value of b is taken as a measure of the *compressibility* of the skin and also characterizes the thinning of the skin in time (mm/log t). Figure 1 shows an example of the measuring procedure.

This method allows simultaneous determination of two characteristics of the skin: (1) compressibility (C) and (2) skin fold thickness (SFT). This is why the method has been designated the CR method.

Equipment

Originally, a light metal clamp that works like a pair of scissors (Fig. 2a) was used. Both tips are tapered to prevent slipping of the instrument on the skin surface. A metal spring is installed in the levering point so that 5.50 p/mm^2 (measured at the tips) must be applied in order to close the instrument. One of the handles is equipped with a gauge (Mitutoyo, Japan) whose pin is pressed inwards when the jaws of the instrument are closed. Values read from the gauge are converted by means of a conversion factor and indicate how much the tips of the jaws are open at a given point of time. The distance of the tips equals the diameter of the grasped skin fold and can be read in mm^{-2}.

Later, the instrument was improved (Fig. 2b). The tips were equipped with rectangular, exchangeable, small blocks. With the help of double-sided adhesive tape the open instrument was attached to the skin so that slipping was effectively prevented. A locking screw was fixed to one of the handles that facilitated various degrees of opening of the jaws. An electronic displacement transducer (Sylvac, Switzerland) was used instead of a gauge. In addition, a switch was installed for the control of start and end of the measuring procedure. During measuring, electronic impulses from the transducer are transmitted to an electric circuit that is connected to a plotter (printer) which automatically prints out the distance of the tips every 0.16 s.

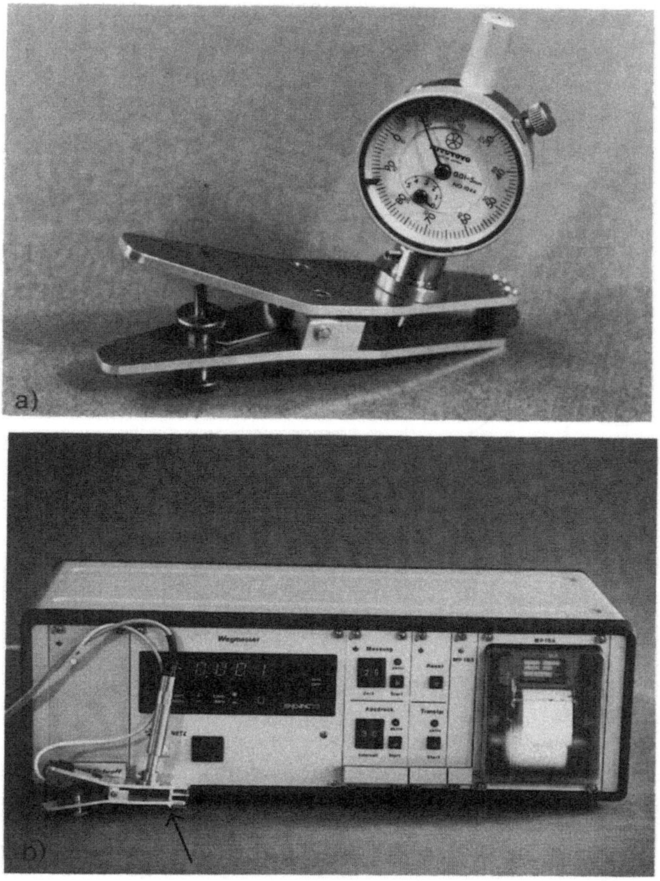

Fig. 2a, b. Instruments used for measurement of skin fold thickness and skin compressibility. Original instrument (**a**). Improved instrument (**b**). *Arrow,* measuring clamp

Closure of the measuring clamp is followed by two phases: (1) a rapid phase during which a skin area of 9 mm (common size) is pressed together in a fold and which terminates after approximately 0.7 s (phase of skin fold formation) and (2) a progressively slower phase during which the skin fold formed in phase 1 is compressed continuously (compression phase). Both phases can be visualized by continuous recording of SFT with the improved instrument (Fig. 3a, b).

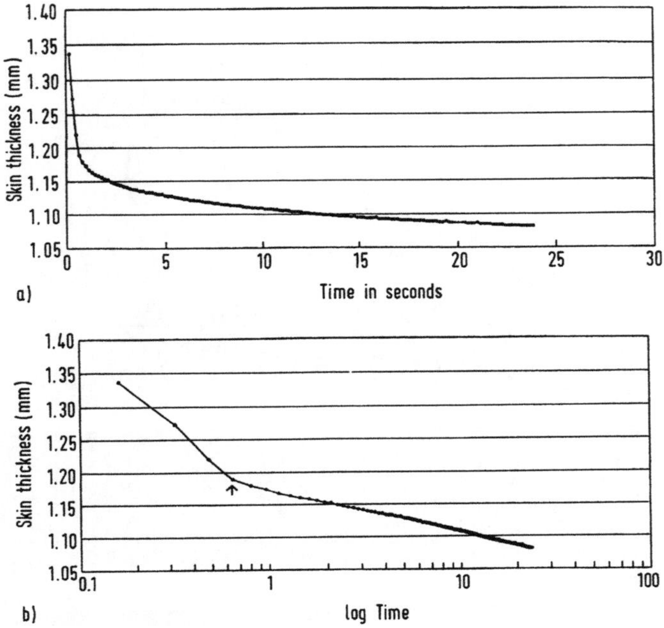

Fig. 3a, b. Sequence of skin fold formation and compression. Skin thickness (mm) was recorded every 0.16 s. The asymptotic course of the curve (**a**) is easily recognized. The curve is transformed into a straight line from 0.5 to 0.7 s onwards if a logarithmic time axis is used (**b**). Transition from fold formation to the compression phase (*arrow*) is also easily recognizable

Results

Comparative Measurements on Identical Skin Areas of Both Forearms

The measurements were performed on 40 volunteers (18 male, 22 female) that were between 20 and 80 years old. C and SFT values of identical skin areas of both arms were compared. The measuring points were: central line of the volar aspect 5, 10, and 15 cm proximal to the wrist.

Statistically, SFT values did not differ significantly (Student's *t* test for paired samples) (Table 1). With regard to thickness, measuring points from proximal to distal were, however, significantly different with the exception of C values between points 15 cm and 10 cm. In this trial, the confidence interval for determination of SFT was 2.96% and 6.86% for C [9].

Table 1. Comparative measurements on identical skin areas of both forearms

Distance to the wrist (cm)	Left		Right	
	SFT (mm)	C (mm/log t)	SFT (mm)	C (mm/log t)
5	2.10 ± 0.26	− 0.274 ± 0.066	2.12 ± 0.30	− 0.272 ± 0.086
10	2.25 ± 0.26	− 0.282 ± 0.068	2.30 ± 0.30	− 0.278 ± 0.064
15	2.32 ± 0.33	− 0.228 ± 0.066	2.20 ± 0.44	− 0.236 ± 0.068

SFT, skin fold thickness; C, compressibility.

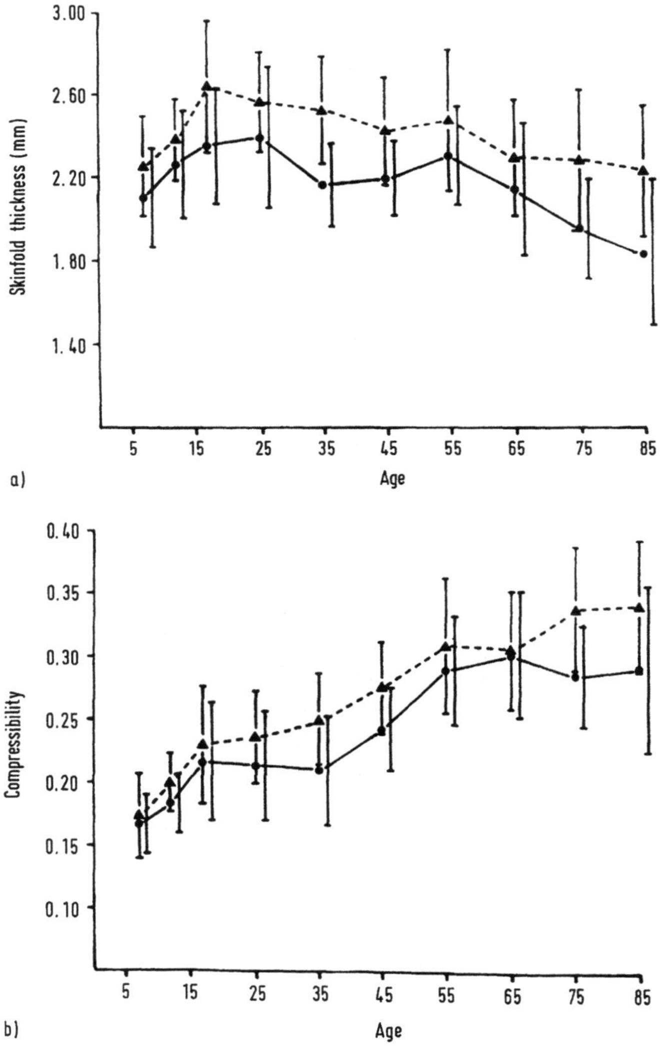

Fig. 4a, b. Skin fold thickness and compressibility values of 340 adults in relation to age. Skin fold thickness is constant between the 20th and 50th year of life and then decreases progressively **(a)**. Values for C increase throughout life (b) Measuring point: central line on the volar aspect of the forearm, 10 cm proximal to the wrist. *continuous line*, women; *broken line*, men

Age-Related Changes of the Skin

Skin fold thickness was determined in 340 individuals between 5 and 89 years of age with unaffected skin. Results were differentiated according to age and sex. Figure 4 shows the results. It becomes clear from the graphs that SFT increases until the 20th year of life and remains constant up to the age of 30 (women) and 40 (men). Diameter of SFT decreases continuously after that. The skin of men is slightly thicker than that of women. Compressibility of the skin does, however, increase continuously throughout life; only women show approximately constant values between the ages of 15 and 35 [10].

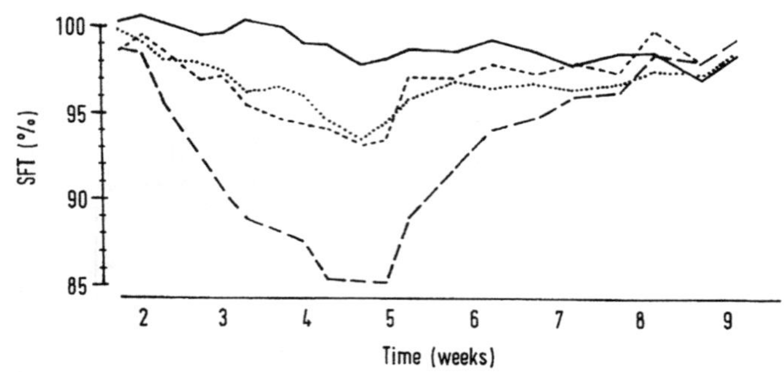

Fig. 5. Decrease of skin fold thickness (*SFT*) after daily application of 1% hydrocortisone (*dotted line*), 0.05 flupredidene-21-acetate (*short broken line*), and 0.05 betametasone-17, 21-dipropionate (*long broken line*); untreated control site, *continuous line*. After termination of corticosteroid application thinning of the skin regressed completely within 2 weeks (during weeks 5–9)

Thinning of the Skin Following Application of Topical Glucocorticosteroids

Samples (0.1 ml) of betamethasone 17,21-diproprionate, fluprednidene 21-acetate, and hydrocortisone (1%) were applied to the volar aspect of the forearms of eight individuals (six female, two male) under occlusion. The corticosteroid samples remained on the skin overnight and were removed in the morning. No treatment was given during the day. SFT of the test areas was measured on four successive days of the first week of the trial period. The means of the obtained values were determined (100%).

The steroids were applied from week 2 through week 4. SFT was determined three times a week and then over another 4 weeks; however, no more corticosteroids were applied. Changes in SFT were calculated as a percent of the baseline value (= 100%).

Figure 5 shows that SFT of the untreated skin areas remains almost constant during the complete trial period. Betamethasone caused thinning of the skin by approximately 15%, hydrocortisone and flumethasone by approximately 5%. After termination of corticosteroid application, almost complete regression of thinning was observed within 2 weeks [12].

Changes During Hemodialysis

Measurements of SFT and C were performed on the dorsum of the hand and two points of the volar aspect of the forearm (5 and 15 cm proximal to the wrist) immediately prior to and 2.5 and 5 h after start of hemodialysis in a total of 83 patients. All patients had been receiving hemodialysis over several years.

Figure 6 shows that SFT decreases significantly during hemodialysis; C was also lower during hemodialysis. The decrease in C values is greater than the decrease in SFT [17].

Changes in UV-Induced Erythemas

Erythemas were induced on the forearms of 11 individuals with a xenon high pressure lamp (150 W). Immediately before and 8 and 24 h after exposure, SFT and C were determined. Only the right forearm was exposed, the left forearm served as control. SFT increased to 122% (24 h): C increased to approximately 130% (Table 2).

Table 2. UV-induced erythemas. Left forearm, control; right forearm, erythema.

Time (h)	SFT (mm)		C (mm/log t)	
	Left	Right	Left	Right
0	1.97 ± 0.31	1.97 ± 0.32	− 0.29 ±0.03	− 0.30 ±0.08
8	2.02 ± 0.33	2.27 ± 0.32	− 0.30 ± 0.04	− 0.34 ± 0.07
24	2.02 ± 0.34	2.41 ± 0.35	− 0.25 ± 0.09	− 0.39 ± 0.07

Left forearm, control; right forearm, erythema

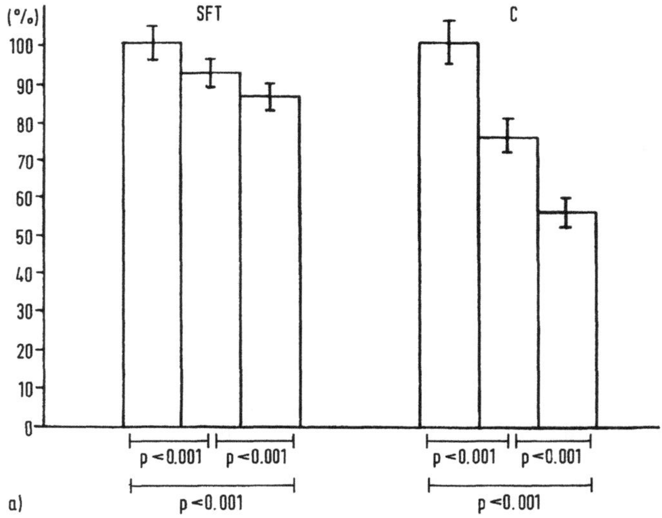

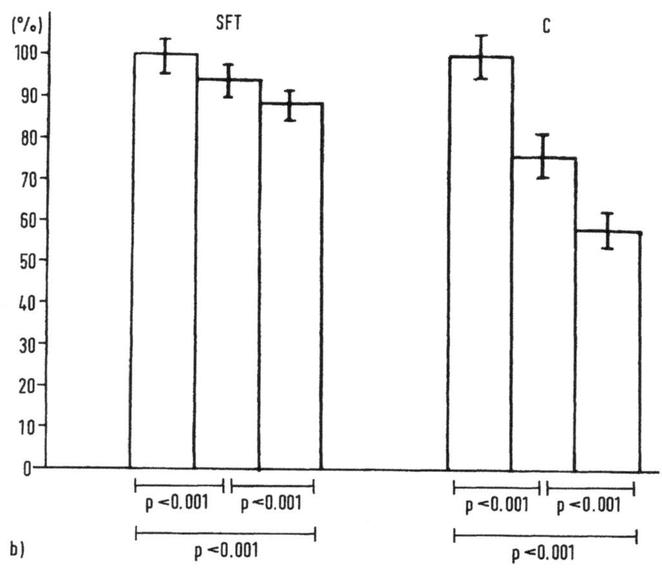

Figs. 6a–c. Skin fold thickness (*SFT*) and compressibility (*C*) values during hemodialysis treatment. *First column*, before treatment; *second column*, 2.5 h after start of dialysis; *third column*, after termination of dialysis. Measuring points: dorsum of the hand (**a**), volar aspect of the forearm, 5 cm (**b**), and 15 cm (**c**) proximal to the wrist

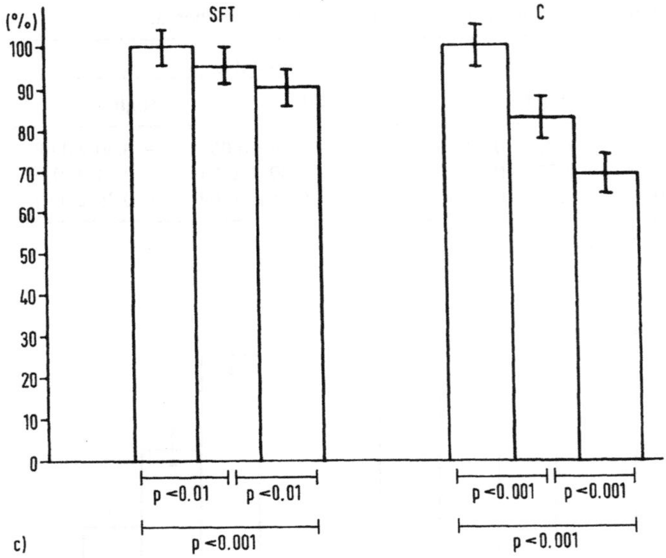

Fig 6c

Measurement of Erythemas

An erythema was induced in 23 individuals by application of a nicotinate-containing oil (Rubriment^{Tn}). While SFT and C values were not different for both test and control skin areas, a highly significant difference ($p \leq 0.001$) was recorded following treatment. The increase of C was greater than the increase of SFT (Table 3). In some persons, slight wheals were observed [2].

Table 3. Measurement of Rubriment erythemas

	Before (%)	Erythema (%)
SFT	1.93 ± 0.31 (100)	2.33 ± 0.42 (121)
C	– 0.230 ± 0.080 (100)	– 0.370 ± 0.349 (161)

Measurement of Positive Epicutaneous Test Reactions

Epicutaneous (patch) tests were performed on the volar aspect of the forearm in 17 women between the ages of 30 and 82 years. The corresponding skin area on the contralateral forearm served as control. SFT and C values were determined before and 24, 48 and 72h after testing (Table 4).

The women had already undergone epicutaneous testing at an earlier date. At that time, a skin area of the back served as the testing site. All patients had shown a positive reaction to one or more allergens.

SFT and C values were only measured in patients that displayed a clear positive reaction. No comparison was made between intensity of the test reaction and SFT and C values (according to the guidelines of the ICDRG) because of the relatively small number of subjects. In this study, the strongest reaction was recorded after 48 h. SFT had then increased to 165% and C to 262% [2].

Table 4. Measurement of positive patch tests

	Patch tests		Control	
Time (h)	SFT (mm)	C (mm/log t)	SFT (mm)	C (mm/log t)
Before	1.60 ± 0.28	− 0.187 ± 0.056	1.58 ± 0.33	− 0.178 ± 0.048
24	2.25 ± 0.55	− 0.435 ± 0.155	1.53 ± 0.19	− 0.191 ± 0.040
48	2.64 ± 0.78	− 0.490 ± 0.238	1.65 ± 0.26	− 0.261 ± 0.061
72	2.30 ± 0.46	− 0.390 ± 0.130	1.62 ± 0.25	− 0.202 ± 0.049

SFT, skin fold thickness; C, compressibility.

Measurement of Wheal Reaction After Scratch Test with an Allergen-Containing Solution

Patients with confirmed atopic allergy were tested on the volar aspect of the right forearm. Identical skin areas on the left forearm served as control. Measurements were performed only when the reaction was clearly positive. The allergenic test solutions were obtained from Bencard (extracts from grass, rye, and house dust mites). The results are shown in Table 5. While SFT increased to 155%, C increased to 288% [2].

Table 5. Wheal reaction after scratch test with an allergen-containing solution

	Control (%)	Test (%)
SFT (mm)	1.99 ± 0.42 (100)	3.08 ± 0.85 (155)
C (mm/log t)	− 0.206 ± 0.081 (100)	− 0.594 ± 0.250 (288)

Discussion

Continuous recording of CT measurements shows that the compression phase starts after approximately 0.5–0.7 s. Subsequently, the skin fold becomes progressively thinner, although the thinning process slows down gradually with time. Earlier investigations have demonstrated that the process of compression was, although extremely slow, still incomplete after 20 min. After the end of the measuring process, an imprint of the measuring clamp is visible on the skin that corresponds to the duration of the measuring process. The impression regresses only slowly. Hence, it can be inferred that the gel-like dermal ground substance is displaced into the surrounding tissue during the compression phase. In simplified terms, the skin can be described as a network of fibers that is filled with a gel-like ground substance. Water is mainly bound to hyaluronic acid; normally, probably less than 1% of the fluid exists as free fluid [1].

An increase of the C value is characterized by a steep decline of compression and is, theoretically, influenced by two factors: (1) a decrease in viscosity of the interstitial gel

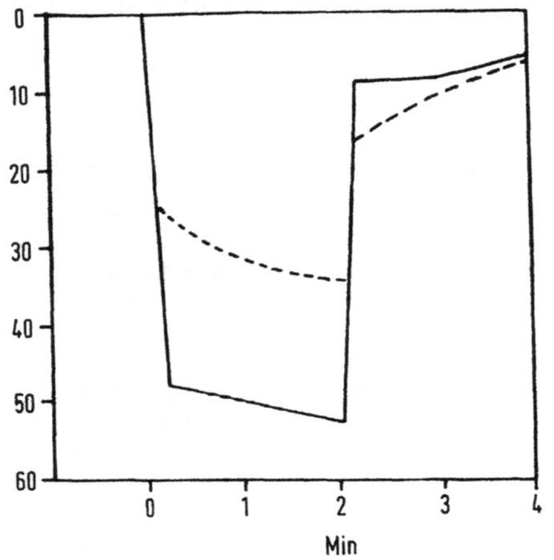

Fig. 7. Schade's elastometry; example of a measuring procedure. The *continuous* line shows normal skin, the *broken line* an edema. The skin is indented forcefully by a weight within a few seconds, a slower phase of compression follows (until minute 2). After removal of the weight, the dent regresses quickly, but incompletely at first. This is followed by a slower phase of complete regression. (From [15])

that is therefore displaced much easier, and (2) an increase in mesh size of the fiber network and no change in viscosity of the interstitial gel. Displacement of the interstitial gel is, however, easier in both cases.

Compressibility of the dermis was methodically studied early in this century by Schade [16] (Schade's elastometry), who described an apparatus that registered the degree and rate of indentation following application of a constant weight (20, 50, or 100 g) to the skin. He and other scientists [7, 15] used the equipment to study tissue induration in different conditions; they showed that marked differences existed between the behavior of normal and edematous tissues regarding depth of indentation and time required for the tissues to return to their original state.

Four quantities were measured: (1) the primary indentation which appears quickly and progresses to (2) the total indentation. The weight impresses the skin only slowly. This phase ends after 2 min in most cases and is followed by (3) the immediate rebound that follows removal of the weight and then by (4) the total rebound (the degree of rebound 2 min after removal of the weight (Fig. 7).

The second and slower phase of indentation of Schade's technique corresponds to the compression curve of the here described CT method. Schade also discovered steeper increases for edematous tissue than for normal tissue. Schmidt-La Baum carried out detailed studies with this technique [15].

Lewis et al. [8] and Robertson et al. [14] used an apparatus that enabled them to continuously record compression curves. They used the technique for measurement of skin indentation by a weight and also for measurement of skin fold compression by a skin fold caliper. The curves they obtained resemble our curves to a wide extent [8, 14].

If an edema (wheal) is present, viscosity will be lower, e.g., because of an increasing quantity of interstitial tissue fluid. At the same time, the mesh size of the fiber network increases due to the increasing volume. These conditions are found in local inflammatory processes of the skin. SFT and C therefore increase. During hemodialysis tissue fluid decreases: SFT and C values decrease due to collapse of the fiber network (smaller mesh size), and viscosity increases.

In contrast to skin thickness, which decrease with age, compressibility increases when the individual becomes older. This finding was unexpected. Similar results were obtained by Kirk and Kvorning [7]. They used Schade's elastometry and also found an increase in the slow phase of indentation and a simultaneous increase in the slow rebound phase. Daly and Odland [3] compressed the skin of the anterior aspect of the tibia with a weight (5 g/mm^2). They discovered that the indentation regressed more slowly in older than in younger persons. The decrease in skin fold diameter in older persons could have two possible reasons: (1) a decrease in ground substance of the dermis causes partial collapsing of the collagenous fiber network or (2) the collagenous fiber network becomes structurally reduced. The increase of C is either due to a decrease in viscosity of the interstitial gel or rarification of the collagenous fiber network. The total amount of collagen decreases about 1% per year through adult life [5]. This explains thinning of the skin with age [5, 6]. A progressive decrease of glycosaminoglycans has also been reported [5]. Pearce and Grimmer [13] however, were unable to demonstrate an age-related decrease in dermal hyaluronate. Instead, they found an increase in relative water content of skin. Hence, ground substance is likely to be reduced. Water content, by contrast, increases so that displacement of interstitial fluid is easier.

Conclusion

The CT method is an easy, inexpensive method for precise measurement of SFT. We routinely use it for studies on steroid-induced thinning of skin. The method also provides insight into alteration of the physicochemical behavior of dermal ground substance. With the CT method, alterations in pathologic skin conditions such as edema or sclerosis can be identified. Application of the CT method is presently restricted to body areas where skin can easily be lifted from underlying tissue.

References

1. Adair TH, Guyton AC (1985) Lymph formation and its modification in the lymphatic system. In: Johnston MG (ed) Experimental biology of the lymphatic circulation. Elsevier, Amsterdam, pp 13–44
2. Dähne-Öchsner U (1982) Eine modifizierte Form der Hautfaltenmessung mit erweitertem Anwendungsspektrum. Dissertation, Medizinische Hochschule Hannover
3. Daly CH, Odland GF (1973) Age related changes in the mechanical properties of human skin. J Invest Dermatol 73: 84–87
4. Dykes PJ, Marks R (1977) Measurement of skin thickness: a comparison of two in vivo techniques with a conventional histometric method. J Invest Dermatol 69: 275–277
5. Fenske NA, Lober CW (1986) Structural and functional changes of normal aging skin. J Am Acad Dermatol 15: 571–585
6. Hall DA, Blackett AD, Zajac AR et al. (1981) Changes in skinfold thickness with increasing age. Age Ageing 10: 19–23
7. Kirk JE, Kvorning SA (1949) Quantitative measurements of the elastic properties of the skin and subcutaneous tissue in yound and old individuals. J Gerontol 4: 273–284
8. Lewis HE, Meyer J, Pandiscio AA (1965) Recording skinfold calipers for the determination of subcutaneous edema. J Lab Clin Med 66: 154–160

9. Lubach D, Koppe R (1984) Die kombinierte Kompressions- und Dickenmessung (KD-Messung) einer Hautfalte. Beschreibung einer neuen Methode. Ärztl Kosmetol 14: 243–251
10. Lubach D, Kunkler A (1984) Die kombinierte Kompressions- und Dickenmessung (KD-Messung) einer Hautfalte. Änderung der Eigenschaften in Abhängigkeit vom Alter. Ärztl Kosmetol 14: 340–344
11. Lubach D (1984) Die kombinierte Kompressions- und Dickenmessung (KD-Methode) einer Hautfalte. Anwendungsbeispiele. Ärztl Kosmetol 14: 388–395
12. Lubach D, Bensmann A, Bornemann U (1989) Steroid-induced dermal atrophy. Investigations on discontinuous application. Dermatologica 179: 67–72
13. Pearce RH, Grimmer BJ (1972) Age and the chemical constitution of normal human dermis. J Invest Dermatol 59: 347–361
14. Robertson EG, Lewis HE, Billewicz WZ, Foggett IN (1969) Two devices for quantifying the rate of deformation of skin and subcutaneous tissue. J Lab Clin Med 73: 594–602
15. Schmidt-La Baume F (1928) Über Dermoelastometrie. Arch Dermatol Syph 156: 383–423
16. Schade H (1912) Die physikalische Chemie der inneren Medizin. Elastizitätsfunktionen des Bindegewebes. Exp Pathol Ther 11: 369–399
17. Wellbrock H (1985) Hautdicke und Komprimierbarkeit der Haut in vivo bei Dialysepatienten und ihre Zusammenhänge mit verschiedenen klinischen Parametern. Experimentelle Untersuchung mittels einer mechanischen Meßmethode. Dissertation, Medizinische Hochschule Hannover

Sebum Analysis Using a Hydrophobic Lipid-Absorbent Tape (Sebutape®)

G. E. Piérard and C. Piérard-Franchimont*

Introduction

Sebaceous glands produce sebum by a holocrine process beginning with the proliferation of cuboidal cells present at the periphery of acini and in intraglandular trabeculae. Cells then move towards the center of the glands and enlarge during lipid synthesis. Finally the cell wall ruptures. The lipid content and the cellular remnants are discharged as sebum into the sebaceous duct and the pilosebaceous infundibulum, which is a large reservoir containing considerable amounts of sebum. This reservoir affects the rate of delivery of sebum to the surface of the stratum corneum, which itself may be considered as a sponge that entraps lipids. Thus the amount of lipids collected at the surface of the skin is the result of many parameters and may not accurately reflect metabolic events in the glands themselves.

Over the years, a wide variety of methods have been developed for measuring the amount of sebum excreted to the skin surface. A number of them, either cumbersome or technically simple, give inaccurate results unless considerable care is taken to avoid the many sources of error.

Most of the available techniques of sebum sampling only yield a single global estimate of the amount of lipids present on a given surface of the skin at one point in time. That test area is always obviously large compared with the size of openings of sebaceous follicles. Thus, any difference among the activity of individual sebaceous follicles remains impossible to evaluate. A few overactive sebaceous follicles producing a sizable amount of sebum would have a disproportionately large effect on measurements of sebum production.

An attempt to overcome that problem consisted in collecting sebum in absorbent papers and staining the material with osmium tetraoxide [3]. This provided pictures with a pore pattern characterized by dots of irregular sizes. However, there was a lack of standardization of the absorbent paper among different laboratories. Moreover, the collection technique involved a long commitment by the patients and considerable skill on the part of the investigator.

A few years ago, progress was made by introducing a method using standardized, hydrophobic, lipid-absorbent tapes (Sebutape, Cuderm Corporation, Dallas, TX). The first reports using this clever and accurate method appeared simultaneously in the literature [4, 6, 7] Since its introduction, it has always been considered as accurate as

* Department of Dermatopathology, University of Liege, CHU du Sart Tilman, B-4000 Liège, Belgium

the popular ground glass photometric method [5, 7] and has largely outdated the solvent extraction and gravimetric methods. Over the years, further refinements of the Sebutape technique were made.

Basic principle of the Lipid-Absorbent Tape Method

Sebutape is an opaque, open-celled, microporous, polymeric film coated on one side with an adhesive layer to tightly adhere to the stratum corneum.

In most studies, sebum excretion is evaluated on the forehead, but such evaluation can be performed on any part of the body, except for hairy areas where close contact to the skin can not be achieved. Ideally, the material has to be affixed to the skin using gentle pressure without interposition of air bubles. When the sebum-absorbent tape is placed on a skin area that can be moved by muscles, the investigator should periodically check for uniform contact between tape and stratum corneum throughout the test.

Subjects should wash the tested area in a normal way during the days prior to the test. We recommend the use of a nonirritant soap, and for standardization purposes we provide volunteers with Cetaphil (Galderma Belgilux, Puurs, Belgium).

The skin must be prepared, prior to the timed collection, by removing sebum from the skin surface. This cleaning procedure must be standardized. We have choosen ethanol 70° or Pannoclean (Pannoc Chemie, Herentals, Belgium).

Unless otherwise desirable for a given study, subjects should be at rest, without sweating, in a room with a controlled temperature of 20° ± 1°C; the relative humidity of the air is of little importance.

The collection time should be standardized depending upon the aim of the study protocol. It usually ranges between 0.5 and 3 h, the best collection time being 1 h [2, 7, 8, 20]. The samples should, where possible, be collected at the same time of the day since there may be circadian variations in the sebum output [21]

During the test, each active sebaceous gland will pour out a certain amount of sebum, which renders the tape transparent at these sites (Fig. 1). The size of the clear spot is proportional to the amount of sebum [5–7]. The number of spots reflects the number of active sebaceous follicles. These parameters can be evaluated by visual inspection alone. Better quantitative evaluations are achieved by computerized image analysis [5, 7, 14, 17, 18] photometry [20], or colorimetry [12].

Quantitative Assessment of the Data

Image analysis is the best method, as it is possible to record the number of spots, their individual size, and their mean size (Fig. 2). The total area of spots (TAS) is linked to the sebum excretion rate, as evaluated by the ground glass photometric method [5, 7].

Photometric evaluation of Sebutape by measuring the intensity of light transmitted through the samples is a rapid approach equivalent to the value of TAS obtained by image analysis [20]. This, however, negates one of the main benefits of the lipid-absorbent tape method, i.e., the evaluation of sebum excretion at each sebaceous follicle on an individual basis.

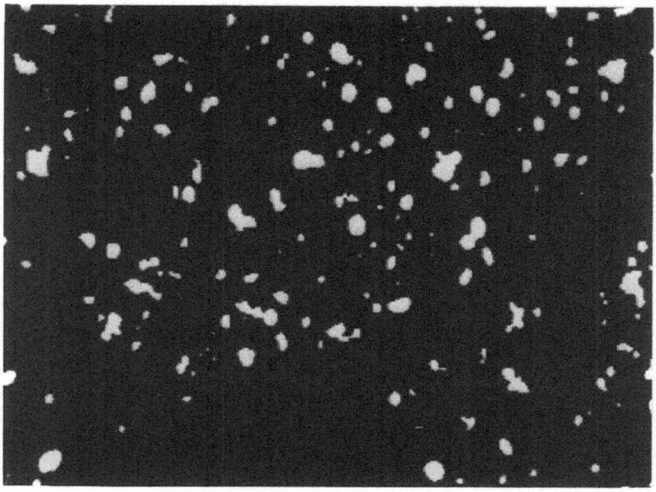

Fig. 1. Typical sebum-sensitive film, *clear dots* represent the amount of sebum collected at the orifice of sebaceous follicles.

More recently, we introduced a novel quantitative approach aiming at collecting data at any time when the Sebutape is still applied to the skin [16]. The principle relies on the measurement of the modifications in color of the tape that occur when it becomes transparent. This shifts the natural white color of the Sebutape to a color closer to that of the skin itself. Reflectance colorimetry (Chromameter CR-200 Minolta, Antwerpen, Belgium) is expressed as ΔE^* ab. The benefit of such an approach is to get multiple measurements without removing the tape and, therefore, to obtain kinetic data regarding sebum output (Fig. 3).

Limitations in the Interpretation of the Method

There are some limitations to the accuracy in the interpretation of the data obtained with the lipid-absorbent tape method. Some are directly related to the material itself, others are biological in nature.

The glue interposed between the lipid-sensitive film and the skin is a limiting factor in the transfer of lipids. This may be of importance when the rate of sebum excretion is low and/or when the duration of the test is short. It is possible to overcome this problem by placing the Sebutape with its original plastic support upside down onto the skin. The material is then held comfortably in position by an elastic head-band. Another possibility is the use of a new sebum-sensitive tape designed without adhesive (Sebum Instant Film, Courage-Khazaka, Köln, Germany).

We have observed a saturation effect occurring on Sebutape when evaluating intense seborrhea during a test period beyond 3 h. The amount of sebum collected over several hours is, in fact, lower than the addition of hourly sebum collections during a similar cumulative period of time (Fig. 4). This is associated with confluence of lipid droplets and inaccuracy in identifying each spot as a single sebaceous follicle. These features are the main reasons why we avoid sebum samplings longer than 1 h with a single Sebutape.

a

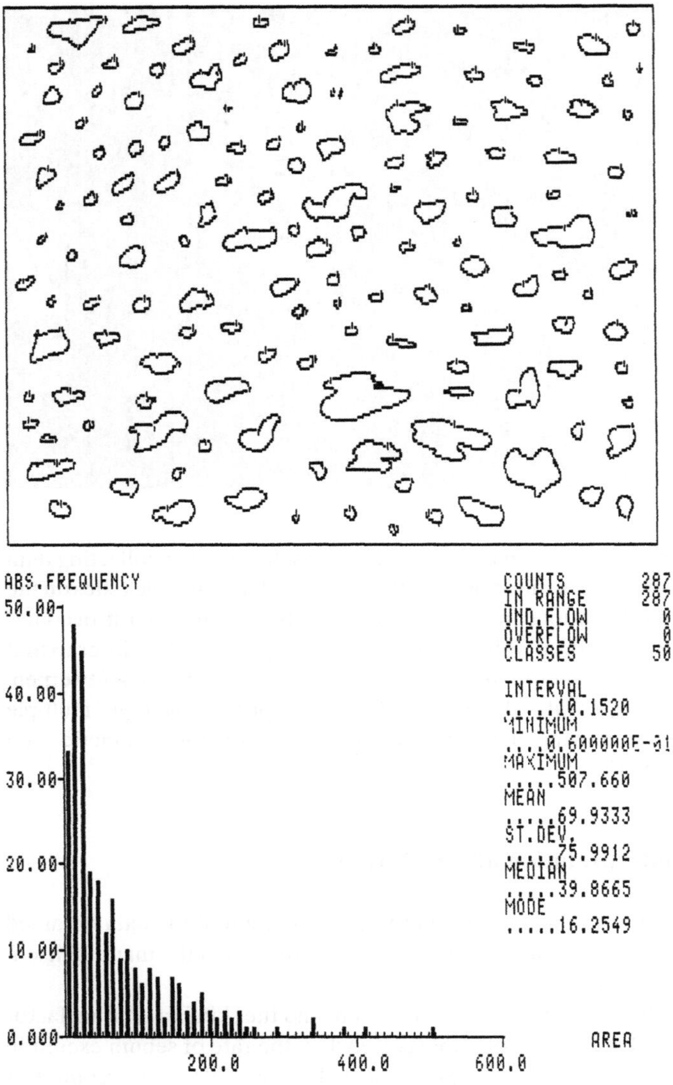

b

Fig. 2 a, b. Image analysis of a sebum-sensitive film. **a** TV scan of the material; **b** histogram of the areas of the spots revealing the uneven amount of sebum collected at each follicle

Some environmental and biological features are sources of error in the interpretation of the collected data. These are critically presented below.

Physiological Variations in the Sebum Output

There are wide interindividual variations in the number and the size of lipid droplets. Moreover, there are often large intraindividual variations in the size of lipid droplets, reflecting heterogeneity in secretion activity and/or the reservoir function of the pilosebaceous follicle. These aspects were critically evaluated in a series of studies.

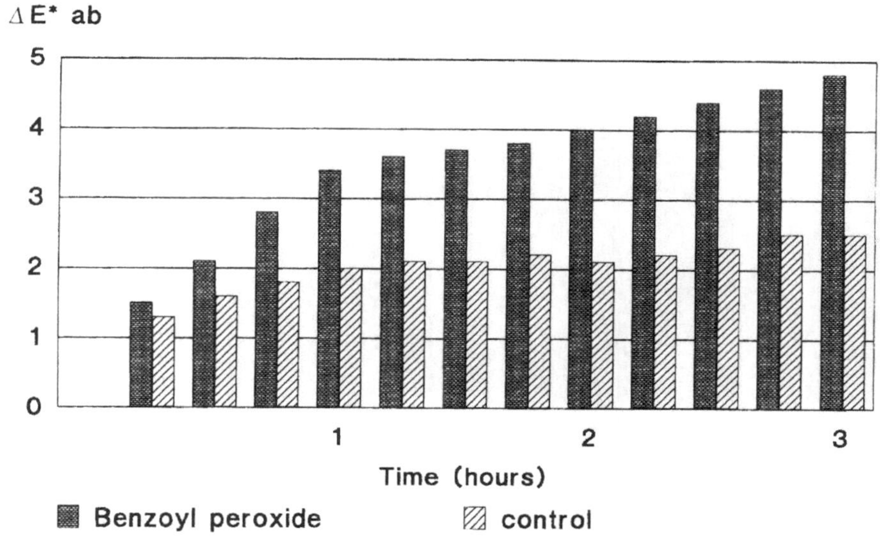

Fig. 3. Variations in Δ E^* ab measured every 15 min by Sebutape placed on the forehead treated or not by benzoyl peroxide for the past month. Sebum excretion is increased at the treated site as Δ E^* ab is higher (close to the skin color) than at the control site (close to the white color of Sebutape)

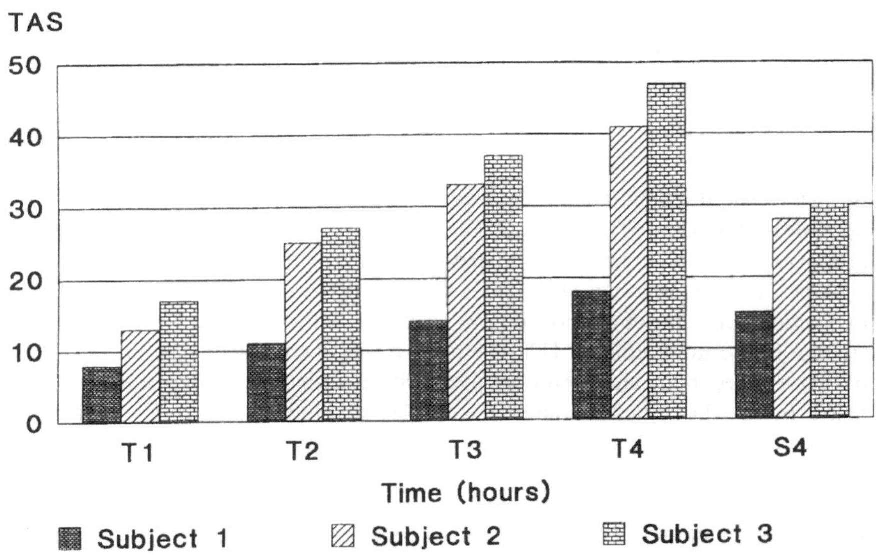

Fig. 4. Cumulative total area of spots (*TAS*) of four hourly collections of sebum (*T1* – *T4*) with Sebutape. The final cumulative amounts of sebum (*T4*) are higher than a single 4 h collection of sebum (*S4*) when the subject is seborrheic (subjects 2 and 3)

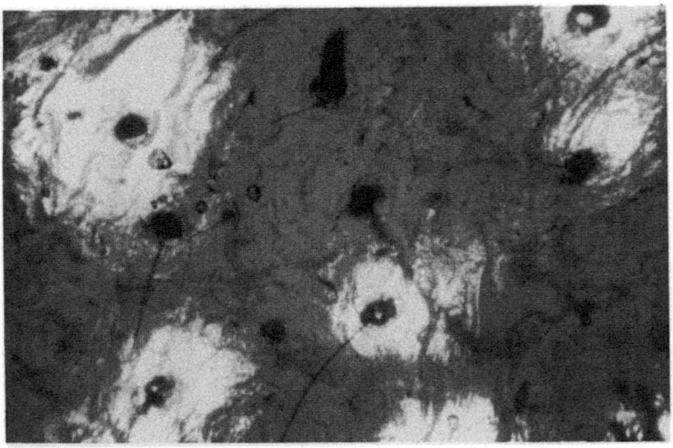

Fig. 5. Superposition of a Sebutape and a cyanoacrylate skin surface stripping taken from exactly the same site of skin. The *white areas* surrounding appendageal openings represent sebum present in active follicles. Other follicles appear quiescent.

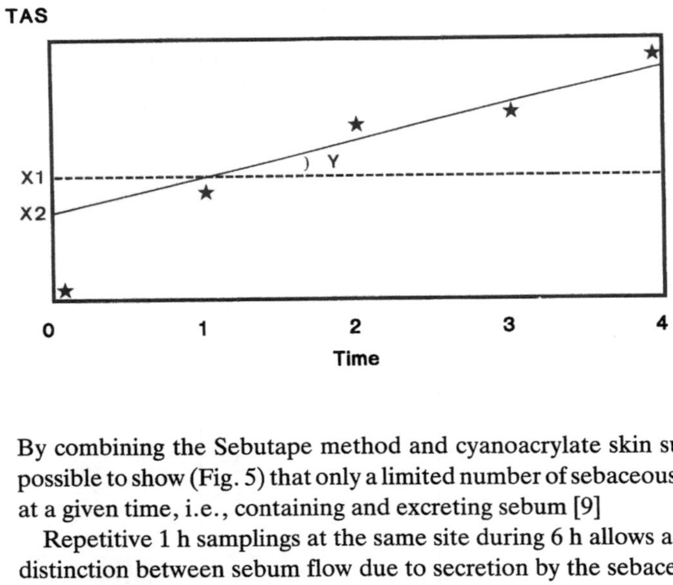

Fig. 6. Cumulative total area of spots (*TAS*) of four hourly collections (T1–T4) of sebum (*) with Sebutape. A significant regression line is usually present from T1–T4. *X1* represents TAS at T1, *X2* is the intercept of the regression line with the TAS axis, and *Y* is the slope of the regression line.

By combining the Sebutape method and cyanoacrylate skin surface biopsies, it was possible to show (Fig. 5) that only a limited number of sebaceous follicles were "active" at a given time, i.e., containing and excreting sebum [9]

Repetitive 1 h samplings at the same site during 6 h allows a rough estimate with a distinction between sebum flow due to secretion by the sebaceous gland and passive storage in the infundibulum [12] The hourly output of collected sebum is maximal during the first hour and then decreases, with irregular variations around a plateau value. In fact, the cumulative amounts of collected sebum usually follow a linear distribution. The slope of the regression line (value Y in Fig. 6) is representative of the true rate of sebum output. The value of TAS obtained at the first collection time (value X1 in Fig. 6) and perhaps the intersect of the regression line with the Y axis (value X2 in Fig. 6) reflect the influence of the sebum follicular reservoir. Therefore, we do not consider that the first hour sampling is spurious, but rather closely reflects the oily clinical presentation of the skin related to both sebum synthesis and its storage and delivery to the skin surface.

There is a positive relationship between the number of active sebaceous follicles and their individual excretion rate. Thus, there is a direct relationship between TAS and the number of active sebaceous follicles [19] There is, however, an upper limit in the number of active sebaceous follicles, and any further increase in TAS is a result of increased sebum flow from some of the secretory units.

There are variations in both the number and size of lipid droplets in the same individual at the same time when several sites of the forehead are explored [7]. These variations are more prominent with increasing seborrhea.

Even when the TAS is roughly kept unmodified for a few weeks, there are large variations in the sebum excretion of each sebaceous unit taken individually. Some follicles quiescent at one moment may be active at another, and vice versa. This suggests the existence of a rhythm in the follicular excretion rate that is unsynchronized among sebaceous follicles [8]. This recalls some aspects of the hair cycle, but it is also possible that these fluctuations do not follow a fixed rhythm.

In addition to a possible rhythm of unknown periodicity, it appears that other fluctuations in sebum excretion may exist. We failed to clearly identify a circadian rhythm which was reported by Verschoore et al. [21].

The ovarian cycle may affect TAS, mostly in strong sebum excretors [18]. The nadir of TAS and, to a lesser degree, of the number of active sebaceous follicles occurs during the week of ovulation. The decline in sebum outflow in the estrogen phase followed by an increase during the luteal phase is probably unrelated to the direct activity of the hormones on sebaceous cells, since the changes occur so rapidly. It is probable that the volume of the follicular reservoir is altered during the ovarian cycle and therefore influences the data.

There is also a seasonal rhythm, perhaps modulated by the ambient temperature [17]. TAS significantly increases in summer compared to spring while the number of active sebaceous follicles is kept unmodified.

Several distinct pattern of follicular sebum excretion have been identified in relation to age [10, 15]. They correspond to the so-called infantile, pubertal, adult, menopausal, and aging phases, distinguished by different densities and by heterogeneity in individual follicular sebum excretion.

Pathological Variations in Sebum Output

There are obvious changes in sebum excretion in a few diseases. The Sebutape technique has been used to study acne [14, 15, 19], hyperandrogenism [13], and Parkinson's disease [10].

Moderate to severe acne is significantly associated with high TAS. The number of active sebaceous follicles, however, remains in the upper range of the normal limit. The intensity of seborrhea turns out to reflect the high sebum output from a small number of "gushers." It must be emphasized that the range of variations of TAS in both normal and acneic subjects is large with much overlap of the values.

Low-grade acne with comedones may have a low TAS indistinguishable from normal values. This is probably related to the secondary regression of sebaceous glands following the formation of horny impactions in the infundibula.

Hyperandrogenism secondary to adrenocortisol hyperplasia and polycystic ovary syndrome, and Parkinson's disease are associated with a significantly increased TAS compared to matched controls. Other endocrinological and neuropathological conditions probably influence the parameters of the Sebutape technique. It could therefore be practical to introduce such a technique in the follow-up of these patients.

Clinical and Pharmacological Influences on Sebum Output

Sebum output at the surface of normal or diseased skin may be altered by chemicals or drugs. The frequent use of some brands of soaps and shampoos may increase TAS without modifying the number of active sebaceous follicles, while other brands have seemingly little or no effect.

Astringents such as those used as antiperspirants tremendously decrease both the number of active sebaceous follicles and TAS. In our experience, these are the strongest topical agents with antiseborrheic activity. Table 1 assesses the different ways that topical and systemic drugs may alter sebum output.

Table 1. Sebutape analysis of drugs influencing sebum output at the level of the total area of spots (TAS) and of the number of active sebaceous follicles (NAF)

	TAS	NAF
Topical		
Aluminium hydroxychloride	− − −	− −
Azelaic acid	+	+
Benzoyl peroxide	++	+
Budesonide	−	0
Clobetasol propionate	− −	0
Erythromycin-zinc	−	+/−
Ketoconazole	0	0
Retinoic acid	++	+/−
Selenium sulfide	++	+
Sodium laurylsulfate	++	+
Spironolactone	0	0
Systemic		
Cyproterone acetate	− −	−
Isotretinoin	− − −	− −
L-dopa	−	+/−
Spironolactone	−	0
Testosterone	++	+

Conclusion

The Sebutape method is unique in many aspects. Some of the reported findings confirm results obtained by older techniques. Other Sebutape data were not comparable with the other approaches and obviously represent a bulk of new information. Hopefully, they will help in clarifying the literature leading to better understanding of some skin and internal disorders. Moreover, the screening of the effect of drugs such as antiandrogens or of some antiseborrheic topical products is now possible by a non-invasive highly reproducible technique. Therefore, the Sebutape technique appears, after 7 years of use to represent significant progress in dermatology and cosmetology.

References

1. Blume V, Ferracin J, Verschoore M, Czernielewski JM, Schaefer H (1991) Physiology of the vellous hair follicle: hair growth and sebum excretion. Br J Dermatol 124: 21–28
2. Cowley NC, Farr PM, Shuster S (1990) The permissive effect of sebum in seborrheic dermatits: an explanation of the rash in neurological disorders. Br J Dermatol 122: 71–76
3. Cunliffe WJ, Shuster S (1969) The rate of sebum excretion in man. Br J Dermatol 81: 697–704
4. Kligman AM, Miller D, McGinley KJ (1986) Sebutape: a device for visualizing and measuring human sebaceous excretion. J Soc Cosmet Chem 37: 369–374
5. Lévêque JL, Piérard-Franchimont C, de Rigal J, Saint Léger D, Piêrard GE (1991) Effect of topical corticosteroids on the human sebum production assessed by two different methods. Arch Dermatol Res 283: 372–376
6. Nordström KM, Schmus HG, McGinley KJ, Leyden JJ (1986) Measurement of sebum output using a lipid absorbent tape. J Invest Dermatol 87: 260–263
7. Piérard GE (1986) Follicle to follicle heterogneity of sebum excretion. Dermatologica 173: 61–65
8. Piérard GE (1987) Is there a rhythm in the secretion rate of sebaceous follicles? J Appl Cosmetol 5: 37–40
9. Piérard GE (1987) Rate and topography of follicular sebum excretion. Dermatologica 175: 280–283
10. Piérard GE (1990) La sécrétion sébacée au cours du vieillissement. In: Meunier L, Michel B, Duntze F, Meynadier J (eds) Vieillissement cutané. Sauramps, Montpellier, pp 101–105
11. Piérard GE, Kligman A (1989) An update about the Sebutape technique. In: Ed. Marks RM, Plewig G (eds) Acne and related disorders. Dunitz, London, pp 111–112
12. Piérard GE, Piérard-Franchimont C (in press) Topical anti-acne drugs. Evaluation of sebum delivery by a combined photometric-multistep samplings with Sebutape. Clin Exp Dermatol
13. Piérard GE, Piérard-Franchimont C (1992) The Sebutape technique as an aid for monitoring androgen-dependent disorders. Eur J Med 1: 109–112
14. Piérard GE, Piérard-Franchimont C, Lê T (1987) Seborrhoea in acne-prone and acne-free patients. Dermatologica 175: 5–9
15. Piérard GE, Piérard-Franchimont C, Lê T, Lapière ChM (1987) Patterns of follicular sebum excretion rate during lifetime. Arch Dermatol Res 279: S 104–S 107
16. Piérard GE, Piérard-Franchimont C, Kligman A (in press) Kinetics of sebum excretion evaluated by the Sebutape-Chromameter technique. Skin Pharmacol
17. Piérard-Franchimont C, Piérard GE, Kligman A (1990) Seasonal modulation of the sebum excretion. Dermatologica 181: 21–22
18. Piérard-Franchimont C, Piérard GE, Kligman A (1991) Rhythm of sebum excretion during the menstrual cycle. Dermatologica 182: 211–213
19. Piérard-Franchimont C, Piérard GE, Saint Léger D, Lévêque JL, Kligman A (1991) Comparison of the kinetics of sebum excretion in young women with and without acne. Dermatologica 183: 120–122
20. Serup J (1991) Formation of oiliness and sebum output-comparison of a lipid-absorbent and occlusive-tape method with photometry. Clin Exp Dermatol 16: 258–263
21. Verschoore M, Poncet M, Blume U, Krebs B, Ortonne JP (1990) Absence de corrélation entre les variations circadiennes hormonales et les variations de l'excrétion sébacée. Ann Dermatol Venereol 117: 225

Colorimetric Evaluation of the Human Skin Blanching Assay

C. Queille-Roussel, L. Duteil, J. Czernielewski, and H. Schaefer*

Introduction

Normal skin color changes occur as consequences of either vascular or pigmentary modifications. Up to now,skin color modifications were usually assessed using various arbitrary visual scales. Numerous attempts to objectively quantify such modifications were performed. Thus, erythema caused by dermal vasodilation can be evaluated by either laser Doppler velocimetry [1] or spectrophotometry [2]. However, vasoconstriction-induced blanching and disturbances of the melanin system (hypermelanosis, e.g., tanning, and hypo-, or amelanosis, e.g., nevus depigmentosa, vitiligo,) have remained difficult to quantify objectively.

Due to its valuable screening abilities, the topical corticosteroid blanching effect was extensively studied. This human skin blanching effect, as described by McKenzie and Stoughton in 1962 [3], is a model used to evaluate new topical steroid formulations prior to their final testing in clinical trials. In fact, the intensity of visually assessed blanching correlates with the clinical efficacy [4]. This bioassay allowed the establishment of relative potency tables for commercially available topical corticosteroid formulations. The European classification has four potency ranks (I: the most potent, IV: the least potent) [5]. Many studies, using quantitative instrumental methods were undertaken to improve the objectivity of this test. Some failed completely, e.g., infrared thermography [6], photoplethysmography [7], and those that succeeded were unsuitable for routine use, being both cumbersome and time consuming (spectrophotometry [8–10], colorimetry [11]). Recently, a hand-held tristimulus colorimeter was developed by Minolta. This device immediately found use for quantifying erythema and tanning [12–14]. For blanching assessment, it seemed to be less useful, since spontaneous variations of normal skin color interact with quantification of the corticosteroid blanching effect, and the amplitude of the blanching phenomena appears to be weak when compared to erythema or pigmentation-induced variations.

The present chapter describes a study [15] undertaken to demonstrate that the Minolta colorimeter could measure a corticoid-induced blanching effect and affirm the rank order of clinical efficacy of the test formulations. Four well known preparations belonging to different potency groups were assessed, and a correlation colorimetry/

* Centre International de Recherches Dermatologiques Galderma (CIRD Galderma), Sophia Antipolis, 06565 Valbonne, France
Centre de Pharmacologie Clinique Appliquée a la Dermatologie (CPCAD), Hôpital Pasteur, 06000 Nice, France

clinical efficacy was sought. In such a case, visual scoring was not indispensable (a single observer would have been questionable in a conventional screening test) but was performed to emphasize the extreme conditions which were selected. Indeed, experimental procedures involving difficulties in visual scoring were deliberately chosen (unoccluded test, early measurements). Results concerning the same methodology and recently reported by other authors are also described in this chapter.

Methods

Subjects

Six healthy male Caucasian volunteers between the ages of 21 and 30 were included in the study. Subjects undergoing either local or systemic treatment were not admitted. Written informed consent was obtained from each volunteer and the protocol was accepted by the local ethics committee (Nice, France).

Products

Four commercial steroid creams were evaluated:

Group I (very high potency): Dermoval cream (Glaxo), clobetasol propionate (0.05% w/w) (CP)
Group II (high potency): Betneval cream, (Glaxo), betamethasone as valerate (0.1% w/w) (BV)
Group III (moderate potency): Tridesonit cream, (Dome/Hollister-Stiers, Miles) desonide (0.05% w/w) (DES)
Group IV (mild potency): Hydrocortisone Astier 1% cream (Astier) hydrocortisone (DCI) 1.0% w/w) (HC)

The vehicle cream Skin Base (Glaxo)was chosen as a negative reference.

Colorimeter Description

The Minolta Chroma Meter CR 200 is a portable instrument with a flexible hand-held probe which can be moved very easily from one site to another (measuring head weight: 651 g). The measured area is 8 mm in diameter. This reflected light colorimeter offers five different color systems for measuring absolute chromaticity. The L^* a^* b^* system recommended by the CIE (Commission Internationale de l'Eclairage 1976) seems to be particularly convenient for skin color assessment. Color is expressed in a three-dimensional space. The L^* value (luminance) gives the relative brightness ranging from total black ($L^* = O$) to total white ($L^* = 100$). The a^* value represents the balance between the red (positive values)and the green (negative values). The b^* value represents the balance between the yellow (positive values) and the blue (negative value). Theoretically, a skin blanching effect should increase L^* and decrease a^*.

Before use, the calibration channel of the colorimeter was brought to standard white plate level (Calibration plate CR-A43). Proper calibration was performed each time the instrument was turned on.

Experimental Procedures

Preliminary assays demonstrated that numerous variables could affect the normal skin color determination. Attempts to control each variable were carried out with extreme caution. To avoid errors related to exerting unappropriate pressure on the skin surface, the measurements on each series of sites were repeated six times. All the measurements were performed by a single trained investigator during the whole study. Since arm position can also modify normal skin color, the subject was kept motionless in a standardized horizontal position prior to each evaluation.

Other parameters such as time, optical properties of vehicles, and site variations were studied using a particular experimental schedule.

The test took place during three consecutive days. On day 1, spontaneous diurnal variations were studied by measuring site color every 2 h from 8 A.M. to 8 P.M. Three circular sites (2.2 cm in diameter) corresponding to the external edges of the probe were outlined with a dermatological dark pencil on the anterior face of each forearm. The distal part of the wrist, the veins, and hair covered areas were carefully avoided.

On day 2, a nonoccluded vasoconstriction test was performed and the blanching observations were continued on day 3. At 8 A.M.(t_O), on day 2, immediately after colorimetric evaluation, 10 μl of each cream were pipetted onto the predetermined skin site at the center of the circle in a double-blind randomized manner and gently massaged for 30 s. One of the sites was left as an untreated control. A nonocclusive protective dressing (a rubber ring covered with a gauze and held in place by Scanpor Norgeplaster) prevented loss of cream during the 2 h application.

At t_O + 2 h, this protection was removed and the excess product was carefully wiped away using a paper tissue. A visual assessment of blanching was made in a double-blind manner by a trained observer, according to the following scores:

0, no changes in skin color; 1, slight (barely visible) blanching; 2, obvious blanching; 3, intense blanching; 4, maximal blanching. Intermediate scores (of a half unit) were used when needed.

Immediately afterwards, colorimetric readings were made as described above. The same investigator used the same method to perform additional identical assessments on day 2 and on day 3, at the same time points as on day 1. Room temperature was kept constant at 21°–22°C and relative humidity at 35%.

Statistical Methods

An analysis of variance was used to evaluate variations due to sites, measurements, hours, and days. Products were compared using the Student-Newman-Keuls test which adjusts for multiple comparisons.

The Fischer-Snedecor *F* statistic resulting from the interproduct comparisons, which reflects overall differences between products, was used as a criterium for comparing discriminative abilities of each variable at each time point. When there is no difference between products, the *F* statistic is close to unity.

Results

Evaluation of Normal Skin Color

The analysis of the results obtained from the day 1 measurements confirmed that there were nonnegligible *intersite variations* showing similar profiles during the day (Fig. 1) and a *diurnal variation in basal values* significantly reproducible over the three consecutive days (Fig. 2).

These observations raised the following question. The blanching test would require adjustments; however, should the colorimetric values be adjusted to the value measured on the site at the same time on the previous day or be adjusted only to the value measured immediately before the application? Statistical analysis showed that intermeasurement variations on each site were small compared to between-site variations. Thus, in additional studies,the number of measurements ($n = 6$) could be reduced ($n = 2$ or 3).

Finally, the application of a neutral vehicle such as Skin Base cream (Base) did not modify in any way the spontaneous diurnal profile (Fig. 3).

The human Skin Blanching Effect

The 2 h topical corticosteroid application performed at 8 A.M. on day 2 ($t = t_0$) subsequently modified the curve profiles on day 2 and even on day 3 in a drug-related manner (Fig. 4). Statistical analysis showed that no additional interproduct discrimination was obtained by adjusting the colorimetric values to the basal values

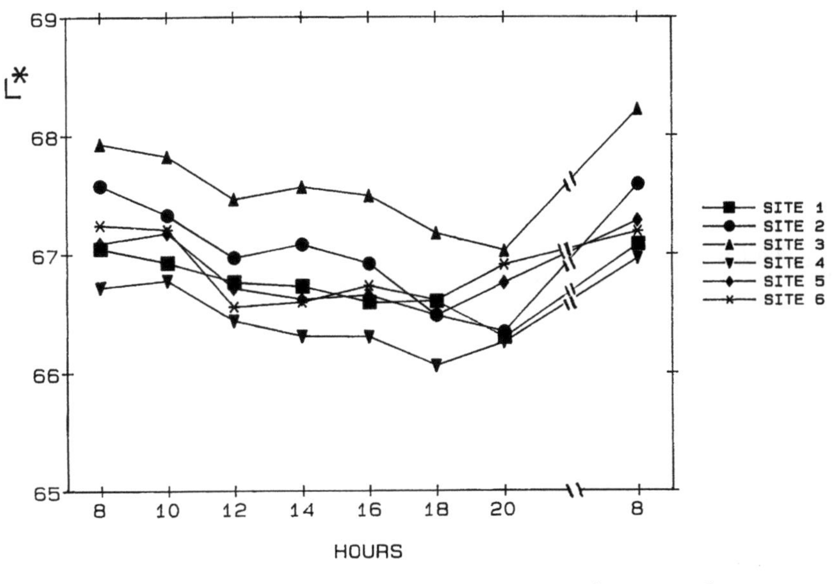

Fig. 1. Intersite variations of L^* colorimetric value during 24 h (mean, n = 6)

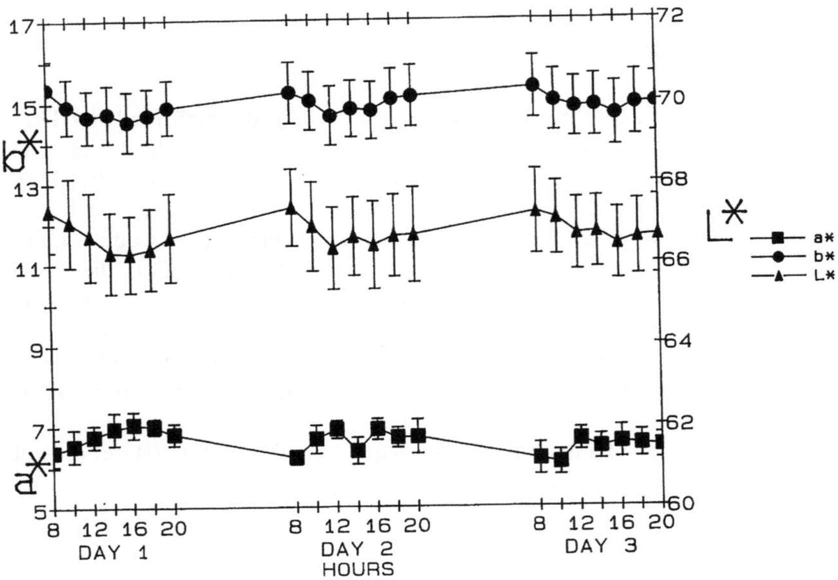

Fig. 2. Diurnal variations of L^*, a^*, b^* basal values (mean ± SEM)

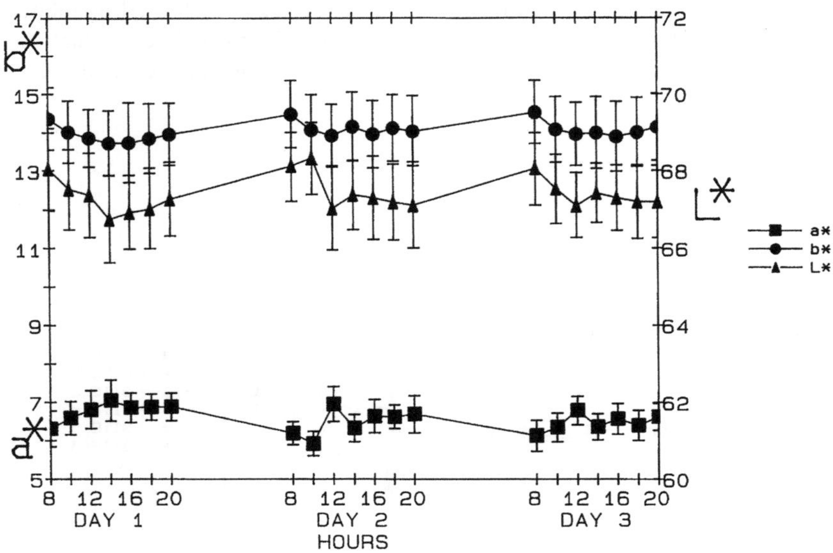

Fig. 3. Diurnal variations of L^*, a^*, b^* measured on vehicle cream treated sites (mean ±SEM)

measured on day 1 at the same hour of day, instead of adjusting them to the immediately preceding application value. Therefore, adjustements were made in the second and simpler manner. Adjusted colorimeter values were expressed as ΔL^*, Δa^*, and Δb^*.

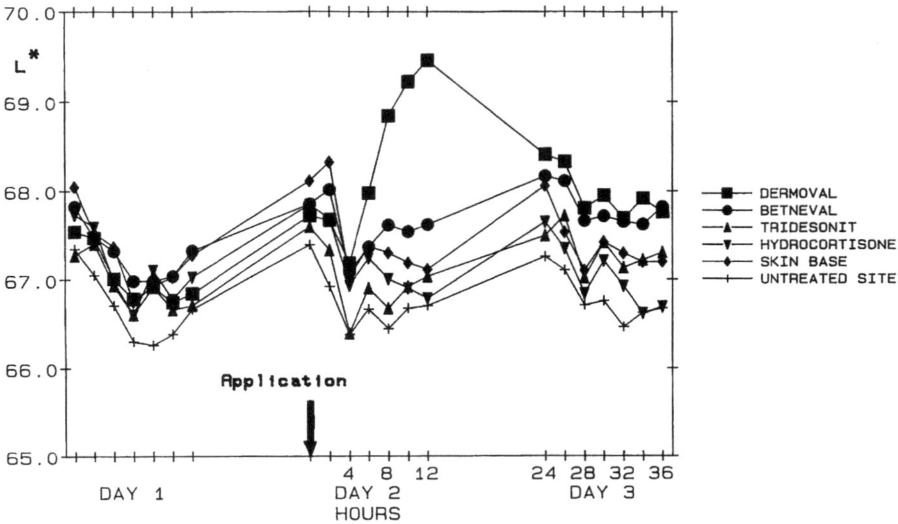

Fig. 4. Absolute L^* values as a function of time. *Day 1*, before treatment;*day 2*, unoccluded application at 8 A.M.; day 3, no application. (mean, n = 6)

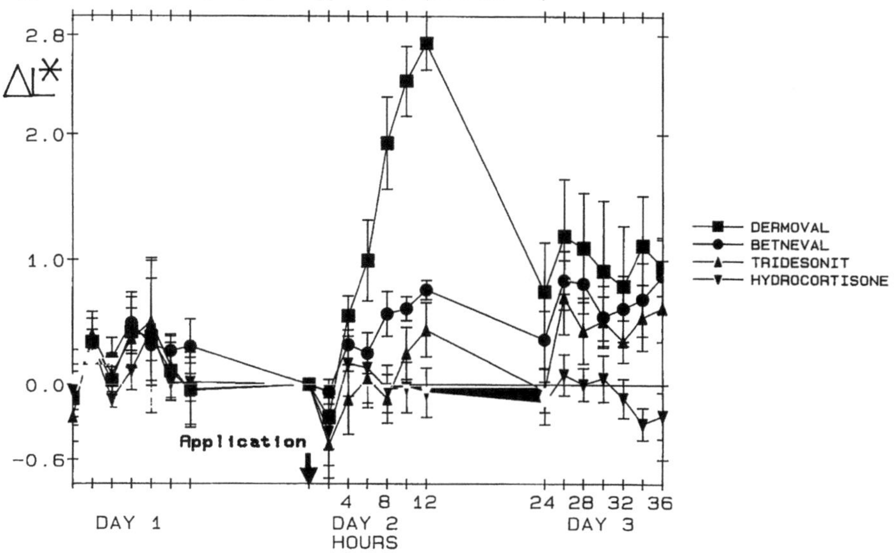

Fig. 5. Adjusted L^* values as a function of time (adjustment from L^* value measured on base cream just before application) (mean ± SEM)

In order to present the results with optimal clarity, graphs were drawn from values which were also adjusted to Base cream values (Figs. 5–7). For the colorimetric parameters L^* and a^*, the classical potency rank order is obviously present 12 h after application. The b^* values are quite unmodified with the exception of CP, which elicits an unexpected inverse effect on day 3 as compared to day 2. Visual scorings (Fig. 8) gave clear-cut blanching only for CP only.

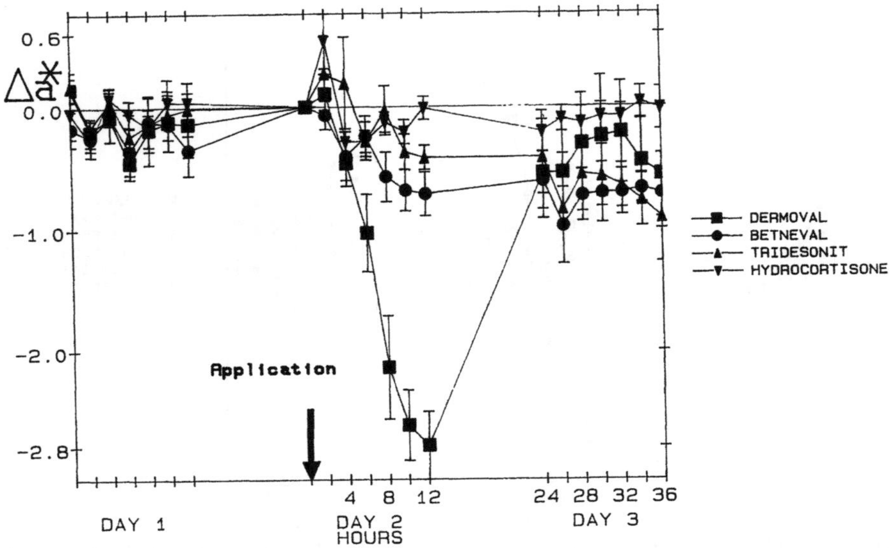

Fig. 6. Adjusted a^* values as a function of time (adjustment from a^* value measured on base cream just before application) (mean ±SEM)

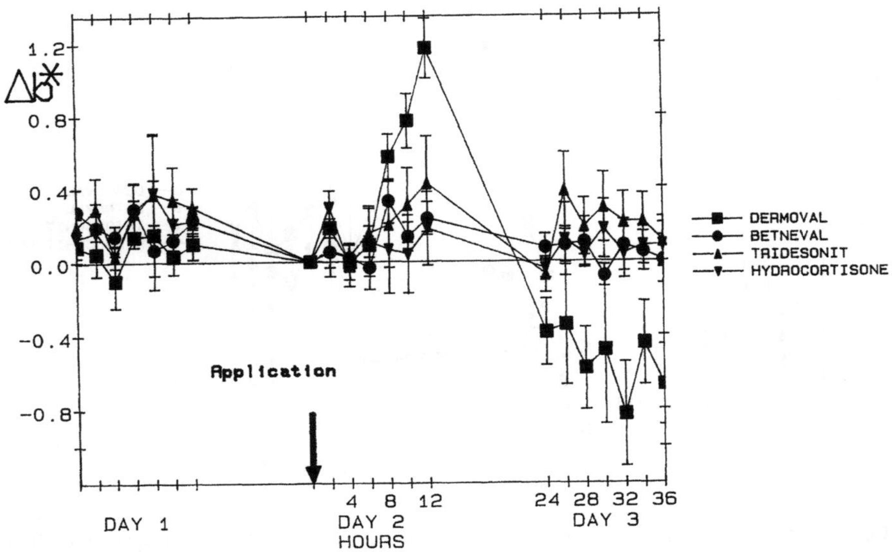

Fig. 7. Adjusted b^* values as a function of time (adjustment from b^* value measured on base cream just before application) (mean ±SEM)

In order to quantify the whole blanching phenomena within the first 36 h following the nonoccluded application, the algebraic sums of mean adjusted values were selected as end results ($\Sigma\Delta L^*$, $\Sigma\Delta a^*$, and $\Sigma\Delta b^*$). The appropriate potency rank order was obtained for $\Sigma\Delta L^*$ and $\Sigma\Delta a^*$ (Fig. 9).

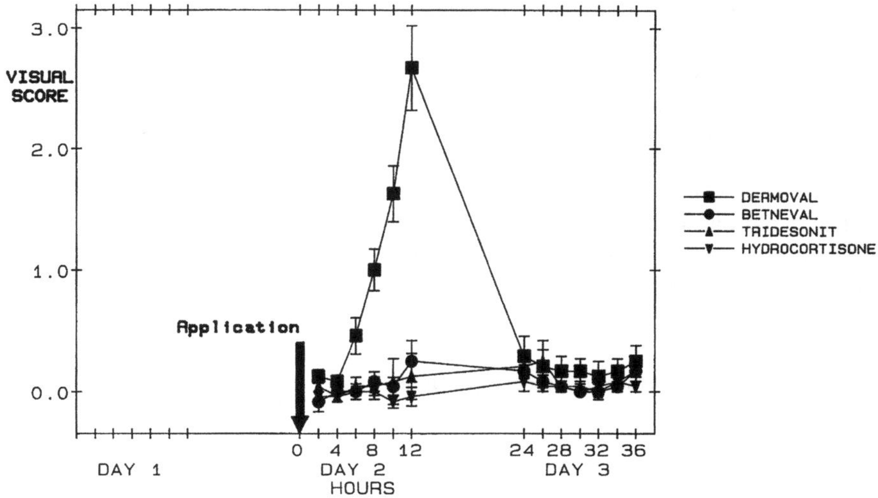

Fig. 8. Visual score means as a function of time (adjusted from base cream scores) (mean ± SEM)

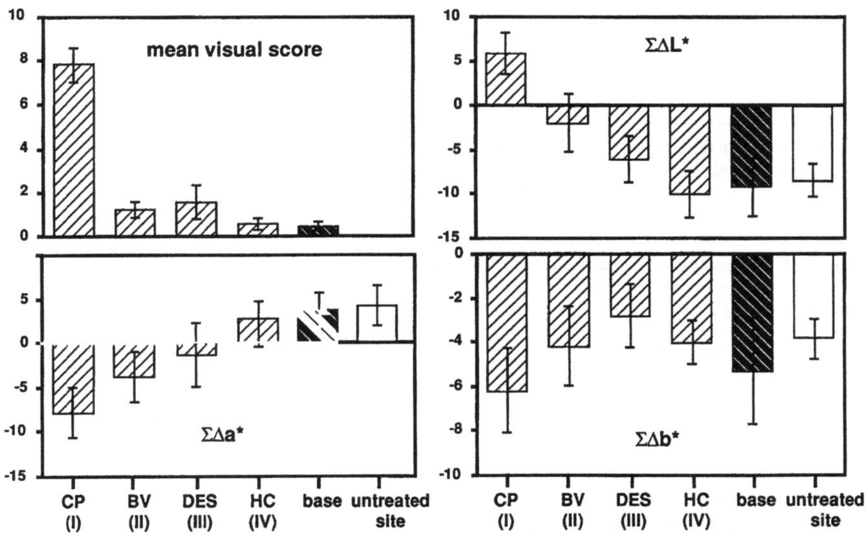

Fig. 9. Algebraic sums (± SEM) of mean visual scores obtained from *t*0 (day 2, 8 A.M.) to *t*36 (day 3, 8, P.M.) and algebraic sums of mean adjusted values (± SEM) of *L**, *a**, *b** measured from *t*0 to *t*36. *CP*, 0.05% clobetasol propionate cream; *BV*, 0.1% betamethasone valerate cream; *DES*, 0.05% desonide cream; *HC*, 1% hydrocortisone cream. Numbers in *parentheses* indicate potency ranking: for explanation, see text

Statistical comparisons of products, performed on ΔL^*, Δa^*, and Δb^*, indicate that, overall, ΔL^* and Δa^* showed discrimination between products of potencies I, II, III and IV although HC is not differentiated from Base cream and from the untreated site (Table 1). A comparison of parameters and time points in terms of discriminative power was made using the *F* statistics from the analysis of variance (Table 2). A large *F* statistic indicates that the differences among products are important. A *F* statistic close to unity would indicate that differences among products represent, in fact, random variations, consistent with experimental variations. It is clear from this table that *F* statistics are greater for ΔL^* than for Δa^* and that *t*O + 12 h is the optimal time point from the design, in terms of its ability to account for differences among these products.

Table 1. Statistical comparisons of products performed on ΔL^*, Δa^*, Δb^*

Time	ΔL^*	*F*	Δa^*	*F*	Δb^*	*F*
$t_O + 12$ h	CP > BV > HC, Base CP > DES, untr.	45	CP < others	39	CP > others	10
Day 2	CP > others	22	CP < others BV < untr.	19	CP > Base	3
Day 3	CP > HC, Base, untr. BV > HC, Base	7	NS	3	CP > others	7
Days 2 + 3	CP > BV > DES, HC, Base, untr.	21	CP < BV, < DES < HC, Base, untr.	14	NS	2

Student-Newman-Keuls test, $p = 0.05$; F, Fischer statistic; CP, 0.05% clobetasol propionate cream; BV, 0.1% betamethasone valerate cream; DES, 0.05% desonide cream; HC, hydrocortisone cream; base, base cream; untr., untreated site; NS, no significant difference.

Table 2. F values at each time point for each colorimetric parameter

Time (t_O + h)	2	4	6	8	10	*12*	24	26	28	30	32	34	36
L^*	3	2	6	20	29	*45*	3	6	6	3	3	8	6
a^*	3	2	5	19	26	*39*	2	3	2	2	2	4	5
b^*	1	0	1	3	6	*10*	3	3	5	3	9	7	8

Further observation of the t_0 + 12 h ΔL^* data (Table 3) shows, that this time and parameter not only form the optimal set of conditions, but also that, for four out of the six subjects, the means of ΔL^* values can be ranked in exactly the same order as the clinical potencies of the creams. For the fourth and the sixth subjects, there is an inversion of the two weakest groups only.

A strict correlation between visual scoring and colorimetric values was not found. As was already noticed in the evaluation of erythema, for a given score, a similar value L^* or a^* was not always obtained. A visual score of 1 in one subject is not always precisely duplicated (score of 1) in another subject, as visual quotation remains a compromise between the absolute intensity of the color observed and the individual rank.

Table 3. $\Sigma\Delta L^*$ values at t_0 + 12 h

Subject	CP	BV	DES	HC
1	0.54 (1)	− 1.01 (3)	− 0.63 (2)	− 1.06 (4)
2	2.14 (1)	− 0.26 (2)	− 0.45 (3)	− 1.03 (4)
3	2.08 (1)	0.01 (2)	− 1.15 (3)	− 1.72 (4)
4	2.56 (1)	0.96 (2)	0.29 (3)	0.12 (4)
5	2.06 (1)	0.30 (2)	− 0.08 (3)	− 0.47 (4)
6	1.05 (1)	− 1.42 (3)	− 1.32 (2)	− 2.20 (4)
Sum	10.43 (1)	− 1.42 (2)	− 3.34 (3)	− 6.36 (4)
Mean	1.74	− 0.24	− 0.56	− 1.06
S.E.M	0.31	0.35	0.25	0.34

Numbers in parentheses indicate rank order.
CP, 0.05% clobetasol proprionate cream; BV, 0.1% Detamethasone valerate cream; DES, 0.05% desonide cream; HC, hydrocortisone cream

Discussion

The colorimetric determination of skin color using the Minolta Chroma Meter offers important new advantages: the device is easy to handle and relatively cheap, the time for each measurement is short, and the space occupied by the measuring head is minimal (no modifications of neighboring sites when measuring). The possible modification of skin color caused by variations in the pressure on the skin could be restricted by using the same trained investigator for all the measurements and by repeating the measurement series each time. Standardization of the forearm position for a few minutes before and during the measurements appeared to be essential. Absolute values exhibited site – and time-related variations.

Colorimetric evaluation of skin color changes induced by topical corticosteroid formulations allows one to recognize their relative clinical potency rank order. Whereas interproduct discrimination was obtained from the statistical analysis of colorimetric values, the visual scoring method did not prove to be as effective. The more discriminant parameter was the luminance (L^*) provided that it had been previously adjusted to its basal value. For a 2 h application without occlusion, under our experimental conditions, the optimal time point was 12 h after application.

Adjustment of colorimetric data, to compensate for the normal skin color variation, has also been suggested by Waring et al. [16] to improve the product differentiation power of this method in the skin blanching assay.

Pershing et al. [17] have recently evaluated the intra- and intersubject variability and power of discrimination of three techniques, visual skin blanching, Minolta Chroma Meter, and tape stripping, to assess the bioavailability of five topical 0.05% betamethasone dipropionate formulations. The tape stripping technique [18] allows quantification of drug content in the treated stratum corneum. In this study the products were applied during 6 h without occlusion on subject's forearms. Skin sites were evaluated 6, 8, 16, 18, 20, and 24 h after drug application. Results showed that the intrasubject variability of the colorimetric parameters (L^*, a^*, b^*) was less than that of the visual skin blanching response or tape stripping techniques. The intersubject variation coefficient was relatively constant over the entire study period for the colorimetric measures L^*,a^*, and b^*, whereas a time-dependent increase was observed for the visual skin blanching assessment. The intersubject variability was lower for L^*, a^*, b^* data than for the two other parameters. Differentiation among the formulations was demonstrated with visual blanching, with the amount of drug in ten tape strips, and with the a^* colorimetric parameter. The best correlation with visual skin blanching assay was obtained with the a* colorimetric component ($r = 0.9508$).

Chan and Li Wan Po [19] recently reported a study concerning the objective comparison, using the Minolta Chroma Meter, of skin blanching response to four proprietary corticosteroid creams of different known clinical potencies. The products were applied on the forearms during a 3 h occlusion period in a six subject study, and a 6 h occlusion in a single subject trial. Colorimetric measurements were performed before (baseline values) product applications and at successive time intervals after occlusion time. Statistical analysis was performed on parameters derived from L^*, a^*, b^* data: area under the time-response curve (AUC), corrected AUC (CAUC) from baseline values, slope of the cumulative L^*, a^*, b^* values over a specified time span (Slope) and its corrected value (Cslope). Product comparisons, performed after analysis of variance, were carried out using Tukey's multiple comparison test to differentiate and rank the group means. Results of product comparisons for the single subject study and for the six subject experiment are consistent with the generally accepted rank order of the clinical corticosteroid potencies. From these results, it seems that parameters related to the L^* component give the best product discrimination, this being in agreement with our results.

In conclusion, the use of the Minolta Chroma Meter allows an objective evaluation of both the cutaneous blanching phenomenon and erythema or tanning.

Nevertheless, before this method can be proposed as a standard protocol in the human skin blanching assay, it needs standardization concerning the time and mode of product application and the type of calculated colorimetric parameters (AUC, Σ, ...). For the human skin blanching assay our results show that adjusted values of colorimetric parameters L^* (luminance) and a^* (redness), obtained from measurements performed 12 h after a 2 h nonoccluded application, give an objective and precise evaluation of topical corticosteroid potency.

References

1. Willis CM, Stephen CJ, Stephen M, Wilkinson JD (1988) Assessment of erythema in irritant contact dermatitis. Comparison between visual scoring and laser Doppler flowmetry. Contact Dermatitis 18: 138–142
2. Mendelow AY, Forsyth A, Feather JW, Baillie AJ, Florence AT (1986) Skin reflectance measurements of patch test responses. Contact Dermatitis 15: 73–78
3. McKenzie AW, Stoughton RB (1962) Method for comparing percutaneous absorption of steroids. Arch Dermatol 86: 608–610
4. Cornell RC, Stoughton RB (1985) Correlation of the vasoconstriction assay and clinical activity in psoriasis. Arch Dermatol 121: 63–67
5. (1983) Dermocorticoïdes (fiche de transparence). Direction de la Pharmacie et du Médicament, p, 13

6. Aiache JM, Lafaye C, Bouzat J, Rabier R (1980) Evaluation de la disponibilité topique des corticoïdes par thermographie. J Pharm Belg 35: 187–195
7. Thune P, The effect of corticosteroids on skin pulse. In Wilson I C, Marks R (eds) Mechanisms of topical corticosteroid activity. Churchill Livingstone, Edinburgh, pp 25–31
8. Altmeyer P, Zaun H (1976) Ergebnisse reflexphotometrischer Bestimmungen der Vasoconstriction nach topischer Applikation: IV. Zeitlicher Ablauf der Vasoconstriction und reaktiven Vasodilatation. Arch Dermatol Res 250: 419–420
9. Feather JW, Ryatt KS, Dawson JB et al. (1982) Reflectance spectrophotometric quantification of skin colour changes induced by topical corticosteroid preparations. Br J Dermatol 106: 436–444
10. Leveque JL, Poelman MC, Legall F, De Rigal J (1985) New experimental approach to measure the skin-reflected light. Application to cutaneous erythema and blanching. Dermatologica 170: 12–16
11. Kiraly K, Soos G (1976) Objective measurement of topiclaly applied corticosteroids. Dermatologica 152 [Suppl 1]: 133–137
12. Seitz JC, Whitmore CG (1988) Measurement of erythema and tanning responses in human skin using a tri-stimulus colorimeter. Dermatologica 177: 70–75
13. Babulak SW, Rhein LD, Scala DD et al. (1986) Quantification of erythema in soap chamber test using the Minolta Chroma (Reflectance) Meter: comparison of instrumental results with visual assessments. J Soc Cosmet Chem 37: 475–476
14. Westerhof W, Van Hasselt B, Kammeijer A (1986) Quantification of UV-induced erythema with a portable computer controlled chromameter. Photodermatology: 3: 310–314
15. Queille-Roussel C, Poncet M, Schaeffer H (1991) Quantification of skin colour changes induced by topical corticosteroid preparations using the Minolta Chroma Meter. B J Dermatol 124: 264–270
16. Waring MJ, Monger L, Hollingsbee DA, Martin GP, Marriott C (1990) Evaluation of the Minolta Chromameter CR200 for the assessment of steroid induced blanching. Pharm Res 7/9 [Suppl]: S50
17. Pershing LK, Lambert LD, Krueger GG, Shah VP (1991) Reproducibility and correlation of the Minolta R chromameter, tape stripping and visual skin blanching in the assessment of bioavailability of topical 0.05% betamethasone dipropionate formulations. In: Scott RC, Guy RH, Hadgraft J, Bodde HE (eds) Prediction of percutaneous penetration: methods, measurements, modelling. IBC Technical services
18. Dupuis D, Rougier A, Roguet R, Lotte C, Kalopissis G (1984) In vivo relationship between horny layer reservoir effect and percutaneous absorption in human and rat. J Invest Dermatol 82: 353–356
19. Chan SY, Li Wan Po A Quantitative skin blanching assay of corticosteroid creams using tristimulus colour analysis. J Pharm Pharmacol 44: 371–378

High-Frequency Ultrasound: A Noninvasive Method for Use in Dermatology

S. EL-GAMMAL[1], T. AUER[1], K. HOFFMANN[1], U. MATTHES[1], R. HAMMENTGEN[2], P. ALTMEYER[1], and H. ERMERT[3]

Introduction

In internal medicine and surgery diagnostic imaging methods have found wide application. This is, among other reasons, due to the fact that organ systems have to be treated which are not directly accessible to the physician. Of the imaging methods in use today, ultrasound has gained particularly wide acceptance, since it is harmless to the patient and can be repeated as many times as necessary.

Since the structures studied are localized several centimeters under the skin, only macroscopic enlargements are necessary. Machines working in the frequency range between 2.5 and 7.5 MHz are commonly used because signal penetration depth is inversely proportional to the frequency of the ultrasound transducer (array).

In dermatological oncology lymph nodes are examined at 5–7.5 MHz in the follow-up of patients with skin tumors [30, 33]. In andrology different conditions of the testes are studied [31, 40].

In the past, dermatologists have showed little interest in noninvasive ultrasound techniques, since their organ of interest – the skin – is easily accessible. Moreover, the ultrasound equipment (including computerized tomography and NMR) was inadequate to study the skin architecture because of poor resolution (about 1 mm). For small skin structures, like hair appendages, and to define depth of tumor penetration (e.g., melanoma thickness), a resolution of better than 100 μm axially is required. New, high-resolution ultrasound imaging systems had to be developed for dermatology. At the beginning only specialized engineering departments and laboratories were able to design, construct, and use such systems. Because the interference of different phenomena (e.g., diffuse scattering, absorption, and angular reflection) can cause artifacts to appear in ultrasound images, it remained hazardous in those days to identify singular structures without histological correlation. Recently, however, commercial, 20 MHz ultrasound imaging systems, which are able to visualize skin sections *in vivo*, have become available. Their routine use in different dermatological clinics has improved our clinical-sonographic dermatological knowledge considerably.

[1] Dermatologische Klinik der Ruhr-Universität, Gudrunstraße 56, 4630 Bochum, FRG
[2] Herzzentrum Nordrhein-Westfalen, Ruhr-Universität Bochum, Georgstraße 11, 4970 Bad Oeynhausen, FRG
[3] Institut für Hochfrequenztechnik der Ruhr-Universität, Universitättsstraße 150 IC6, 4630 Bochum, FRG

Transducer Technology and Technical Equipment

Today, single transducers (and not transducer arrays) are used in high-resolution ultrasound. These transducers work in pulse-echo mode as transmitter/receiver and are focused.

Resolution describes the minimum distance between two point sources which can be discerned as being distinct. The lateral resolution is defined by the shape of the ultrasound beam and the axial resolution by the bandwidth of the ultrasound signal. By increasing the center frequency of the transducer, resolution improves, but the depth of signal penetration diminishes, due to frequency-dependent signal attenuation in biological tissue (about 1 dB/MHz per cm). Fortunately, the structures of interest in the skin lie only a few millimeters beneath the skin surface. Frequencies between 20 and 80 MHz should, consequently, be of interest in dermatology. Presently, no general biological phantom has been accepted in dermatology. Note that experimental data suggest that the center frequency is lower in biological tissue than in the metal plates or point sources used in material science to define the transducer characteristics [15].

Figure 1 shows a circuit diagram of the DUB 20 (Taberna pro medicum, Lüneburg, FRG) and Dermascan C (Cortex Technology, DK). Both systems use a 20 MHz ceramic transducer and are well suited for routine clinical purposes and have been described elsewere [4, 24, 42]. These systems have a lateral resolution of about 200 μm and an axial resolution between 80 and 100 μm.

The experimental 50 MHz ultrasound imaging system (Fig. 1c) uses a point-focused ultrasound transducer, built on a polymer base, which has a center frequency of 40 MHz and a bandwidth (−6dB) of 30 MHz [26]. Using this PVDF (polyvenylendifluoride) transducer technology an ultrasound transmitter receiver could be developed which is not much bigger than the 20 MHz ceramic transducers commercially available but which has a much better lateral and axial resolution. The ultrasound beam width in the focus area was 125 μm (lateral resolution) and the axial resolution was 37.5 μm in biological tissue [26]. The ultrasound transducer has a diameter of 3 mm, a radius of curvature of 12 mm, and a focal point approximately 11.5 mm in water. A water path was used as coupling medium between the transducer and the skin, without membrane or contact gel. The active transducer has incorporated a wideband sender and a receiver preamplifier, thereby minimizing the number of external electronical parts since only a trigger signal is required.

Figure 1c shows the circuit diagram of the 50 MHz experimental system. The transmitter is initially triggered and the returning echo signal preamplified (Fig. 2a) and converted into voltage oscillations. The strong signal attenuation in biological tissues makes the use of a TGC (time-gain-control) amplifier necessary to amplify the backscattered echo signals by 8 dB, according to the time elapsed (assuming 1600 m/s) over a distance of about 4 mm. Analog-to-digital conversion of the voltage oscillations was accomplished using a transient recorder (Sony Tektronix RTD 710; sampling frequency: 200 MHz; quantization levels: 1024). Moving the transducer laterally, oscillation curves were collected at adjacent points by an IBM Model 80 computer using a databus and stored line by line as a radio frequency (RF) picture. The RF images were demodulated using envelope detection. To visualize small changes in gray levels in the low frequency (LF) image, we used a false color coding of the 255 gray-levels, which is similar to the standard DUB20 color table.

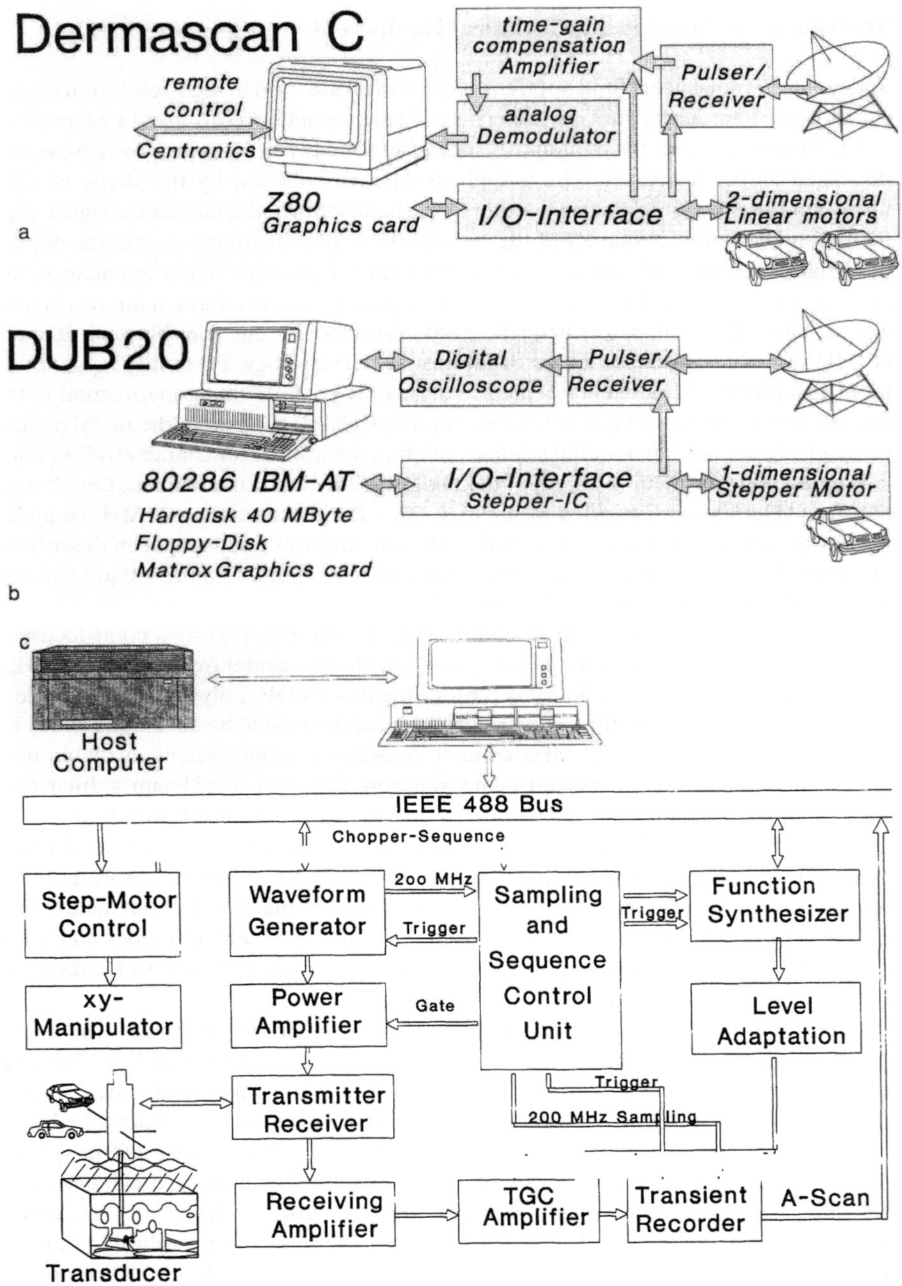

Fig. 1a–c. Technical setup of commercially available 20 MHz B scan ultrasound equipment for dermatology. **a:** DUB20 (Taberna pro medicum, FRG) **b:** Dermascan C (Cortex Technology, Denmark). Data processing diagram of the different units of 50 MHz ultrasound computer imaging system (from [16])

Photography

Special precautions are necessary, to obtain high quality photos from a computer screen. An autofocus camera (e. g. Minolta 9000), a KR3 filter, a telezoom objective of 200 or 300 mm, and a tripod are needed. Since the computer monitor emits in the UV spectrum, a KR3 filter should be used to reduce the blue color component in the images. Furthermore, because the surface of most computer monitors is spherical, the edges are further away from the focus plane than the center point of the screen. Since the focal plane of the camera is also spherical, both effects sum up. To reduce this image distortion, a telezoom objective of 200–300 mm is sufficient. The camera is placed on a tripod about 1.8–3 m away from the monitor. Focusing on the monitor image is done in two steps: first, the autofocus equipment is used at high magnification in the upper left corner. After switching on "manual," the focus is controlled in the three other corners of the monitor. Note, that the monitor has to be tilted in most cases. Second, the correct magnification is chosen with the telezoom and the autofocus is again activated on the center of the image. This procedure is necessary because two thirds of the focal depth lie behind the focal plane, whereas one third lies in front of the focal plane. By using a long exposure time (e.g., 15 s), a diaphragm aperture of 11 can be used; the focal depth is then sufficient to obtain sharp monitor edges.

A-, B-, and C-scan

After generation by the ultrasound transducer, the acoustic wave is propagated through the water path. The first structure which is struck by the acoustic wave and which has a different impedance is the epidermis. At the boundary between these two different media, part of the acoustic energy will be reflected while the rest of the energy will be transmitted through the boundary, continuing to travel through the tissue. Different phenomena, like absorption, diffuse scattering, and reflection, modify the back-scattered echo signal. In the transducer, the received echo signal is transformed into voltage oscillations, which can be amplified and further processed in different ways (Fig. 2a):

1. A (amplitude)-scan: This mode involves direct visualization of the voltage oscillation curve on an oscilloscope. For distance measurements, the time spans between the acoustic pulse and the returning echo are transformed into spatial distances, assuming a constant sound speed in different tissues. Note that this assumption is partly responsible for some of the inexactitudes about skin measurements compared with caliper or post-mortem measurements. In fact, sound speed actually varies by about 10% in different biological tissues of the skin [45]. Note that in other structures, e.g., bone, sound velocity is about twice as fast as in soft tissues.

When the first, high-frequency, A-scan ultrasound was used in dermatology [1], the interpretation of the voltage oscillation curve was reduced to thickness measurements of the cutis, subcutaneous fatty tissue, and muscle fascia. In those years, the corium-subcutis interface was especially prone to misinterpretation due to fatty tissue inlets or hair follicle structures. With the advent of two-dimensional, high-resolution, ultrasound imaging systems, topographic information became available, facilitating the interpretation of images.

2. B (brightness)-scan: By moving the transducer laterally in one direction (e.g., *x*-axis), grossly parallel to the skin surface, multiple A-scans can be obtained. Every A-scan is then demodulated by detecting the envelope of the voltage oscillation curve. The amplitude of the envelope curve is then transformed into a brightness modulation. Multiple rotated B-scan sections are obtained when moving a transducer linear-laterally over a plane pitched by the *x*- and *y*-axis. Figure 2a shows two orthogonally oriented B-scan sections (*x*-, *y*-axis).
3. C (computed)-scan: If two motors are used to move the transducer over a total surface area, a tomographic horizontal section of the skin can be computed. Using a time window, only echoes from a certain skin depth are selected for this section.

Figure 2b–s shows different orthogonal sections (registered at 50 MHz) through the 2x2 (lateral direction) x 4 (axial direction) mm tissue bloc of *in vivo* skin from the lower arm of a young woman. The B-scan sections in Fig. 2b–d are perpendicular to the B-scan sections in Fig. 2e–g; Fig. 2h–s represents C-scan sections through the same tissue cube at different skin depth. Note the apparently randomly scattered undulating echo lines in the middle of the B-scan sections (Figs. 2b–g). In the C-scan sections, however, these structures have a globular shape (Fig. 2l–q). This region corresponds to the corium (Fig. 3). The echo reflexes of the corium (Figs. 2, 3) therefore form discus-shaped, undulating, partly irregular-shaped ovaloids grossly parallel to the skin surface.

Collagen seems to be the main source for the echo reflexes in soft tissue. Fields and Dunn [18] could demonstrate that the supporting tissue has a thousand times higher bulk modulus or "stiffness" than the surrounding parenchyma. Since collagen and other proteins form the connective tissue skeleton in soft tissue, one would expect that different organs show a different back scattered pattern. In skin cancer, tumor tissue can replace normal collagen tissue thereby forming regions of reduced echogenicity. In a fresh skin scar, which is accompanied by an increase in collagen fibers, one should expect more echo reflexes. We observed, however, that a three month old skin scar is echo-poor. This finding illustrates that the orientation of the collagenous fibers in space also strongly influences the sonographic pattern of the corium: In a scar or wound, the new collagenous fibers are unordered, the region therefore remains echo poor. Scanning electron microscopy studies [6] show that the orientation of the collagen fibers in the corium of the skin changes under different tension forces. Brown [6]

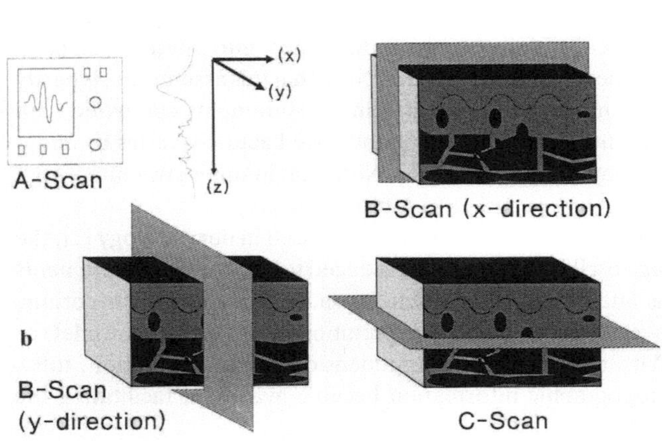

Figs. 2a–s. A-, B-, and C-scan. The A (amplitude)-scan is a solitary, amplitude-modulated, echo signal which has been transformed into a distance representation. B (brightness)-scans use many A-scans which are aligned with each other forming a two-dimensional picture. Every A-scan is reduced to a single line by transforming the echo signal amplitude ▶

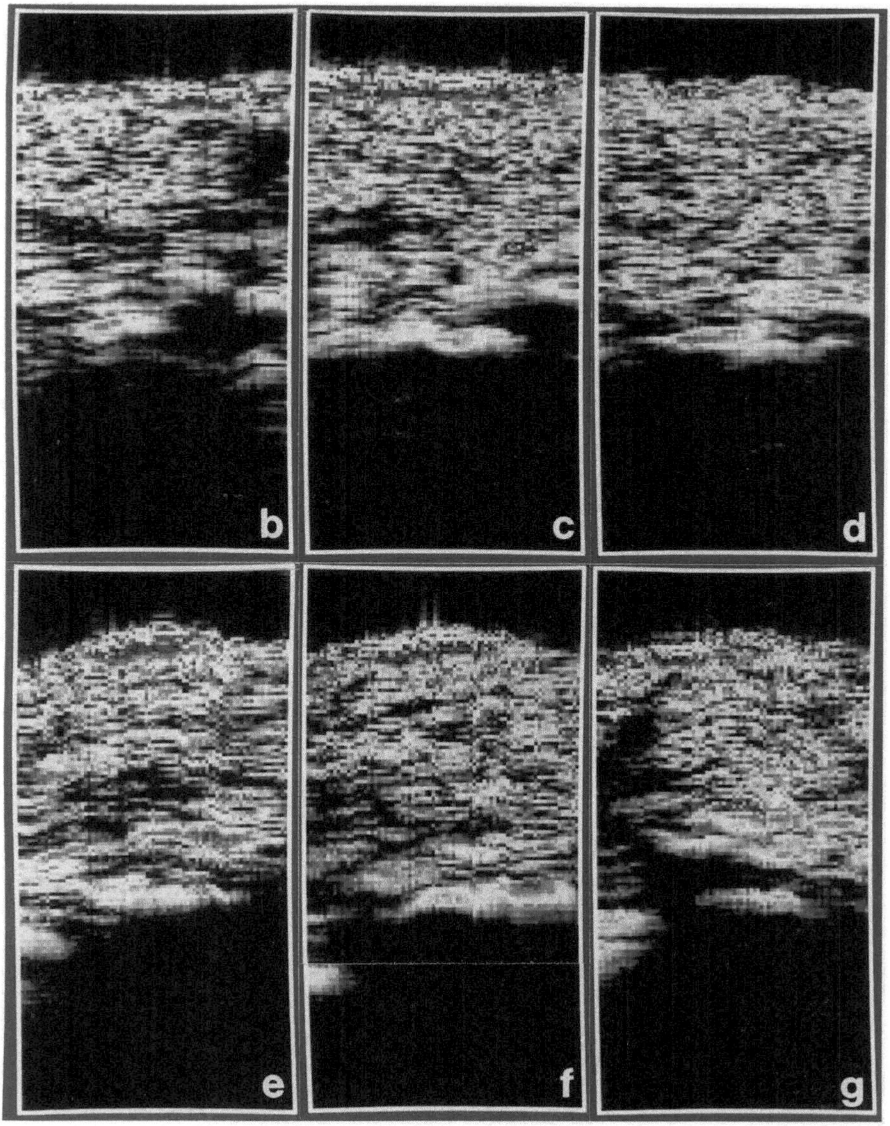

into a brightness modulation of the points along the line. C (computed)-scan is defined as a horizontal section through the skin. The two B-scan planes and the C-scan plane are orthogonal to each other (from [16]). **b–s** Different sections through a 2x2x4.8 mm tissue bloc of normal skin. A false color gray level coding (black-green-red-yellow) was used. **b–g** Two groups of orthogonally oriented B-scan sections, with their section plane at 0.5 (**b**), 1.0 (**c**), 1.5 (**d**), and 0.5 (**e**), 1.0 (**f**), 1.5 (**g**) mm. Note the undulating echo lines in the corium which become larger at greater distance from the skin entry echo. **h–s** C-scan sections at different levels. Every section is 5μm thick according to the time window used. The distance of the sections from the upper corner of the tissue bloc is 0.4 (**h**), 0.5 (**i**), 0.6 (**j**), 0.8 (**k**), 1.0 (**l**), 1.25 (**m**), 1.5 (**n**), 1.75 (**o**), 2.25 (**p**), 2.5 (**q**),

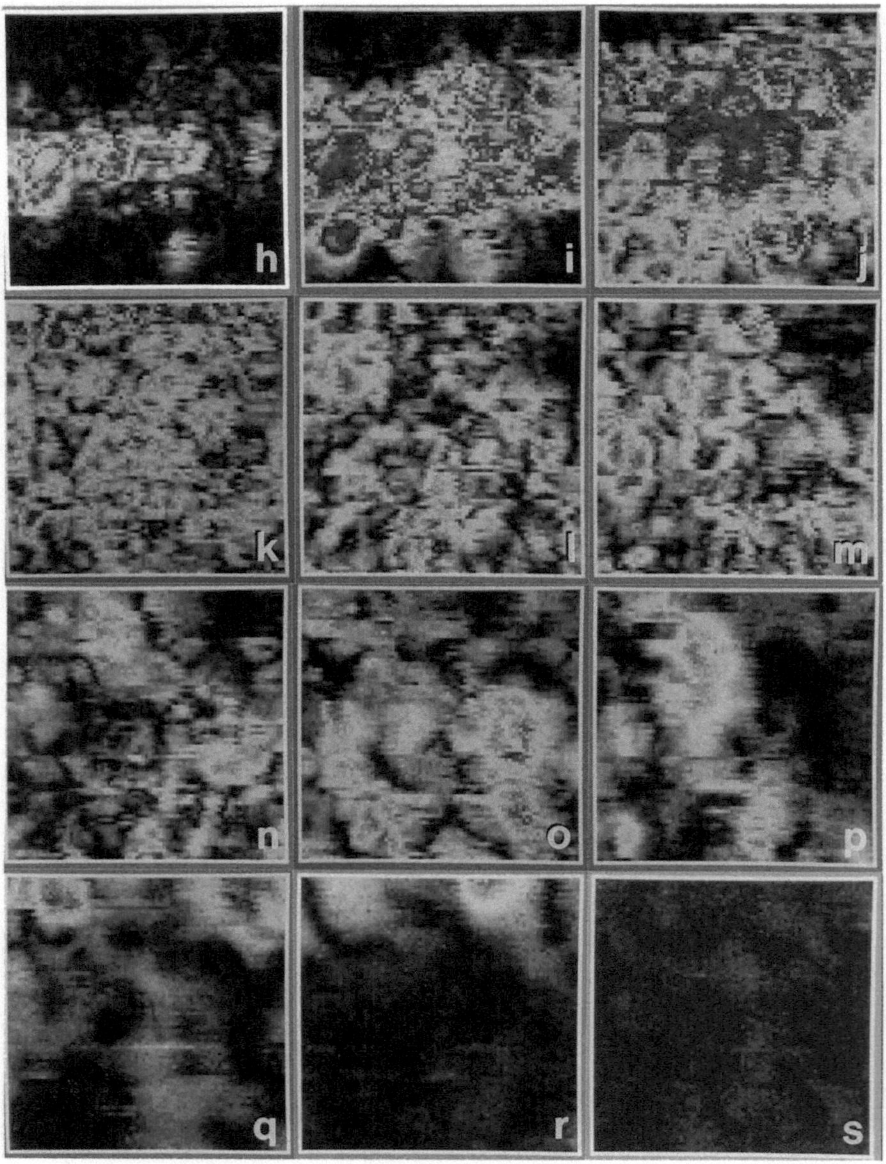

2.75 (**r**), 3.25 (**s**) mm. Note the globular aspect of the skin entry echo (**h–j**). Small globular and irregular shaped echoes predominate in the upper corium (**k–m**), the middle of the corium shows fewer echo globules (**n, o**). In the lower part of the corium big globular structures are again visible (**o–q**). In fact, this finding is not as obvious in the B-scan sections (**b–g**) due to the slightly oblique orientation of the corium/subcutis border. The subcutaneous fatty tissue (**s**) exhibits nearly no echo signal (from [16])

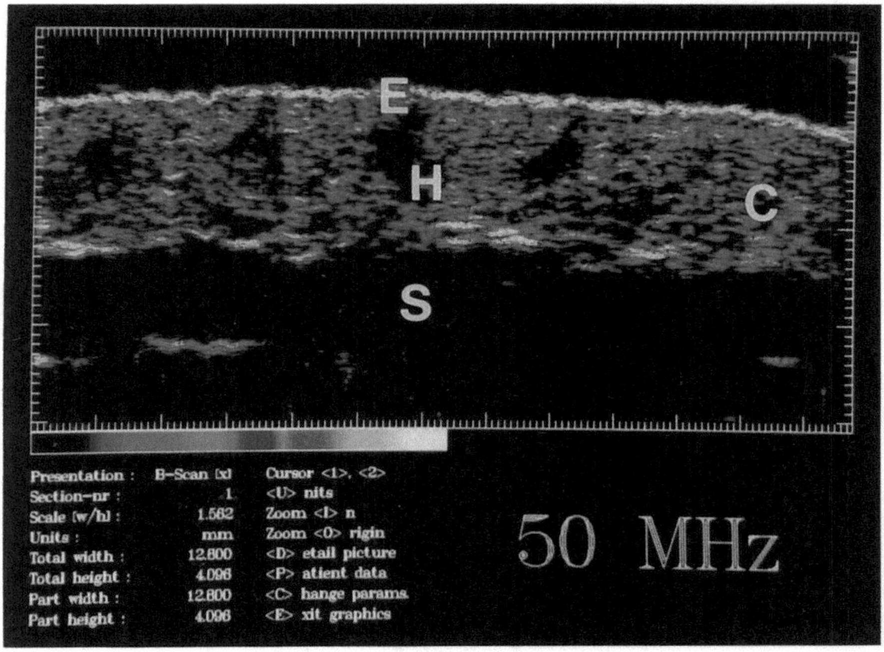

Fig. 3. Normal skin examined using 50 MHz ultrasound. E, skin entry echo; C, corium; S, subcutaneous fatty tissue; H, hair follicle. The *ruler* at the borders is divided in 1/10 mm units; the distance between the two longer *bars* is 1 mm.

observed that the dermal fibers reorientate, straighten, and become aligned and compacted in response to the increasing strain. This effect could explain the higher echogenicity of the skin during tension that is observed in ultrasound [13]. Since the wavelength of the ultrasound signal is in the dimensions of the studied structures, reflection, absorption, and scattering phenomena produce interference patterns in the gray level picture. These patterns can change their spatial distribution, especially when movement (heart contraction, respiration) occurs. We therefore can conclude that the concentration, spatial orientation, and packing of collagen fibers indeed strongly influence the back scattered pattern in soft tissue.

Normal Skin Architecture

Figure 3 shows a 50 MHz ultrasound image of the skin on the lower arm of a 25 year old man. An echolucent region is seen at the top of the image; this is demarcated by an echo-rich line (E). Beneath, a loosely texture with apparently randomly scattered echo signals is seen (C). A quite sharply defined echo poor structure (H) leaves at an angle of about 50° from the echo-rich line downwards through C. Its structure is sharply delimited at its lower border. Beneath C, a nearly echolucent region (S) follows; it sometimes exhibits sparse linear obliquely oriented reflex bands, depending on the skin region studied.

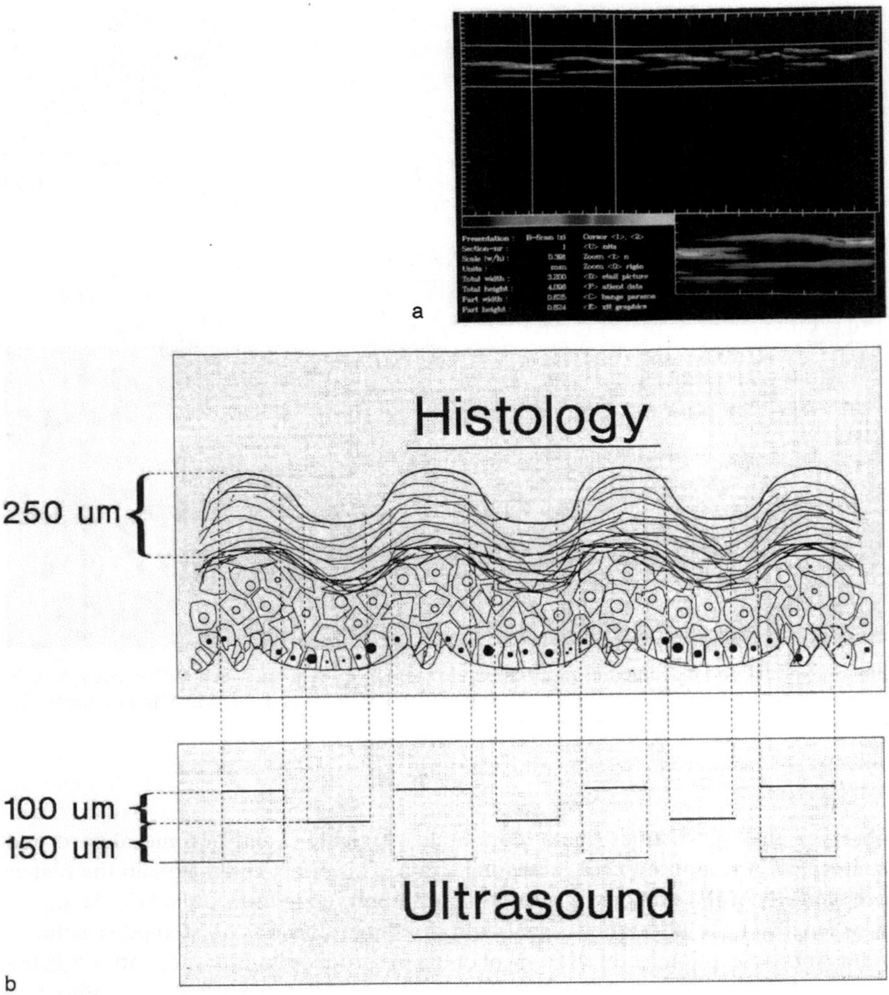

Fig. 4a, b. Analysis of the normal skin of the palms perpendicular to the ridges. **a** Two echo-rich lines 250 μm beneath each other are shifted periodically up and down. The period is about 0.5 mm. The four white lines delimit a rectangle within the picture which has been further enlarged in the inset. **b** Comparison of histology and ultrasound. The upper echo-rich *line segments* correspond to the water/stratum corneum interface, the echo rich *line segments* beneath originate from the stratum corneum/stratum Malpighii interface. The mean height difference between the crest and valley is about 100 μm (from [15]).

Correlating histology shows that the above described areas in the ultrasound image correspond to the water path (echo-lucent region), the corium (C) and the subcutaneous fatty tissue (S). Between the water path and the corium lies an echo rich line (E).

It is interesting to notice that the fatty tissue in high-resolution ultrasound is echolucent. In this region a few, elongated, echo-rich structures oriented diagonally or parallel to the skin surface are often seen. Correlating histology shows that these structures correspond to connective tissue septa, with nerve and vessel routes. Note that the skin anatomy differs greatly in different body regions [2, 19]. We shall now concentrate on the echo-rich line (E). From an anatomical point of view, one would expect that this line should correspond to some part(s) of the epidermis. To analyze epidermal substructures, low analog signal amplifications are necessary, thereby reducing signal depth.

Since the skin on the palms and soles is very thick, it should be well suited for further examinations of the epidermis. Note the ridge pattern of the palm (Fig. 4). It is evident that the shape of the skin in the ultrasound picture is greatly influenced by its orientation according to the ridges. To eliminate overmodulation of the echoes from the echo-rich line (E), the A-scan signal preamplification was further reduced and sampling in lateral direction occurred every 20 μm. When the ultrasound picture dissects the ridges perpendicularly (Fig. 4a), two, interrupted, disconnected, echo lines beneath each other alternate with a shifted echo line (Fig. 4b). The alternating bands are about 250 μm wide, i.g., the mean distance between neighboring ridge crests is 0.5 mm on the palms.

We can conclude for normal ridged skin (Fig. 4) that only the crest and the valley of the ridges are seen as singular echo bands. In the region between them the ultrasound beam is reflected obliquely, so that no echo signal reaches the transducer. As expected, the echo texture of the corium has disappeared at this amplification.

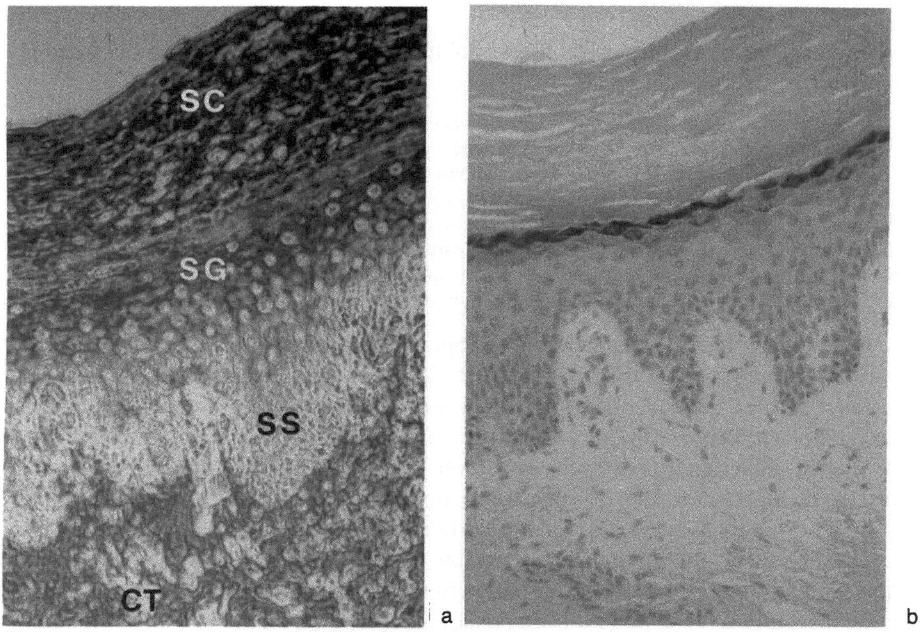

Fig. 5. Acoustic microscopy at 1.1 GHz of normal skin from the sole of the foot. **a** 1.1 GHz image, deparaffinized paraffin section, SC, stratum corneum; SG, stratum granulosum; SS, stratum spinosum; CT, connective tissue in the upper corium, x 250. **b** Histological reference section, H and E, x 250

By simply reducing the analog signal preamplification, analysis of the palms and the soles demonstrates that the skin entry echo is composed of several layers (Fig. 3). The skin entry echo ceases to be an undefined, echo-rich line [29, 38, 39]. It is interesting to note that the acoustic microscope has revealed two layers of different echogenic behavior within the epidermis [14, 32].

Using the acoustic microscope, the elastic properties of cellular structures in a 6–10 μm thick skin section can be studied. The section is placed on a glass slide; the magnification is between x 125 and x 2000 [32]. Figure 5 shows an acoustic and optical micrograph of normal skin. In the upper region of Fig. 5a, the total reflection of the glass slide is seen, appearing white. The stratum corneum, keratinocytes, and connective tissue in the upper corium are echo-poor, i.e., dark. The stratum spinosum, granulosum, and lucidum can be distinguished in the epithelial band. The stratum spinosum is considerably more echo-rich than the stratum granulosum.

Our findings *in vivo* are in agreement with those from acoustic microscopy. Fine granular structures resembling metal powder only increase the entry signal and make the slopes of the ridged skin apparent [15]. The border of the upper interrupted echo line therefore corresponds to the border between water and stratum corneum. By comparing these ultrasound images with histology, it becomes apparent that the echolucent zone beneath corresponds to the stratum corneum. The border between the stratum corneum and stratum Malpighii produces a less intense echo-rich line. Beneath, the stratum spinosum is echolucent. The border to the corium is, in most cases, diffuse.

Inflammatory Diseases

Figure 6 summarizes the general high-resolution ultrasound phenomena observed in pathological skin conditions.

The ultrasound image of psoriasis vulgaris reveals an irregular skin entry echo with focal reflex enhancements above (Fig. 7a). This is followed by a nearly completely wide echolucent band (ELB) beneath. Note the two distinct echo shadows (dorsal signal attenuation) passing through the corium. In fact, the 50 MHz machine allows us to zoom and amplify an image section (see inset) to further analyze the skin entry echo. Figure 7b shows the corresponding histologic section, which is characterized by hyperkeratosis, focal parakeratosis, and a regular elongation of the rete ridges. In the stratum corneum, small aggregations of neutrophilic granulocytes are seen. The upper corium and the dermal papillae exhibit a perivascular lymphocytic infiltrate.

By applying the image interpretation approach described in the preceding section, we can easily classify the echo-rich structures above the epidermis in psoriasis as hyperkeratotic zones and squamae. The comparison with histology shows us that this assumption was right. Furthermore, focal epidermal hyperkeratoses produce a stronger, focal, echo-rich signal. In psoriasis the lower border of the skin entry echo is irregular in the regions where the histological section shows very elongated and enlarged psoriatric dermal papillae. The focal hyperkeratotic zones we had discussed before are causing a signal attenuation (echo shadow) of the deeper skin layers. In normal sonograms the signal is strongly amplified to view deeper structures, thereby merging these structures in to a wide skin entry echo. Thus the term "skin entry echo" indicates that the above mentioned layers (Figs. 5, 6) have joined to form a single echo line. It is remarkable that hyperkeratosis is observed as an echo-rich structure and that focal normal epidermis stripes show a focal echo-rich line.

a. ultrasound phenomena of the epidermis

water path (echo-poor/echo-rich spots [hairs? water contamination?])
skin entry echo (split, widened, level jumps, interrupted, absent)
upper border of the skin entry echo
  shape (regular/irregular/echo-rich spots)
  orientation (linear/bumping upwards/"pagode-shaped")
*echolucent line beneath entry echo (present/absent)

b. ultrasound phenomena of the corium

upper corium (echo-poor to echolucent band [ELB]/echo-rich)
  corium texture (echo-rich/echo-poor/echolucent area [ELA])
  echo distribution within the corium (regular/irregular/gradient)
hair follicle complex (existent/missing)
  border (sharp/unsharp)
  orientation (oblique/straight)
lower corium (reduced/enhanced echo signal)
corium-subcutis-border (sharp/unsharp, regular/irregular, straight/bumping downwards)

c. ultrasound phenomena of the subcutaneous fatty tissue

fatty tissue lobules
  texture (echo-poor/few or multiple echo reflexes)
  size and shape (enlarged/normal/small)
connective tissue routes (sparse/multiple, normal width/widened)

d. ultrasound phenomena of skin tumors

tumor region (echo-rich area/echo-poor to echolucent area [ELA])
tumor borders (sharp/unsharp)
border region (regular/irregular, normal/echo-rich/*small undulating lines)
subtumoral echo signal (attenuation/reduced/enhanced)

Fig. 6. Classification of high-frequency ultrasound phenomena. (*) Additional phenomena using the 50 MHz equipment.

Recently, several other inflammatory dermatoses such as lichen planus, chronic eczema, and mycosis fungoides were studied using 20 MHz [24, 42] and 50 MHz [15]. All these dermatoses show an echo-poor to echolucent band in the upper corium. As has been put forward by Murakami and Miki [35], "dense inflammatory infiltrates, hypertrophic sebaceous glands and epithelial or mesenchymal tumour cell nests within the dermis were clearly demonstrated as echolucent masses or zones within a relatively dense dermal echo. However they all looked alike." Using 50 MHz, multiple, fine, undulating, green reflex lines in the border regions of the inflammatory infiltrate are seen. Here the inflammatory infiltrate is not so dense [14].

To study connective tissue diseases and pathological changes in the corium, the resolution of 20 MHz systems is sufficient. The progression and regression of scleroderma plaques, for example, under therapy can be followed easily [8, 24, 26, 41]. Especially in patients in whom the connective tissue layers involved lie deeper (e.g., in sclerofascia) are simple methods like the observation of a lilac ring insufficient. Until recently, the doctor had to rely upon deep punch biopsies and indirect methods such as biochemical blood examination (antibodies, etc.). Using high frequency ultrasound the lesions can now be studied directly [41].

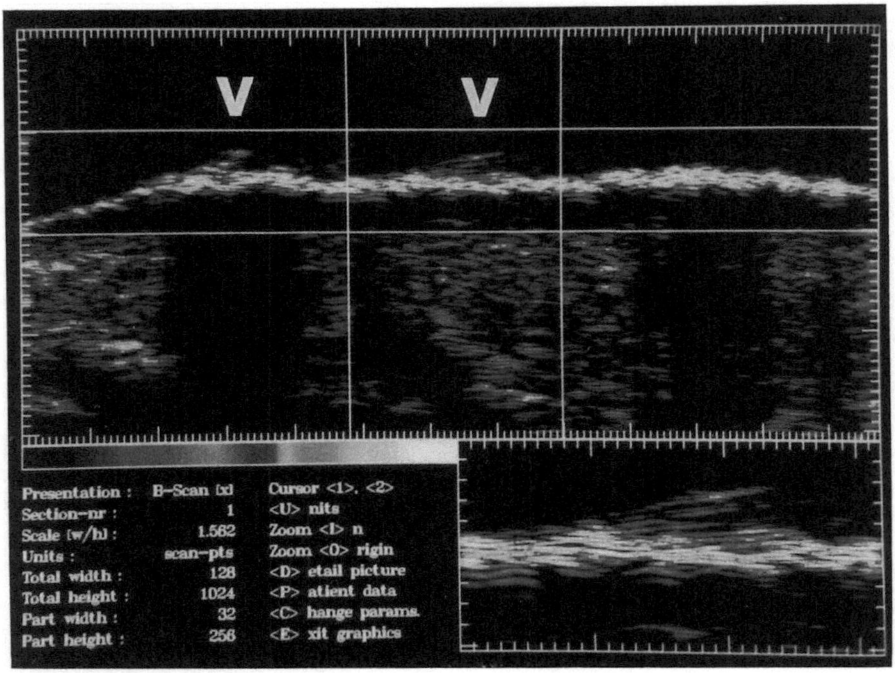

a

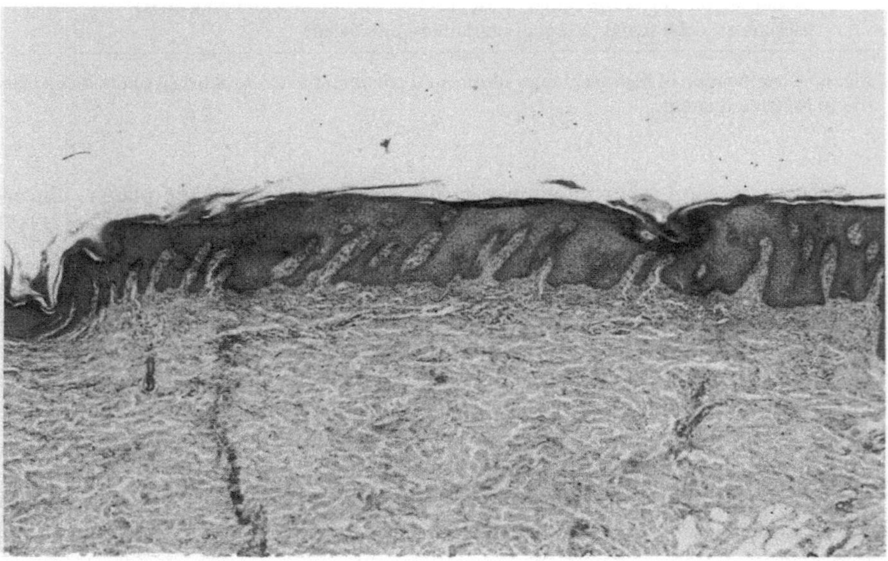

b

Fig. 7 a, b. Psoriasis vulgaris. **a** The sonographic picture (50 MHz) shows an irregularly thickened skin entry echo with echo-rich lamellae *(arrows)* protruding into the water path. Note the echo shadows emanating beneath the skin entry echo. In the upper corium an echo-poor band is seen. **b** The histologic section shows hyperkeratosis, focal parakeratosis, and a regular elongation of the rete ridges. In the upper corium and dermal papillae a perivascular inflitrate is observed.

Skin Tumors

Of all skin conditions, tumors have received the greatest attention from the different research groups using high-frequency ultrasound.

Malignant melanoma is, in a first approximation, a homogenous, spindle-shaped, echo-poor tumor [3, 29, 34]. Using 50 MHz with a higher magnification and amplification one observes, however, that this is not true. Instead, solitary, round, nearly echolucent regions, which can be correlated to the tumor convolutes in the histologic section, can be seen. The peri- and subtumoral inflammatory infiltrate corresponds to areas of multiple, undulating, reflex-rich, green lines [17].

However, since at present no generally accepted amplification values are available, the results are not reproducible on different machines, especially when the analog amplifiers do not function linearly. Different authors therefore argue quite logically [23, 35] that tumor parenchyma and infiltrate cannot be differentiated in particular when using 20 MHz ultrasound. In our experience dense infiltrates and tumor masses melt together also in 50 MHz ultrasound images. After diagnosis, the maximal tumor thickness is determined to define the minimal operative security distance. The tumor thickness is also one of the main factors used to classify high-risk and low-risk tumors concerning their metastatic potential [16]. In fact, 20 MHz sonography is well suited for measurements of depth of tumor penetration. However, 20 MHz sonography cannot differentiate between tumor and infiltrate. It therefore tends to measure "too thick" tumors. Nonetheless very thin tumors (melanoma in situ) may also be missed due to insufficient resolution [25].

Concerning semimalignant basal cell carcinoma, the axial and lateral expansion of the echo-poor area (corresponding to the tumor parenchyma, stroma, and infiltrate) can be delimited easily [23] as long as no actinic elastosis is present [3, 43]. Once again the 20 MHz machine, however, cannot discriminate between infiltrate and tumor since both structures are summed into an echo-poor area [43]. It is therefore in many clinical situations no longer necessary to make circular biopsies to determine the lateral borders of the basal cell carcinoma.

Different skin tumors can be studied as long as they are limited to the corium [23]. All these tumors show a more or less echolucent area in a region of multiple, apparently randomly scattered, corial echo reflexes. However, apart from a few exceptions, it would be rather hazardous to use tumor texture for differential diagnosis or to demark the tumor parenchyma and infiltrate. We have to accept that 20 MHz sonography is presently mainly suited to defining the location of a large tumorous process within the corium and to judge certain ultrasound phenomena, such as depth at which signal attenuation or enhancement along the borders of the tumor's process occurs.

Experimental Methods

Ultrasound is well suited for the follow-up of different inflammatory diseases and experimental (Multitest Mérieux, allergic skin reaction) skin conditions (Fig. 6). In these situations, changes in the echolucent band or area occur over time.

In follow-up studies, the acoustic tissue parameters have to be kept constant to obtain comparable ultrasound images. It is kown that the ultrasound image is influenced by

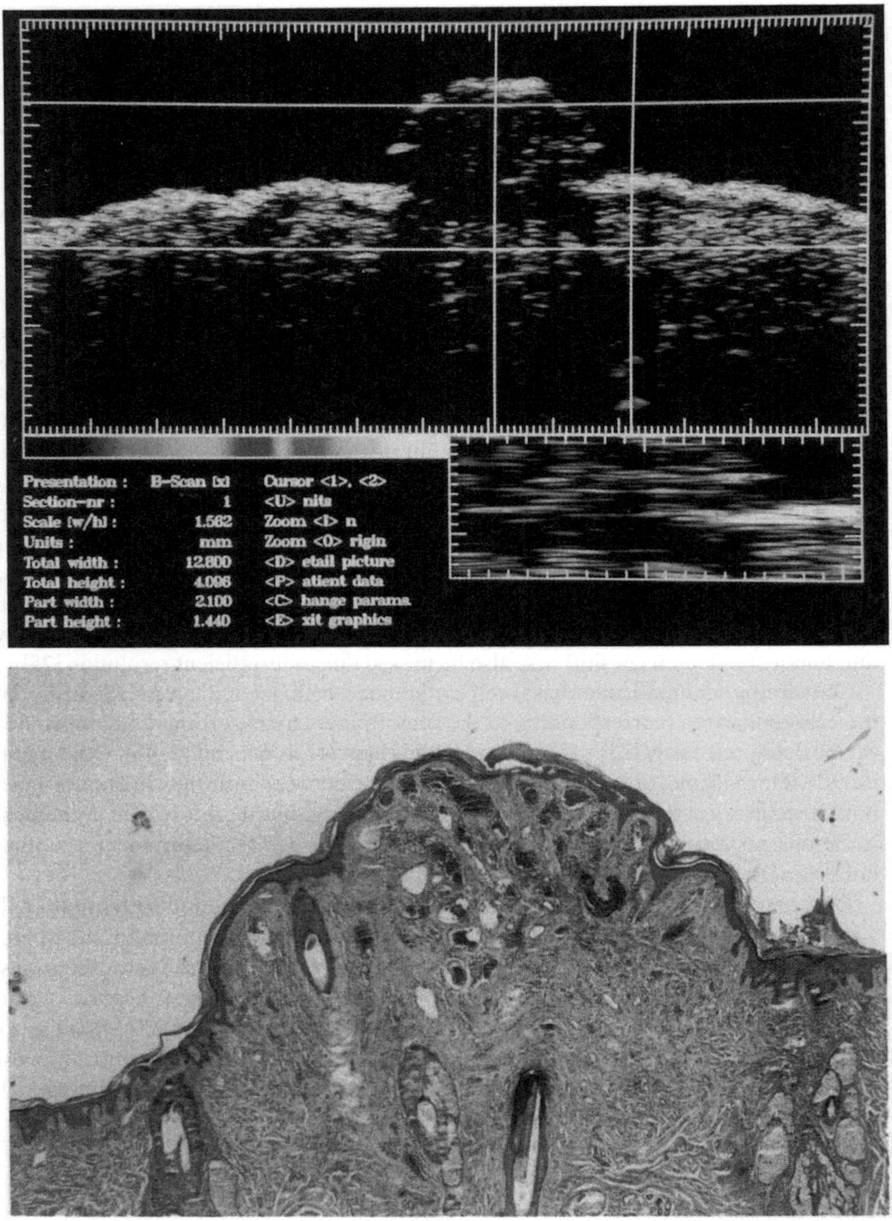

a

b

Fig. 8. Senile haemangioma. **a** The sonographic picture (50 MHz) shows an echo-rich skin entry echo with an echo-poor area protuding into the water path. The lateral borders of the tumor exhibit a "pagode-shaped" skin entry echo. Beneath the tumor, incomplete echo shadows are observed; the surrounding corial structure is normal. Remark multiple echo-rich spots within the angioma. **b** correlating histology exhibiting multiple small vessels with thrombosis.

different physical variables such as skin elasticity, tissue and water bath temperature, epidermis moisture, skin oiliness, and external ointment application [14, 17]. In order for the acoustic parameters to provide a unique signature for a specific tissue type, these parameters must also be determined or kept constant to obtain comparable results.

Intravascular Ultrasound

It should be noted that high-frequency sonography of the skin has many unique advantages over other disciplines, e.g., endosonography [9, 20] or angiosonography [16]. Since the skin is directly accessible, it is possible to register an ultrasound picture and take a biopsy from the corresponding skin region to directly compare the ultrasound image with a histological section. It is expected that this kind of comparison will promote other fields using high-resolution ultrasound, in which image interpretation has posed problems.

Recently, 20 MHz intravascular sonography (IVUS) has become possible. A miniaturized catheter with a 20 MHz ultrasound transducer is used for this technique. A motor rotates an ultrasound transducer over 360°, as in a radar system. Vessel wall lamination can be visualized (Fig. 9), and arteriosclerotic plaques and other pathological conditions can be examined directly [16, 20].

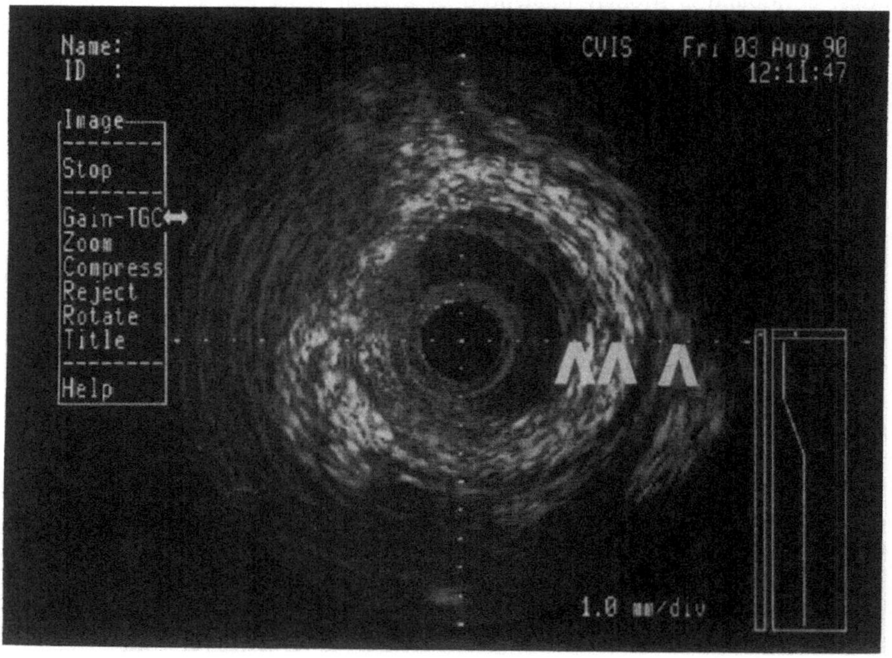

Fig. 9. Intravascular ultrasound. 20 MHz sector scan image of an artery in vitro, using a 3 mm thick catheter with a motor rotating the transducer over 360°, as in a radar system. Note the three layers of the vessel wall: intima, media, adventitia *(arrows)* (from [16])

Three-Dimensional Reconstruction Methods

By correlating *in vivo* ultrasound pictures with histological sections taken from the very same skin region, different, smaller, anatomical or pathological structures can also be discerned in ultrasound. During this period of knowledge aquisition, we have become increasingly aware that different skin structures have a specific shape in space and are oriented in a particular way. The loss of skin tension and elasticity modifies a structure's histological shape and appearance compared with *in vivo* methods. Our knowledge of the skin architecture has therefore to date been based upon "histological artifacts". It is thus important to study the existing, living three-dimensional architectures of different anatomical skin structures and pathological conditions to understand a structure's shape and orientation in vivo.

Two different reconstruction methods are principally available today. They are characterized by the order in which the data preprocessing and image analysis take place. *Voxel reconstruction methods* apply image analytical methods and filtering on the complete data set prior to image viewing. As a consequence, fast computers with a huge memory are needed for this type of three-dimensional image processing.

Voxel reconstruction methods have found wide application in computer tomography (CT) [21], to study mainly bone anatomy [22, 44] and magnetic resonance imaging (MRI), study in particular brain anatomy [7, 27]. In contrast to CT and MRI, in which structures have a specific texture and rather sharp, angle-independent boundaries, ultrasound is strongly influenced by angular reflection properties at tissue boundaries and absorption phenomena due to tissue layers above the structure of interest. In ultrasound, tissue boundaries produce different artifacts (e.g., a structure border may vanish when it is obliquely oriented in relation to the ultrasound beam), which make voxel reconstructions difficult to interpret, since all these artifacts are included in the ultrasound B-scan picture and may give a higher contrast than the structure of interest. For small structures, such as echo reflexes within the corium, sections along the three orthogonal axes can help in the interpretation of the orientation of these reflexes (Fig. 2).

The second procedure, *structure boundary reconstruction*, reduces data prior to reconstruction. Often the interaction between only a few biological structures is of interest. The image information can then be reduced to the essential: a few contours and some point clouds. This condensation to the main image elements affords quite sophisticated image analysis. One of the best image analytical systems of this type that is available is our own visual perception system.

Note that the contours of a structure are greatly influenced by the orientation of the section plane. Our mind can therefore be easily illusioned about the true shape of a structure when simple line reconstructions are used. Computer modeling should therefore include surface reconstruction procedures, since biological structures are delimited by surfaces [11]. Although the program ANAT3D was primarily developed on an Atari Mega ST4 computer using a digitizing graphics tablet to enter structure contours, a version running under Microsoft Windows 3.1 is now available. The latter version uses a frame grabber to instantaneously digitize the video image, thereby making an intermediate paper copy obsolete. Combined with image preprocessing and filtering for structure boundary extraction, the time necessary for a

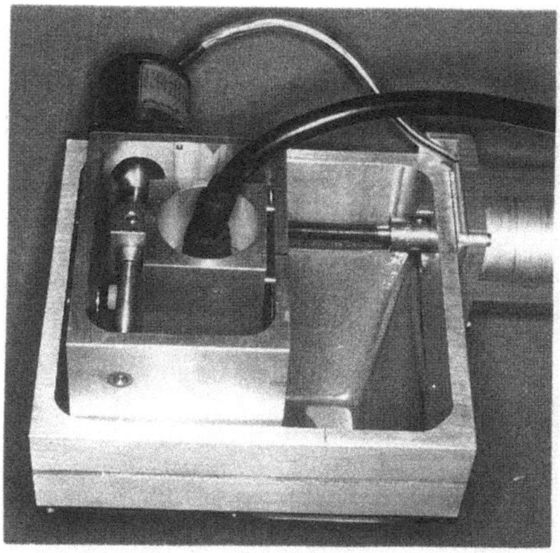

a

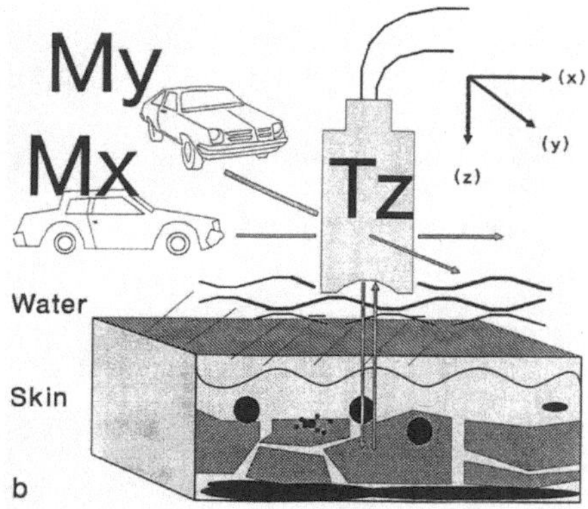

b

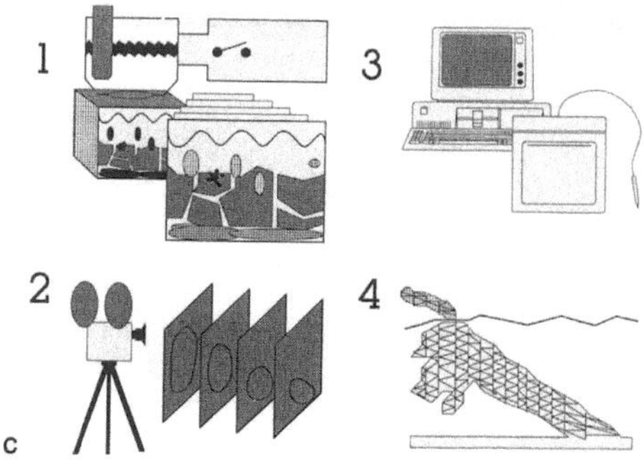

c

Figs. 10a–c. The applicator. **a** Photographic top view of the applicator showing the transducer and the perpendicularly oriented stepper motors (from [14]). **b** The orientation of the three axes of the orthogonal coordinate system in the applicator. **c** Reconstruction procedure using serial B-scan ultrasound sections. In a first step (*1*), many serial sections of the skin were obtained using an applicator with two stepper motors. All sections were photographed one by one from the monitor and projected onto a drawing tablet using a slide projector (*2*). All structures of interest within each section were then copied onto paper, named by a system of indices, and entered into the Atari Mega ST4 computer using a digitizing tablet (*3*). The program ANAT3D finally reconstructs a three-dimensional surface model which can be studied from any arbitrary view point (*4*) (from [17])

three-dimensional computer reconstruction can be significantly reduced so that this method is more suitable for routine diagnostics [16, 17]. Figure 10c summarizes the different steps.

Methods

Two computer-controlled stepper motors were used to move the focused, active, 50 MHz PVDF transducer parallel to the skin surface. For hair follicle reconstructions, equidistant, 50 μm, B-scan sections were processed. Although this oversampling is redundant, it helps in defining precisely the borders of the hair appendages. The parallel B-scan sections in sequence were then photographed from the monitor. The contours of all structures of interest within each section were copied on to paper, using a slide projector (Paximat, Braun, FRG). The corners of the picture were marked as fiducial points. Finally, all structures were named by a system of indices. The digitizing tablet

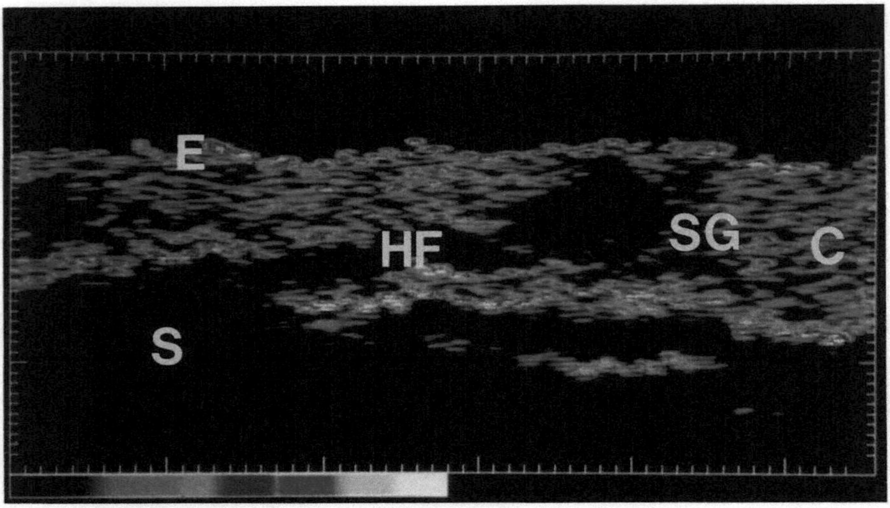

b

Figs. 11 a–c. Vellus hair follicle of a young woman, lower limb. Longitudinal section (**a**), line model (**b**), and surface reconstruction (**c**) of an anagen hair follicle. *E* entry echo; *C*, corium; *S*, subcutaneous fatty tissue; *H* hair; (*HF*) hair follicle; *SG*, sebaceous gland (**a**) Note the obliquely oriented hair follicle (*HF*) passing through the corium (*C*) (from [16]). **c** The in-depth shaded wire frame presentation mode makes it easy to follow structures within structures. The front (*SC*) plane of the hair follicle was omitted, thereby exhibiting the interior of the hair follicle. The hair (*H*) can only be followed discontinuously. Note the lobular structure of the sebaceous gland (*SC*)

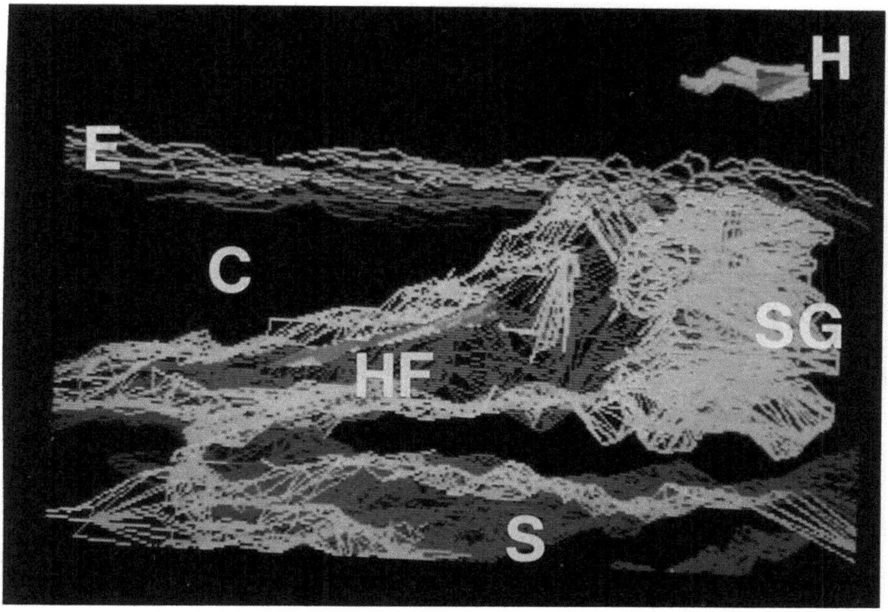

Fig. 11c

(1st CRP Koruk, FRG) was calibrated using the fiducial points to correct for the different axial and lateral scaling. This calibration was necessary for the computer to be able to convert all point coordinates into SI units, ranging from 10^{-37} to 10^{37} m. Finally, the contours of different structures were entered into an Atari Mega ST4 computer (Atari Corp, Sunnyvale, CA, USA) as single points (*x*/*y* coordinates) interconnected by lines (polygons) using a cross-hair button cursor. The program ANAT3D orders all sections by their *z* coordinate and adapts single sections within the section series. The further processing steps have been described elsewere [12, 17].

For the final reconstruction, all structures of interest within the structures list and all sections necessary within the section series are selected. For every single structure, the user decides whether it is to be reconstructed as a surface model, a wire frame model, a line contour model, or a point cloud. Combining these different presentation modes, structures within structures may easily be studied. Analogous to any viewing instrument (TEM, LM, SEM), the structures selected are scaled to study them at a reasonable magnification. The object is then rotated over any user-defined arbitrary axis (x, y, z). As the user spends most of the time looking at different views and structural combinations, a special effort is necessary for maximum comfort and speed during this period. We implemented perspective three-dimensional red-green stereo pictures for real time object manipulation. Once the optimal view has been found by the user, the computer is told to redraw all structures using depth shading and/or a virtual light source. Volume and surface calculations are available.

Figure 11a exhibits a longitudinal section of a vellus hair follicle on the lower limb of a young woman. In the ultrasound B-scan picture, the thickness of the skin entry echo is about 50–70 μm.

Respiration artifacts are seen because the registration of a 3D tissue bloc is time consuming. The hair above the skin surface has not ben sectioned in this plane and therefore cannot be observed. The corium is about 1.5 μm thick. At this body location, the border between corium and subcutis is sharp. The hair follicle canal in the corium can be easily followed. Figure 11b exhibits a contour line three-dimensional reconstruction of the entire hair follicle and sebaceous gland. In comparison to Fig. 11c, it can be easily seen that only shaded surface reconstructions readily allow visualization of the anatomy. This gland is more echo-rich and less well delineated with respect to the surrounding corium than is the hair canal (Fig. 11a). Note the echo-rich ovaloid structure in the water path, which is seen discontinuously as an obliquely oriented hair in the follicle canal (H). The follicle canal is oriented at an angle of about 30° within the corium. This value was measured after correcting the unequal scaling in the lateral and axial directions. A connective tissue septum is seen in the upper part of the subcutis.

Using ultrasound, structure boundary three-dimensional models are superior to voxel reconstruction models because ultrasound artifacts due to reflection, absorption, and attenuation can be eliminated. We suggest that a structure boundary reconstruction system should include different possible presentation modes for every individual structure. Transparency algorithms are elegant but very time consuming [37]. By combining different presentation modes for different structures in an object, structures within structures are easily analyzed. Figures 11c and 13a,b show that the combination of different modes improves structure interpretation considerably. Furthermore, by selectively omitting structures, the region of interest can easily be studied from any perspective. Hair follicles have already been identified as echo-poor structures in the dermis [1, 10]. However, the sebaceous gland could not be clearly delimited and differentiated from the hair canal [35, 38]. By combining high-resolution, 50 MHz, ultrasound, B-scan sections and 3D reconstruction techniques, it is possible to study the spacial interrelationship of different structures of the hair complex [27]. This additional information makes it possible to differentiate between the hair canal and the sebaceous gland (Fig. 11c) due to their location and echogenicity. The hair canal is a sharply demarcated structure passing through the corium. The sebaceous gland is not sharply bordered and shows diffuse inner reflexes. Using structure boundary reconstructions, the lobular structure of the sebaceous gland in vivo is revealed. Due to skin tension and elasticity, the sebaceous gland has a flatter shape *in vivo* than observed in histology. The hair itself cannot be followed continuously from the skin surface into the hair canal, since where it is oriented obliquely to the ultrasound beam it cannot be detected. We think that the echo-rich structures within the hair canal belong to the hair.

Figure 12 shows a macroscopie view of a comedo and acne papule. 30, equidistant, 100 μm, B-scan, 50 MHz section were used for this reconstruction. Figure 12c shows an echo-rich saddle within the echo-poor area. Figure 12d exhibits a hair within the water coupling medium accompanied with a strong dorsal signal attenuation. The three-dimensional reconstruction reveals that the comedo is a tent-shaped echo-poor structure in the corium (Fig 13). Figure 14 shows a three-dimensional reconstruction of the same comedo using 7 μm thick histological sections; this comedo perforated during histological manipulation.

We can conclude that high-resolution ultrasound is well suited to study noninvasively different pathological conditions of the skin. 3D reconstruction methods can enhance image interpretation considerably since new topographical information becomes available. This additional information can either be used for volume and surface calculations or as a tool to accomplish follow-up studies of exactly the same skin region.

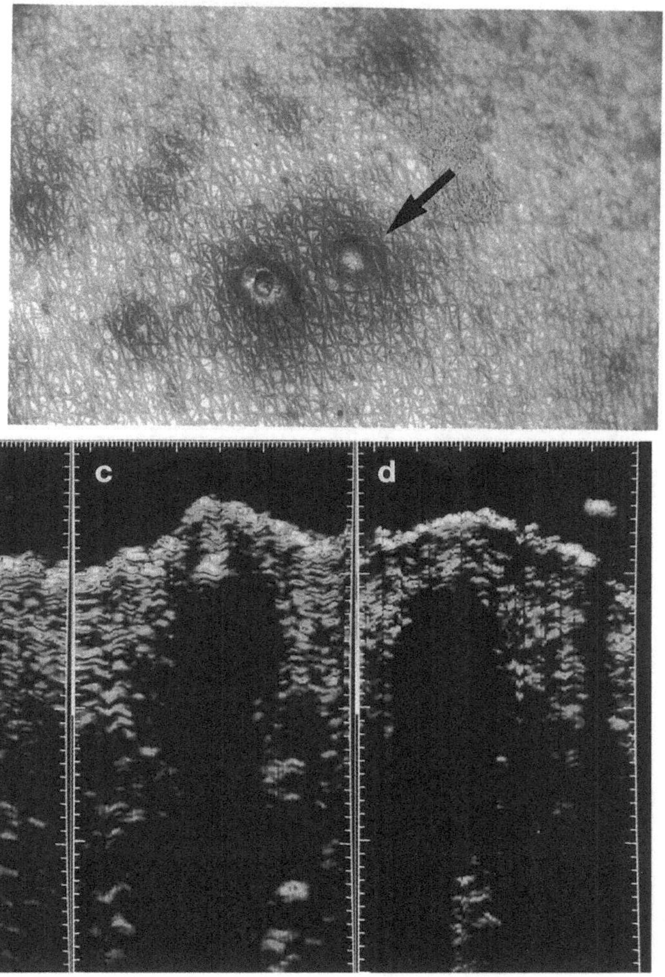

Fig. 12 a–d. Macroscopic view (**a**,*arrow*)and 50 MHz B-scan ultrasound images (**b–d**) of a comedo and acne pustule. B-scan sections at 100 μm distance in sequence. **b** 0.7 mm; **c** 1.5 mm; **d** 2.4 mm. Echolucent area with in-depth signal attenuation. Note the echo-rich saddle in the middle of the comedo. **d** A hair lying above the skin showing in-depth signal attenuation. The distance between the small marks at the upper *border* is 100 μm.

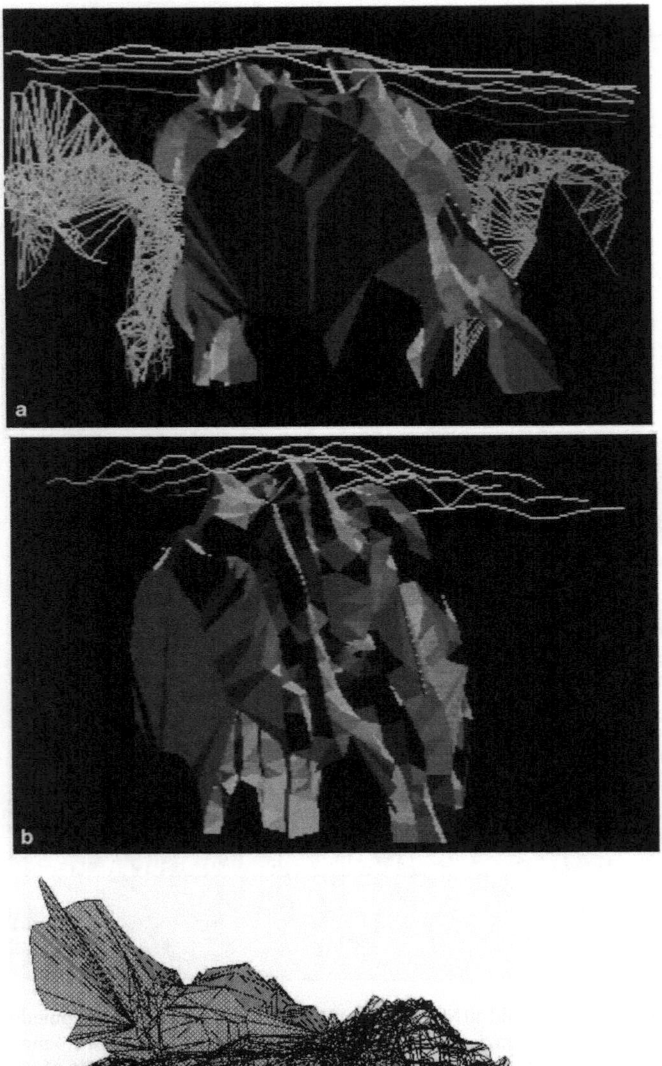

Fig. 13a, b. Ultrasound three-dimensional reconstruction of a comedo with acne pustule on the back of a patient. **a** Half-opened echolucent area with neighboring echo-poor domes. Note the saddle in the middle. On the back, the border between the corium and subcutaneous fatty tissue is not sharp in ultrasound. **b** The three-dimensional model turned towards the side. The echolucent area is dome-shaped.

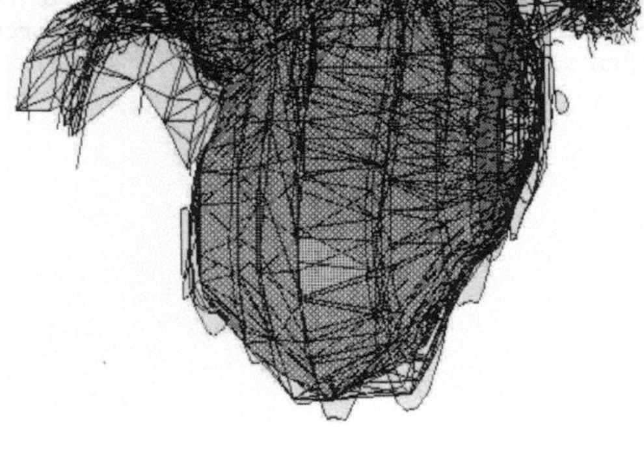

Fig. 14. Histological three-dimensional reconstruction of the comedo with acne pustule shown in Fig. 12. Due to excision, fixation, and shrinkage artifacts, the comedo has partly perforated comedo (Gray-shaded surfaces) epithelial sac (wire frame mode).

Conclusion and Outlook

Already today, 20 MHz ultrasound imaging systems promise additional preoperative information about the extension of tumorous and inflammatory diseases below the skin's surface. For correct image interpretation, however, histology is often indispensable. High-resolution ultrasound is also well suited for the follow-up of patients with inflammatory diseases and experimental skin conditions, since it is noninvasive and can be easily repeated.

In the future, we will therefore need multifrequency ultrasound equipment in dermatology to study the different parts of the skin adequately (Fig 1): 5–7.5 MHz could be used for lymph nodes, 20 MHz for dermal and subcutaneous structures, and 40–100 MHz for epidermal and upper dermal processes. Finally, epiluminescent microscopy can close the gap between ultrasound and macroscopy by exhibiting the skin surface architecture and supporting the analysis of pigment anomalities (Table 1).

Table 1. Applications listed according to frequency spectra of ultrasound in dermatology. Epiluminescent microscopy closes the gap between macroscopy and ultrasound

Method	Application
5–15 MHz:	Fatty tissue Arteries, veins Lymph nodes Musculature
15–30 MHz:	Subcutaneous fatty tissue Corium Arterioles, venules
40–100 MHz:	Epidermal structures Mucosa Upper corium
Epiluminescent microscopy:	Skin surface Mucous surface Pigmentation

References

1. Alexander H, Miller DL (1979) Determining skin thickness with pulsed ultrasound. J Invest Dermatol 72: 17–19
2. Altmeyer P, Hoffmann K, Stücker M, Goertz S, el-Gammal S (1992) General phenomena of ultrasound in dermatology, In: Altmeyer P, el-Gammal S, Hoffmann K (eds) Ultrasound in dermatology. Springer, Berlin Heidelberg, New York, pp 55–80
3. Breitbart EW, Rehpennig W (1983) Möglichkeiten und Grenzen der Ultraschalldiagnostik zur in vivo Bestimmung der Invasionstiefe des malignen Melanoms. Z Hautkr 58: 975–987
4. Breitbart EW, Hicks R, Rehpennig W (1986) Möglichkeiten der Ultraschalldiagnostik in der Dermatologie. Z Hautkr 61: 522–526
5. Breslow A (1975) Tumor thickness, level of invasion and node dissection in stage cutaneous melanoma. Ann Surg 182: 572–575

6. Brown IA (1973) A scanning electron microscopic study of the effects of uniaxial tension on human skin. Br J Dermatol 89: 383–393
7. Cline HE, Dumoulin CL, Hart HR, Lorensen WE, Ludke S (1987) 3D reconstruction of the brain from magnetic resonance images using a connectivity algorithm. Magn Res Imaging 5: 345–352
8. Cole CW, Handler SJ, Burnett K (1981) The ultrasonic evaluation of skin thickness in scleroderma. J Clin Ultrasound 9: 501–503
9. DiMagno EP, Buxton JL, Regan PT, Hattery RR, Wilson DA, Suarez JR, Green PS (1980) Ultrasonic endoscope. Lancet 9: 629–631
10. Dines KA (1984) High frequency ultrasound imaging of the skin, experimental results. Ultrasound Imaging 6: 408–434
11. el-Gammal S (1987) ANAT3D: a computer program for stereo pictures of three-dimensional reconstructions from histological serial sections. In: Elsner N, Creutzfeld O (eds) New frontiers in brain research. Thieme, Stuttgart, p 46
12. el-Gammal S, Altmeyer P, Hinrichsen K (1989) ANAT3D: shaded three-dimensional surface reconstructions from serial sections. Applications in morphology and histopathology. Acta Stereol Suppl 8: 543–550
13. el-Gammal S (1990) Experimental approaches and new developments in high frequency ultrasound in dermatology. Zentralbl Haut Geschlechtskr 157: 327
14. el-Gammal S, Auer T, Hoffmann K, Matthes U, Altmeyer P (1992) Möglichkeiten und Grenzen der hochauflösenden (20 und 50 MHz) Sonographie in der Dermatologie. Akt Dermatol 18: 197–208
15. el-Gammal S, Hoffmann K, Auer T, Korten M, Altmeyer P, Höss A, Ermert H (1992) A 50 MHz high-resolution imaging system for dermatology. In: Altmeyer P, el-Gammal S, Hoffmann K (eds); Ultrasound in dermatology. Springer, Berlin Heidelberg New York, pp 293–320
16. el-Gammal S, Hoffmann K, Höss A, Hammentgen R, Altmeyer P, Ermert H (1992) New concepts and developments in high-resolution ultrasound. In: Altmeyer P, el-Gammal S, Hoffmann K (eds) Ultrasound in dermatology. Springer, Berlin Heidelberg New York, pp 395–438
17. el-Gammal S, Hoffmann K, Kenkmann J, Altmeyer P, Höss A, Ermert H (1992) Principles of three-dimensional reconstructions from high-resolution ultrasound in dermatology. In: Altmeyer P, el-Gammal S, Hoffmann K (eds) Ultrasound in dermatology. Springer, Berlin Heidelberg New York, pp 351–380
18. Fields S, Dunn F (1973) Correlation of echographic visualizability of tissue with biological composition and physiological state. J Acoust Soc Am 54: 809–812 L
19. Görtz S, Hoffmann K, el-Gammal S, Altmeyer P (1990) High frequency B-scan sonography and skin thickness measurements of normal skin. Zentralbl Haut Geschlechtskr 157: 319
20. Hammentgen R, Godder V, el-Gammal S, Meine M, Bergbauer M, Ricken D (1992) Intravascular ultrasound. In: Altmeyer P, el-Gammal S, Hoffmann K (eds) Ultrasound in dermatology. Springer, Berlin Heidelberg New York, pp 92–100
21. Herman GT, Liu HK (1979) Three-dimensional display of human organs from computed tomograms. Comput Graph Image Proc 9: 1–21
22. Hirschfelder H (1989) Dreidimensionale (3D) Oberflächenrekonstruktion aus computertomographischen Schnittbildern. Orthopädie 18: 18–23
23. Hoffmann K, el-Gammal S, Altmeyer P (1990) B-scan Sonographie in der Dermatologie. Hautarzt 41: W7–W16
24. Hoffmann K, el-Gammal S, Gerbaulet U, Schatz H, Altmeyer P (1992) Examination of circumscribed scleroderma using 20 MHz B-scan ultrasound. In: Altmeyer P, el-Gammal S, Hoffmann K (eds) Ultrasound in dermatology. Springer, Berlin Heidelberg New York, pp 233–245
25. Hoffmann K, el-Gammal S, Winkler K, Jung J, Pistorius K, Altmeyer P (1992) Skin tumours in high-frequency ultrasound. In: Altmeyer P, el-Gammal S, Hoffmann K (eds) Ultrasound in dermatology. Springer, Berlin Heidelberg New York, pp 177–197
26. Höss A, Ermert H, el-Gammal S, Altmeyer P (1992) High frequency ultrasonic imaging systems. In: Altmeyer P, el-Gammal S, Hoffmann K (eds) Ultrasound in dermatology. Springer, Berlin Heidelberg New York, pp 22–31

27. Hu X, Tan KK, Levin DN, Galhotra S, Mullan JF, Hekmatpanah J, Spire JP (1990) Three-dimensional magnetic resonance images of the brain: application in neurosurgical planning. J Neurosurg 72: 433–440
28. Kenkmann J, el-Gammal S, Hoffmann K, Altmeyer P (1990) A 50 MHz ultrasonic imaging system for dermatology – 3D reconstructions of the hair complex. Zentralbl Haut Geschlechtskr 157: 330
29. Kraus W, Nake-Elias A, Schramm P (1985) Diagnostische Fortschritte bei malignen Melanomen durch hochauflösende Real-Time-Sonographie. Hautarzt 36: 386–392
30. Kraus W, Nake-Elias A, Schramm P (1986) Hochauflösende real-time-Sonographie in der Beurteilung regionaler lymphogener Metastasen von malignen Melanomen. Z Hautkr 61: 9–14
31. Leopold GR, Woo VL, Scheible W, Nachtsheim D, Gosnik R (1979) High-resolution ultrasonography of scrotal pathology. Radiology 131: 719–722
32. Matthes U, Höxtermann S, Hoffmann K, el-Gammal S, Bruschke E, Altmeyer P (1992) Acoustic microscopy in dermatology: normal skin structures and tumours. In: Altmeyer P, el-Gammal S, Hoffmann K (eds) Ultrasound in dermatology. Springer, Berlin Heidelberg New York, pp 321–333
33. Mende U, Petzoldt D, Tilgen W, Schraube P (1992) Comparison of ultrasound with clinical findings in the early detection of regional metastatic lymph nodes in patients with malignant melanoma. In: Altmeyer P, el-Gammal S, Hoffmann K (eds) Ultrasound in dermatology. Springer, Berlin Heidelberg New York, pp 115–125
34. Miyauchi S, Tada M, Miki Y (1983) Echographic evaluation of nodular lesions of the skin. J Dermatol 10: 221–227
35. Murakami S, Miki K (1989) Human skin histology using high-resolution echography. J Clin Ultrasound 17: 77–82
36. Myers SL, Cohen JS, Sheets PW, Bies JR (1986) B-mode ultrasound evaluation of skin thickness in progressive systemic sclerosis. J Rheumatol 13: 577–580
37. Newman WF, Sproull RF (1979) Principles of interactive computer graphics. 2nd edn. McGraw-Hill, Auckland
38. Querleux B, Leveque JL, de Rigal J (1988) in vivo cross-sectional ultrasonic imaging of human skin. Dermatologica 177: 332–337
39. Schwaighofer B, Pohl-Markl H, Frühwald F, Stiglbauer R, Kokoschka EM (1987) Diagnostic value of sonography in malignant melanoma. Fortschr Geb Röntgenstr. 146: 409–411
40. Schwenk WB, Schwenk WN (1989) Sonographie des Skrotalinhaltes. In: Braun B, Günther R, Schwenk B (eds) Ultraschalldiagnostik. Lehrbuch und Atlas. Ecomed, Munich
41. Serup J (1984) Decreased skin thickness of pigmented spots appearing in localized scleroderma (morphoea) – measurement of skin thickness by 15 MHz pulsed ultrasound. Arch Dermatol Res 276: 135–136
42. Serup J (1992) Ten year's experience with high-frequency ultrasound examination of the skin: development and refinement of technique and equipments. In: Altmeyer P, el-Gammal S, Hoffmann K (eds) Ultrasound in dermatology. Springer, Berlin Heidelberg New York, pp 41–54
43. Stücker M, Hoffmann K, el-Gammal S, Altmeyer P (1992) The acoustic characteristics of the basal cell carcinoma in 20 MHz ultrasonography. In: Altmeyer P, el-Gammal S, Hoffmann K (eds) Ultrasound in dermatology. Springer, Berlin Heidelberg New York, pp 203–216
44. Vannier MV, Gado MH, Marsh JL (1984) Three-dimensional CT reconstruction images for craniofascial surgical planning. Radiology 150: 179–184
45. Wessels G, Weber P (1983) Physikalische Grundlagen. In: Braun B, Günter R, Schwenk B (eds) Ultraschalldiagnostik. Lehrbuch und Atlas. Ecomed, Munich

Part II: Clinical Applications

Objective Assessment of Human Skin Reaction to Sun and UV–B*

S. EL-GAMMAL[1], K. HOFFMANN[1], P. STEIERT[1], J. GASSMÜLLER[2], AND P. ALTMEYER[1]

Introduction

Skin color and its changes in time are important in clinical dermatology. Experience shows, however, that the perceived skin color is influenced by many properties, such as (a) the skin surface (e.g.: humidity, oiliness, squamae), (b) the temporary blood perfusion of the skin, (c) structures in the corium and the corium/subcutis interface, (d) skin temperature [17], (e) previous sun exposures [6], and (f) the quite important ambient light conditions during examination. It has therefore been good practice in dermatology to judge skin color under standard natural illumination conditions, i.e., indirect sun light. It is interesting to note that the light energy spectrum of interest (100–3000 nm) has a maximum depth penetration in the visible and infrared (IR–A) range [9]. This nonlinear effect is, to a great extent, due to the energy absorption curve of water, which shows a steep minimum between 400 and 550 nm [14]. Moreover, because the penetration of light varies for different frequencies, the perceived color of deep lying structures can even be modified, a typical example is the "blue" aspect of the blue nevus.

Skin color changes in time, resulting from drug effects (e.g.: corticosteroids, sunscreens) in experimentally induced erythema and/or different skin diseases has been one of the major concerns of skin colorimetry. Many authors have dealt with experimental setups in which a pigmentation was not expected to occur, thereby avoiding the problems of exact color measurement and determining only the amount of redness [2, 10, 18, 23].

Different methods of skin color measurement have been proposed, replacing the filters or color plates used in the past [review: 4]. We used the Minolta CR200 colorimeter, which is supposed to "see" color like the human eye.

This study focuses on a clinically relevant system of sun reactive skin type classification. Haußer and Vahle [13] could show that the ability of UV energy to induce a "sunburn" erythema has a maximum in the UV-B range. Furthermore, skin tanning seems to have a protective effect against sunburn. We therefore tried to characterize the energy filtering capabilities of natural and tanned skin under UV–B exposure by studying the color changes.

---

[1] Dermatologische Klinik der Ruhr-Universität, D-4630 Bochum, FRG
[2] Humanpharmakologie II, Schering AG, D-1000 Berlin, FRG
* This publication contains substantial results from the dissertation of P. Steiert

Methods

Colorimetry

Color measurement instruments which analyze the whole color spectrum are suitable for dermatology when they comply the following conditions: (a) they should perceive skin color like the human eye does, (b) they must have a very stable light source which is controlled by the measuring unit, (c) the measured skin area should be small and must not be submitted to pressure or tangential forces during registration, (d) the surrounding temperature must not fluctuate, (e) the measurements should be registered fast and automatically.

The Minolta CR 200 Colorimeter (Minolta, Japan) (Fig. 1) complies with these conditions. It uses a pulse xenon arc lamp and six silicon photocells, three to measure the source illumination, three for the reflected light (Fig. 2). Different filters select the value pairs for blue (450 nm), green (550 nm), and red (600 nm). A microcomputer corrects the three measured value pairs according to the CIE (Commission Internationale d'Eclairage) Colorimetric Standard Observer Curve. Wilhelm and Maibach [21] observed a low variability in measuring different skin surfaces repeatedly. They found, however, a considerable variation in measuring untreated skin at daily intervals. It is therefore advisable, to exchange the plastic ring (Fig. 1, arrow) for a thinner black ring, with six to eight tiny feet, 2 mm thick and 5 mm in diameter, on the far periphery of the ring, to avoid direct contact with the skin and to minimize the pressure of the measuring window on the skin [16].

The three measured values are then integrated in a color which can be described by three aspects: (1) lightness (brightness) or "gray value", (2) the basic color or "hue", and (3) saturation (vividness) or "chroma". These color parameters can be converted to different color representation systems, such as the CIE Yxy color triangle, the Munsell notation, and the *Lab* system. The *Lab* color ovaloid is a simple and rational

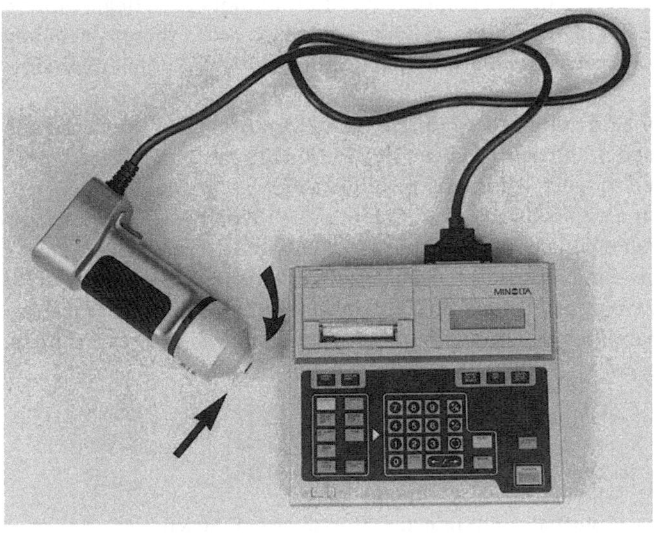

Fig. 1. Minolta tristimulus Chroma Meter CR200, consisting of a microprocessor-controlled panel and a hand-held probe (weight 1032 g). By pressing the button at the base of the probe, a Xenon arc lamp light pulse is emitted. The probe head has a round measuring field of 8 mm diameter at its tip. The transparent plastic ring should be exchanged for skin color measurements (*arrow*)

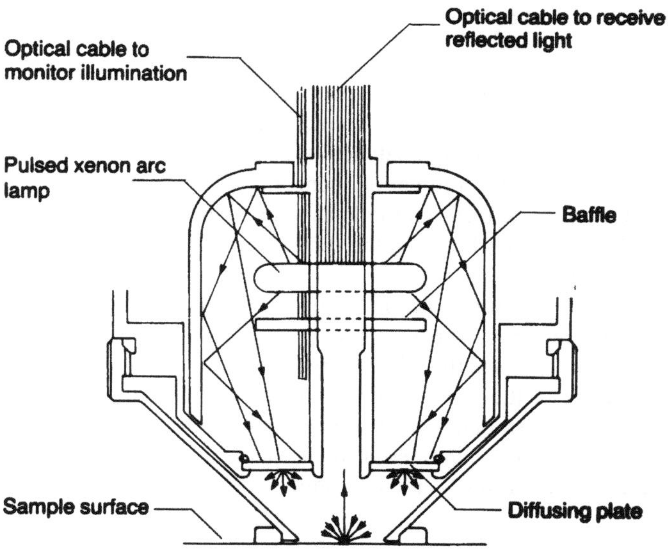

Fig. 2. Optical setup of the Minolta CR200 Chroma Meter probe head

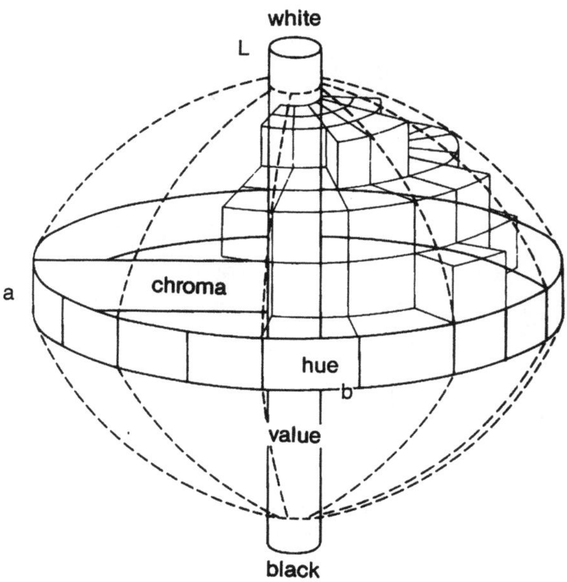

Fig. 3. The *Lab* color representation system forms a 3–D ovaloid, in which all possible colors are included. *L* is the lightness factor and is oriented vertically, ranging from black to white; *a* and *b* are represented horizontally; *a* deterines the hue and chroma along the green-red axis and *b* the same aspects along the blue-yellow axis. By moving in a radial direction the chroma of the color changes; by moving circularly its hue changes.

way of representing colors. *L* stands for lightness (brightness) of the color, *a* for its hue (oriented circularly) and chroma (oriented radially) on the green-red axis, and *b* for the same aspects on a blue-yellow axis (Fig. 3). The green/red and blue/yellow axes are oriented horizontally; the vertical axis represents the lightness factor, which varies from 0 (black) to 100 (white).

UV–B Provocation

Erythema and tanning are the cardinal macroscopic responses of human skin to ultraviolet radiation. Using photoprovocation procedures, the skin reaction to UV energy can be studied under standardized conditions. While some devices reduce the energy dose in the different skin patches (e.g., using gray filters) keeping the time constant, other systems keep the energy constant and reduce the exposure time (e.g., using covering plates). Both methods have in common that the cumulative UV–A and/or UV–B dose varies between the different skin patch areas (100% down to 0% of the primary emitted energy).

We used a photoprovocation apparatus which has wire meshes of variable thickness to reduce the energy prior to UV–A or UV–B filtering (Fig. 4). The apparatus emits different energies in the UV spectrum through the seven rows of holes (Table 1). After applying twice the minimal erythema dose (MED)in the UV-B spectrum, the skin color within the seven patch areas was measured after 7, 12 and 24 h. A few subjects had sensitive skin and exhibited a slight edema in several skin patch areas after 24 h. In these individuals the 24 h-color value was rejected.

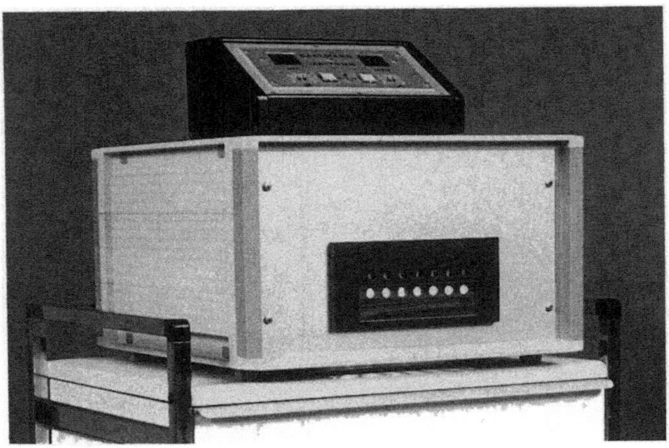

Fig. 4. Photoprovocation apparatus. Two lamps with a separate timing circuit are used (UV-B, UV–A). Every lamp emits its light through seven holes in a row. Before reaching the skin patch area, the energy has been reduced stepwise using grids and filtered appropriately. For photoprovocation, the gluteal region is placed directly in front of the holes.

Table 1. The cumulative total energy for every skin patch area is calculated by multiplying the cumulative emitted light energy with the corresponding field factor. Example: UV–B 0.177 J/cm^2/min for 20 s: field 2 = 0.0513 J/cm^2

Field	*Factor*
1	1.00
2	0.87
3	0.75
4	0.60
5	0.45
6	0.32
7	0.18

Subjects

A total of 382 Central European subjects (179 male, 203 female) ranging from 8 to 86 years were studied in winter. The skin color was measured several times in two UV-exposed regions (forehead and back of the hand) and two non-UV-exposed regions (gluteal region and back of the foot). Three measurements on the same spot were always averaged.

Unsing a questionnaire, the subjects were classified into skin type classes I – IV (Table 2). This working classification of sun reactive skin types, as introduced by Fitzpatrick et al., is based on the history of an individual's tendency to sunburn and to tan, along with some racial parameters [11]. This classification is therefore highly subjective.

Finally, 20 subjects took part in a UV-B photoprovocation study to evaluate the effect of erythema on skin color.

Table 2. The working classification of sun reactive types

	Sun-reactive	
skin type	*Sunburn*	*Tanning*
I	Always	Never
II	Always	Sometimes
III	Sometimes	Always
IV	Never	Always

This classification system, introduced by Fitzpatrick et al. [11], is based on the tendency to sunburn and to tan, as remembered by the individual along with some racial parameters. We studied Central European subjects who fitted into the skin type classes I–IV

Chroma 3D software

To visualize skin color changes, we reconstructed the three-dimensional *Lab* color ovaloid. The computer program CHROMA 3D is an ad-on for the program ANAT 3D previously published [7, 8]. This precise color determination is essential for subtle analysis of the complex changes occurring simultaneously in several axes in space (three-dimensional vector).

The color model can be rotated over any user-defined axis in space, while being projected onto the computer monitor (see el-Gammal et al., this volume).

Results

Natural Skin Colors

The natural skin color due to UV exposure in winter was studied in 382 subjects who were further classified into the sun reactive skin type classes I–IV [11] based on their response to a questionnaire. Table 3 compares the natural skin color of the forehead, dorsum of the hand, gluteal region, and back of the foot within those skin type classes. General trends are seen: in the UV-exposed regions (forehead and dorsum of the hand), the *L* value was lower than in the nonexposed regions (gluteal region and dorsum of the foot).

The red saturation is higher on the dorsum of the hand than in the gluteal region. Furthermore, the L gray value decreases from skin type I to IV, whereas a and b increase. However, the standard deviation is quite large, in particular in skin type IV, making a classification into skin types by simple color measurement impossible. A different classification approach for sun-reactive skin types was therefore necessary.

Table 3. Comparison of the *Lab* values of the forehead, dorsum of the hand, back of the foot and gluteal region in 382 Central European subjects in winter.

	Forehead	Dorsum of hand	Gluteal region	Back of foot
I				
L	67.51 ± 3.68	72.58 ± 4.63	73.87 ± 4.50	71.03 ± 3.51
a	11.34 ± 3.74	10.70 ± 2.04	5.98 ± 2.10	6.43 ± 2.24
b	13.10 ± 3.11	10.80 ± 2.36	9.01 ± 2.41	6.09 ± 3.23
II				
L	62.34 ± 3.85	61.22 ± 4.12	70.08 ± 3.40	67.71 ± 3.80
a	13.12 ± 3.56	11.12 ± 2.14	6.99 ± 2.15	7.25 ± 2.37
b	13.14 ± 2.40	14.64 ± 2.77	12.71 ± 2.92	11.40 ± 2.93
III				
L	59.08 ± 4.25	57.65 ± 4.21	66.30 ± 5.07	63.17 ± 5.90
a	14.17 ± 3.05	11.80 ± 2.24	8.63 ± 2.79	8.41 ± 2.49
b	15.12 ± 2.18	16.60 ± 2.52	15.02 ± 3.41	13.95 ± 3.16
IV				
L	58.12 ± 4.64	53.57 ± 5.21	61.42 ± 6.36	55.90 ± 12.08
a	13.68 ± 2.48	12.84 ± 1.55	9.79 ± 1.91	10.96 ± 2.31
b	16.31 ± 1.35	17.70 ± 1.66	17.72 ± 2.96	15.36 ± 2.46

According to a questionnaire were classified into sun reactive skin types I ($n = 8$), II ($n = 69$), III ($n = 291$), IV ($n = 14$). Note the strong overlap of the L, a, and b values subjects when analyzing the mean and standard deviation

Photoprovocation and UV–B Erythema

Figure 5 shows the skin color changes which occurred under UV-B exposure in summer and in winter on the back of the same subject. Skin color was measured in the different skin patch areas after 7, 12, and 24 h. All values were found to fit on a regression line oriented in space. Figure 5 shows two orthogonal side projections of this line (*aL* and *ab* diagram). When comparing skin reactions in summer and in winter, only a parallel shift of the line was observed, whereas the slope of the line remained nearly constant.

The regression lines of the other Central European subjects, who were registered in winter, were entered into the computer program CHROMA 3D using different colors to distinguish skin types I to IV (Fig. 6). By rotating the *Lab* color ovaloid, it can be shown that the four sun reactive skin types exhibit regression lines which have a specific slope and shift. The exact spatial orientation of the regression lines can be studied in different projections (Fig. 6a–d). The colorimetric dose-response regression lines of the sun-reactive skin types I–IV, viewed from a perspective corresponding to the *ab* diagram, did not exhibit any apparent order.

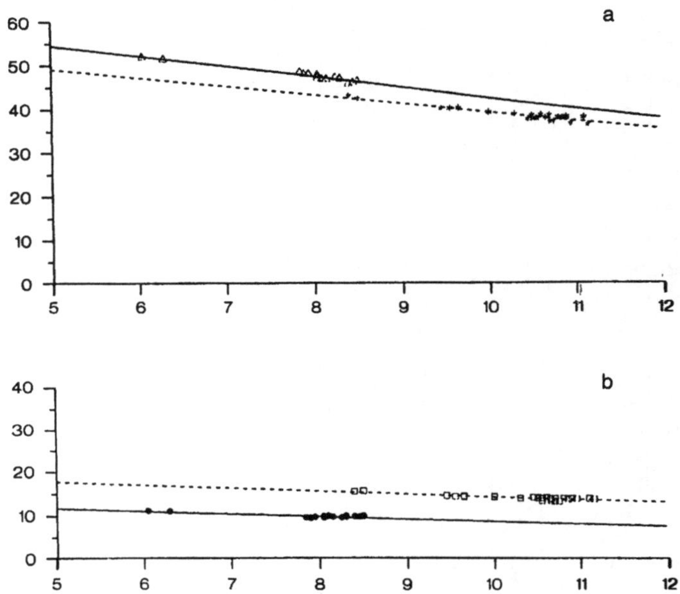

Fig. 5a, b. Colorimetric dose-response curve to UV–B provocation of a single subject in winter (*continuous line*) and in summer (*dotted line*) **a** *a* value (*x*-axis) plotted against the *L* value (*y*-axis). Note that the regression line has shifted downwards, whereas its slope angle has remained nearly constant **b** *a* value (*x*-axis) plotted against the *b* value (*y*-axis). The regression line has shifted parallel upwards.

The colorimetric dose-response values to UV-B provocation, when plotted in a projection corresponding to an *aL* diagram, are all located on regression line with a negative slope angle (arctan *x*). This slope angle decreases continuously in skin types IV (Fig. 6b), varying between any value greater than 0° (never sunburn) and smaller than 90° (always sunburn).

In most cases, the subjective classification into sun reactive skin types by the subject corresponded to our classification using the slope angle in the *aL* diagram. However, some subjects obviously gave inplausible answers. This was especially true for the sun-reactive types II and III.

Discussion

The results can be summarized as follows:

1. Objective measurement of skin colors is possible. However, in Central Europeans, a clinically relevant classification into sun reactive skin types should be accomplished using photoprovocation tests, since their natural skin color exhibits a strong variability due to sun exposure (even in winter), thereby producing a strong overlap within the skin type groups.
2. The erythema observed after UV-B provocation correlates well with changes of the *a* value in the *Lab* color representation system.
3. The slope of the *Lab* color regression line after UV-B provocation is well suited to define skin sensibility to sunburn. In particular the slope angle in the *aL* diagram is a good indicator to sun reactive skin sensitivity and is expected to be better suited for clinical purposes than the working classification of sun reactive types introduced by Fitzpatrick et al. [11].

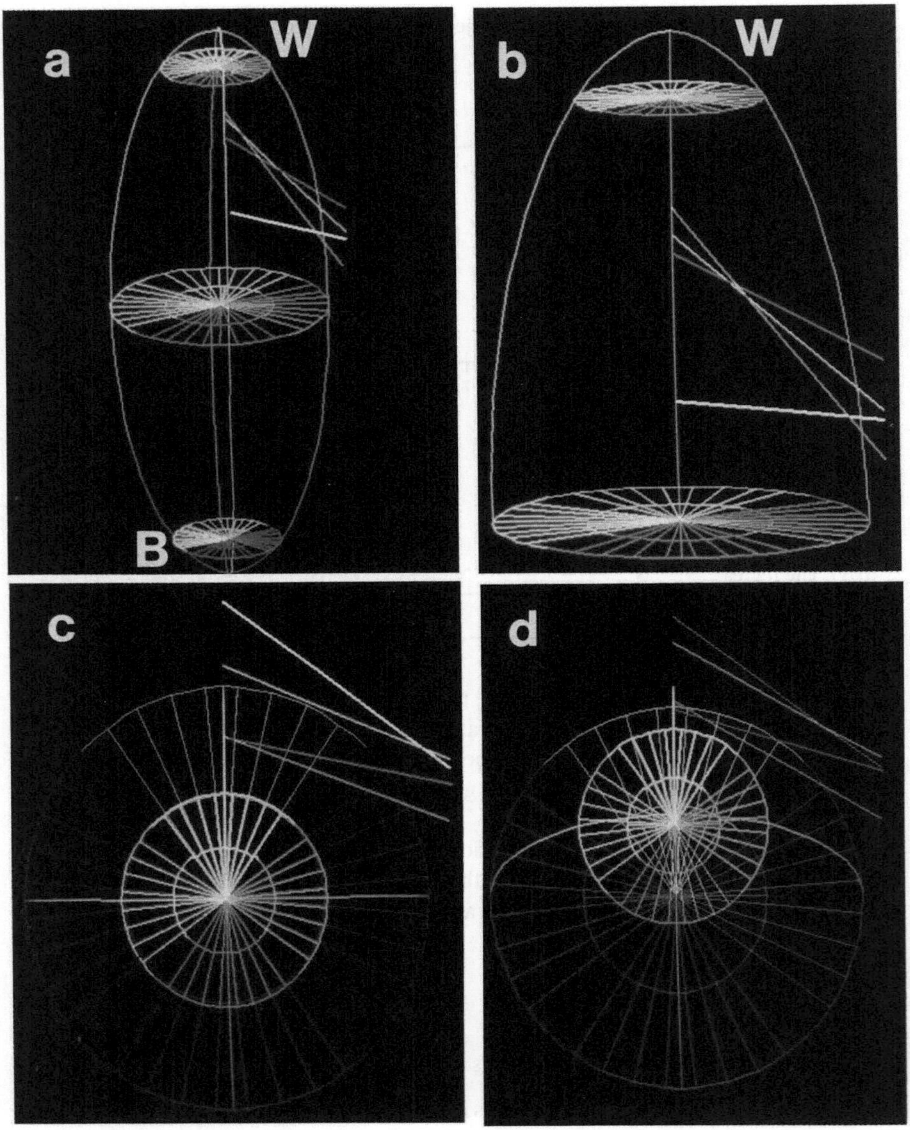

Fig. 6a–d. Colorimetric dose-response curve to UV–B induced erythema in subjects with sun reactive skin types I–IV. The three-dimensional *Lab* color ovaloid, created with the program CHROMA3D, has been depth shaded to improve the perspective. The horizontal color wheel with the basic colors green, yellow, red, and blue; the lightness factor varies between black (*B*) and white (*W*). Representative regression lines of sun reactive skin type I (*red*), II (*green*), III (*blue*), and IV (*white*) from a pool of 20 subjects. **a** The two concentric rings in the *middle*, *upper*, and *lower* level correspond to *a* and *b* values of 10 and 20, respectively. The vertical ovaloids move along the value 20 shell. Note that skin types I–IV differ in the slope of their regression line. **b** Only the upper part of the *Lab* ovaloid is represented; this perspective projection corresponds to an *a L* diagram (e.g., Fig. 5a). Note that skin types I–IV differ in the slope of their regression line. **c + d** Top view down onto the *Lab* ovaloid. This view corresponds to an *a b* diagram (e.g., Fig. 5b). Note that there is no apparent order in this perspective.

Erythema

It is generally accepted that the erythema is mainly due to a accumulation of blood in the capillaries. Melanin which is integrated in epidermis, interferes when skin vessels are observed. Although pigmentation is of indirect significance for inflammatory diseases, it can cause an systematic error in quantitative photobiology. Tanning and erythema overlap. Hemoglobin and oxyhemoglobin contribute little to the absorbance in comparison to the other skin pigments [4]. Therefore, a precise quantification of erythema is difficult even with highly developed instrumentation.

We observed an interdependence between the three color parameters, since, with increasing cumulative UV radiation, the skin redness (*a*) increased, whereas the yellow component (*b*) and color lightness (*L*) decreased. Our results confirm that the *a* value of the Minolta Chroma Meter is a good indicator of skin erythema [3, 19].

After inducing an erythema by sodium lauryl sulfate at six different concentrations, Wilhelm and Maibach [21] observed the same interdependence between the *Lab* values, stating that the *a* value correlated best with the dose of the irritant and with the visual score.

Skin Pigmentation

In 1934, Bode published light remission curves of the skin under different experimental conditions. Using a Zeiss photometer and monochromator, he disassembled a white light source into the color spectrum and measured the gray filter adjustment which was necessary to render the color of the skin and a Baryt white plate identical. Some 22 points between 400 and 700 nm wavelength were measured. All remission curves showed a peak at 500 and 630 nm and a third small peak at 560 nm. Deep depressions were observed at 545 and 575 nm, due to the absorption bands of oxyhemoglobin. In comparison to normal skin, he observed in red skin a shift of the 500 nm peak to lower levels (26%) and remarked that this greater absorption in the blue-green spectrum is responsible for the red color shift. In another experiment he compared the remission curves of white anemic skin and pigmented skin. According to Bode [4], pigmentation is characterized by a relative shift of the entire curve to lower levels, i.e, the total light reflection is diminished.

These observations led to the theory that skin pigmentation behaves like a gray filter. Different erythrometers and melanometers are based on this theory.

Attempts to characterize melanin compounds chemically and physically were not very successful, because the UV-visible absorption spectrum of melanin shows no specific absorption bands [22]. Some research groups have assumed that epidermal melanin absorbs much like DOPA-melanin, which is soluble in water and easily analyzed. Kollias and Baqer [15] have proposed that human melanin absorbs visible radiation through two distinct mechanisms: one that is in effect over the entire visible range and is linear in wavelength and one that is evident at wavelengths in the range of 400–500 nm and is expontential in frequency. By comparing the diffuse reflection spectra of DOPA-melanin in solution (low molecular weight) and as a powder (high molecular weight) with the skin absorption curves, they concluded that melanin must exist in two distinct states in the skin.

The Cumulative UV–B Dose

In a recent study, Breit [5] analyzed spectral remission curves of normal skin in different experimental settings. A collar used for blood pressure measurement was applied to the upper arm and inflated slowly up to 200 mm Hg. First the venous pressure and later the arterial pressure were exceeded; blood was therefore trapped in the lower arm. This resulted in a darkening, i.e., the entire remission curve moved downwards (2%–8%). After injection of physiological 0.9% NaCl solution into the upper corium and waiting for the disappearance of the reflex erythema, the remission curve at this artificial urtica had moved upwards (2%–8%). Changes of the skin remission spectrum, observed after applying three times the MED UV-B were studied after 2 and 7 h. After 2 h the remission curve had moved downwards by 5% in the range beneath 600 nm and exhibited two peaks at 545 and 575 nm (approximate absorption spectra of oxyhemoglobin). After 7 h the depression below 600 nm had become more prominent, whereas above 600 nm the remission values were even higher than on the contralateral normal skin. Breit [5] explained this effect by the development of a local edema. These findings emphasize that skin color is highly sensitive to different physical effects, which have to be kept constant during measurement. Furthermore, since the edema falsifies color measurements, the applied, cumulative UV-B dose must either be below the dose producing an edema or the measurements have to be made within the first few hours. In the present study those 24 h color measurements after UV-B-provocation were rejected when an edema could be palpated. As has been shown by Breit [5] an edema can obviously modify color perception significantly.

Sun Reactive Skin Type Classification

Haake et al. [12] studied a population consisting of Fitzpatrick's skin types I to III and found no correlation between the MED and skin color. These findings were confirmed by Westerhof et al. [20], observed a greater than threefold difference between the highest and lowest MED values in each skin type, reflecting the large variation of individual MED values. They speculated that either the skin type did not accurately estimate UV sensitivity or that MED is not a sensitive method to measure the skin response to UV provocation. Westerhof et al. [20] concluded that the lack of a close relationship of Fitzpatrick's skin types with the dose-response curves for erythema and pigmentation shows that Fitzpatrick's skin types are an inadequate predictor of skin UV reaction. These findings are further supported by Alsins et al. [1] who could show that the minimal blister dose (MBD) varies less between individuals than the MED at 313 mm.

We suggest measuring the dose-response regression line to UV-B provocation. This curve is of clinical relevance because it measures the human skin reaction to UV provocation over a longer time period. However, because skin colorimetry is presently not widely available, MED determination will also continue to be used in the future to assess UV-B skin sensitivity.

However, for sophisticated phototesting, such as determination of the protection provided by sunscreens, the response curve of the skin better reflects changes in UV sensitivity. We believe that the dose-response curves for erythema and pigmentation describe most accurately the tendency of an individual's skin to sunburn or to tan. The skin color dose-response curve to evaluate sunburn can be easily determined 12 h after UV–B radiation and should become a standard in phototesting.

For further simplification we suggest using the angle of the regression line (arctan x) in the aL diagram as a direct measure of the individual's sunburn sensitivity. This angle can vary between some value greater than 0° (never sunburn) and smaller than 90^0 (sunburn at infinitely small energy quantities).

References

1. Alsins J, Claesson S, Fischer T, Juhlin L (1975) Development of high intensity narrow-band lamps and studies of irradiation effect on human skin. Acta Derm Venereol (Stockh) 55: 261–270
2. Altmeyer P (1977) Modification of experimental UV Erythema by external steroids – a reflex photometric study. Arch Dermatol Res 258: 203–209
3. Babulak S, Rhein L, Scala DD, Simion A, Grove GL (1986) Quantification of erythema in a soap chamber test using the Minolta Chroma (Reflectance) meter: comparison of instrumental results with visual assessments. J Soc Cosmet Chem 37: 475–479
4. Bode HG (1934) Über spektralphotometrische Untersuchungen an menschlicher Haut unter besonderer Berücksichtigung der Erythem- und Pigmentmessung. Strahlentherapie 51: 81–118
5. Breit R (1987) Rötung und Bräunung durch UV-A. Spektrales Remissionsverhalten und farbmetrische Analyse der Hautreaktionen des Menschen unter UV-Bestrahlungsanlagen. Zuckschwerdt, Munich, pp 36–110
6. Clark P, Stark AE, Walsh RJ, Jardine R, Martin NG (1981) A twin study of skin reflectance. Ann Hum Biol 8: 529–541
7. el-Gammal S (1990) Anat3D: on-line computer demonstration of shaded three-dimensional models under Microsoft Windows. In: Elsner N, Roth G (eds) Brain – Perception – Cognition. Thieme. Stuttgart, p 530
8. el-Gammal S, Altmeyer P, Hinrichsen K (1989) Anat3D: Shaded three-dimensional surface reconstructions from serial sections. Applications in morphology and histophathology. Acta Stereol 8: 543–550
9. el-Gammal S, Hoffmann K, Steiert P, Gaßmüller J, Dirschka T, Altmeyer P (1991) Objective assessment of intra- and interindividual skin colour variability: an analysis of human skin reaction to sun and UVB. In: Marks R, Plewig G, (eds) Environmental threat to the skin. Dunitz, London, pp 99–115
10. Emden J, Schaefer H, Stüttgen G (1971) Vergleich physikalischer Parameter von Hautdurchblutungsänderungen nach epikutaner Applikation von Nikotinsäurebenzylester. Arch Dermatol Forsch 241: 353–363
11. Fitzpatrick TB, Pathak MA; Parrish JA (1974) Protection of human skin against the effects of the sunburn ultraviolet (290–320 nm). In: Fitzpatrick TB et al. (eds) Sunlight and man-normal and abnormal photobiological responses. University of Tokyo Press, Tokyo, p 751
12. Haake N, Buhles N, Altmeyer P (1987) Sensitivity of human skin to UV-light, practicability and limits in clinical diagnosis. Z Hautkr 62: 1505–1509
13. Haußer KW, Vahle W (1921) Sonnenbrand und Sonnenbräunung. Wiss Veröff Siemens Werken 6: 101–120
14. Helfmann J (1989) Nichtlineare Prozesse. In: Berlien HP, Müller G (eds) Angewandte Lasermedizin, Lehr- und Handbuch für Praxis und Klinik. Ecomed, Munich
15. Kollias N, Baqer AH 1987) Absorption mechanisms of human melanin in the visible, 400–720 nm. J Invest Dermatol 89: 384–388
16. Lees FC, Byard PJ, Relethford JH (1978) Interobserver error in human skin colorimetry. Am J Phys Anthropol 49: 35–37
17. Little MA, Sprangel CJ (1980) Skin reflectance relationships with temperture and skinfolds. Am J Phys Anthropol 52: 145–151

18. Rampini E, Rastelli A, Cardo P (1978) Comparative study of the vasoconstrictor activity of halopredone acetate in a modified McKenzie test. Eur J Clin Pharmacol 14: 325–329
19. Seitz JC, Whitmore CG (1988) Measurement of erythema and tanning response in human skin using a Tristimulus Colorimeter. Dermatologica 177: 70–75
20. Westerhof W, Estevez-Uscanga O, Meens J, Kammeyer A, Durocq M, Cario I (1990) The relation between constitutional skin color and photosensitivity estimated from UV-induced erythema and pigmentation dose-response curve. J Invest Dermatol 94: 812–816
21. Wilhelm KP, Maibach HI (1989) Skin color reflectance measurements for objective quantification of erythema in human beings. J Am Acad Dermatol 21: 1306–1308
22. Wolbarsht ML, Walsh AW, George G (1981) Melanin, a unique biological absorber. Appl Opt 20: 2184–2186
23. Zaun H, Altmeyer P (1973) Ergebnisse reflexphotometrischer Bestimmungen der Vasokonstriktion nach topischer Steroidapplikation. Arch Dermatol Forsch 247: 378–386

Mechanical Measurements in Assessing Aging

H. G. Vogel*

Introduction

The age of an individual is estimated by his appearance, and particularly of his skin. In a negative sense age is related to the wrinkles and flaccidity of the skin. On the positive side youth is related to soft skin with high turgor. It seems reasonable to estimate age by measuring the mechanical properties of skin. In this respect, many attempts have been made using various methods, with contradictory results. A critical judgement seems necessary on the methods hitherto used.

Survey of *in vivo* Methods

Historically, one of the first attempts to measure the mechanical properties of skin was made in 1912 by Schade, who used an apparatus consisting of a loaded rod applied perpendicular to the skin, measuring the excursions after loading and unloading. Already this author described the relaxation phenomenon in human skin in vivo. The refined apparatus was called an elastometer [72]. The method was used later on by Schmidt-LaBaume [73–75] for various purposes, although not for systematic investigations of the influence of maturation and aging. The technique and an apparatus called an indentometer were further developed by Dikstein and coworkers [28–30] and Lanir et al. [49, 50]. Several investigators have used this type of method [67]. Suggestions for standardization were made by Barbanel and Payne [11].

Instead of continuous pressure, a method involving a sudden impact on to the skin has been developed as ballistometry, counting the number of rebounds with decreasing amplitude [6, 81]. Since no mathematical data in terms of stress or strain can be calculated the results are difficult to compare with those from other methods.

Instead of pressing down on the skin, elevation of the skin has been used, either with suction cup systems [4, 5, 7, 8, 22, 31, 39, 59, 60] or levarometry as described by Dikstein and Hartzshtark [29] Lanir et al. [50]. Due to the complexity of these systems a comparison with other methods is hardly possible.

A further approach is the torsional tests, as described by Finlay [33, 34], Sanders [69], Barbanel and Evans [10], Agache et al. [1], Leveque et al. 53], and Aubert et al. [7]. These systems consist of a rotating disk usually surrounded by a guard ring. A special apparatus called "twistometer" has been developed by de Rigal and Leveque 65].

---

* Hoechst AG Geschäftsbereich Pharma Postfach 800320 6230 Ffm 80, FRG

The results depend largely on the degree of the torque and the geometry of the apparatus, making comparisons of the results of various authors rather difficult.

Tensile tests are standard methods in mechanics and give the most reliable results in physical terms. They can be used *in vitro* and *in vivo*. For *in vivo* stretching, tabs are glued on the surface of the skin. In most cases, the displacement of the tabs is uniaxial, in one direction vs the body axis. The geometry, e.g., size of the tabs and distance between them and the separation rate have to be standardized [11]. Such methods have been used by Gilson et al.[37], Burlin et al. 16–19], Thacker et al. [80], Wijn 123], Brakkee et al. 13], Jagtman [43], Vogel [100], Vogel and Denkel [115–117], Berardesca et al. [12], Manschot and Brakkee [55, 56], Baker et al. [8], and Ballou et al. [9]. These methods allow not only the registration of stress-strain behavior but also analysis of relaxation and the hysteresis phenomenon. By these methods data obtained *in vivo* can be compared with those found *in vitro* [95, 100, 115]. Moreover, a special phenomenon can be studied by this means: the *in vivo* recovery or the restitutio ad integrum of mechanical properties of skin after repeated load 111, 113, 117].

In contrast to all other methods, tensile tests most clearly show the anisotropy of skin which can be demonstrated both in *in vitro* experiments [63, 97, 98, 101, 105, 106, 110] and *in vivo* studies [111, 113–115, 117, 124].

Experimental Results

In vitro Studies in Rat and Human Skin

Many experimental studies have been performed with skin strips from animals *in vitro*. In order to extrapolate from these studies to the clinical situation in humans, one has first to compare the results of *in vitro* studies of animal and of human skin. If these results are in agreement, one can try to compare *in vivo* studies in animals with data in humans, even if they were obtained with different methods.

Stress-Strain Experiments

Ultimate Values

Even simple stress-strain experiments *in vitro* have to be standardized. In all our studies we prepared the skin strips as follows [84, 86]: Subcutaneous fat tissue was removed from flaps of skin. Skin thickness was determined by using calipers. A dumb-bell-shaped 4 mm wide specimen was punched and fixed between the clamps of an Instron® instrument allowing a gauge length of 30 mm. Usually, the strain rate was 5 cm/min. Care was taken to prevent exsiccation during measurement. The experiments were performed at room temperature.

In the basic stress-strain experiments, curves such as those shown in Fig. 1 are obtained. During initial elongation the measured load remains at zero for a short period of time, if preloading during clamping has been avoided. The stress-strain curve than ascends according to an exponential function. This part can be analyzed by a special approach in rat skin [118]. The relative extensibility at low loads had a maximum in adolescents rats (2 months) indicated by a low modulus of elasticity at this part.

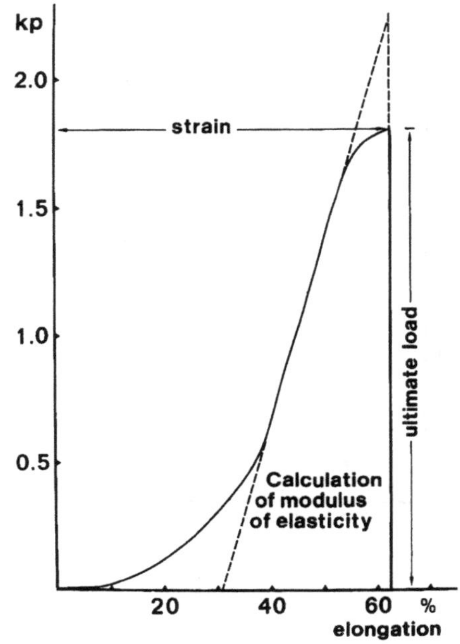

Fig. 1. Stress-strain curve of skin strips *in vitro* (original recording)

With higher extension degrees, the stress strain curve, becomes an almost straight line, indicating the dependence on Hook's law. From this part the ultimate modulus of elasticity can be calculated. The point of rupture indicates the values for ultimate strain and ultimate load. By dividing with the initial cross-sectional area the ultimate stress values can be calculated.

The age-dependence of ultimate values in rats skin has been evaluated in several studies [85, 86, 89–94, 98, 99, 102, 104–106, 112, 114, 118, 121, 122]. Directional variations have been found in rat skin obtained either perpendicular or longitudinal to the body axis, indicating that in adult animals extensibility is much higher perpendicular than longitudinal to the body axis [105]. Figure 2 gives a survey of ultimate values of rats of different ages, ranging from very young animals (1 week) to old animals (24 months). Age is depicted on a logarithmic scale on the abscissa; body weight, skin thickness, and ultimate strain on a linear scale and ultimate load, tensile strength, and modulus of elasticity on a logarithmic scale on the ordinate. Body weight increases steadily until the age of 12 months, followed by a significant decrease during the period of senescence up to 24 months. Surprisingly, skin thickness decreases during early maturation from 1 to 4 weeks, followed by an increase during late maturation until 12 months, ending with a decrease during senescence up to 24 months. Ultimate strain is different longitudinal and perpendicular to the body axis. Perpendicular to the body axis ultimate strain increases during maturation, achieves a maximum already at the age of 4 months, and decreases later on. In contrast, longitudinal to the skin ultimate strain does not show the maturation-dependent increase; however, an age-dependent decrease is noted. In this way, the curve for ultimate strain of perpendicular samples crosses the curve of longitudinal samples at an age of 5 weeks. Ultimate load,

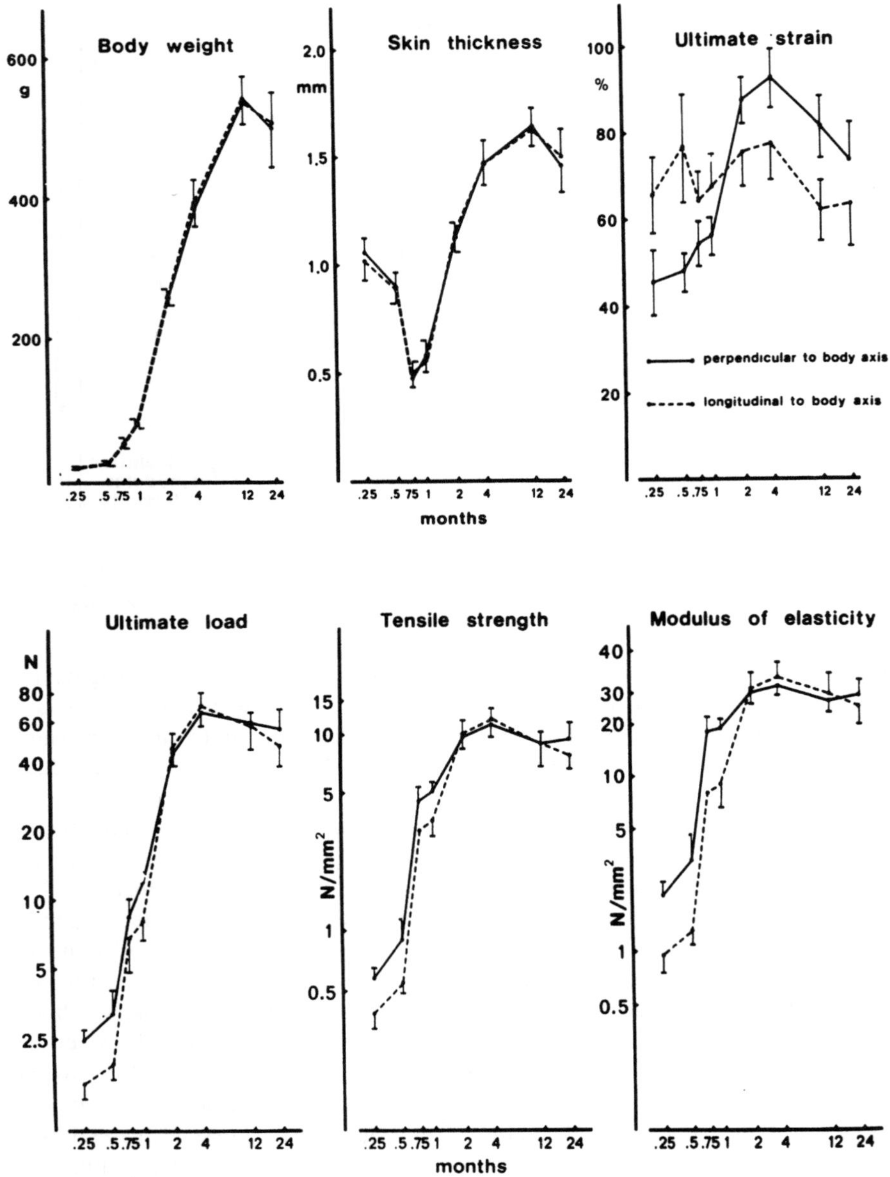

Fig. 2. Ultimate values (body weight, skin thickness, ultimate strain, ultimate load, tensile strength, modulus of elasticity) of rat skin perpendicular and longitudinal to body axis

tensile strength, and modulus of elasticity are higher in very young animals perpendicular to the body axis. In both directions a maximum is achieved at the age of 4 months, in some studies after 12 months. The decrease until 24 months was significant. The differences in ultimate strain between longitudinal and perpendicular direction have to be explained by orientation of the collagenous network and not by the presence of the muscular layer in rat skin [110]. Higher values of ultimate load, tensile strength, and ultimate modulus of elasticity were found in old rather than in young rats independent of strain rate, ranging from creep velocities ($5.\ 10^{-3}$ cm/min) up to speeds approximating free fall (3.10^4 cm/min) [85].

Higher values of tensile strength in 15 months old rats than in young (70 days old) rats have also been found by Mendoza and Milch [57]. In other studies [36] the breaking strength of skin rings on the legs of rats increased with age, whereas extensibility showed a maximum after maturation.

With the same method and the same apparatus two studies in human cadaver skin were performed [42, 108]. In the first study skin samples were obtained above the sternum and from the inner thigh, in the second study only from the sternum. A total of 104 specimens were analyzed in the first study, a total of 348 in the second one. The age of the deceased patients ranged from newborn to 97 years. Due to the death rate, less skin samples were available from young patients than from old people. Most samples were from patients between 40 and 85 years. The evaluated parameters showed generally a steep increase during maturation and a slight but continuous decrease during senescence. Therefore, two concurrent exponential functions have been used for computer calculations. The most appropriate constants were calculated and the curves plotted on an *XY*-recorder (Fig. 3a). Skin thickness reached a maximum between 20 and 30 years. Thereafter, a continuous decrease was noted. Ultimate strain showed a maximum at the same time and thereafter a continuous decrease. Ultimate load showed a similar pattern (Fig. 3b). After a sharp rise during maturation, a maximum was found between 20–25 years, followed by a continuous decrease during aging. Tensile strength exhibited a sharp incease during early maturation and achieved a maximum already at 10–15 years. Therafter, the decrease was evident. Likewise, modulus of elasticity showed a sharp increase during maturation with a maximum at about 10 years. The subsequent decrease was almost linear with age. Evaluation of all data with a similar mathematical approach resulted in the same shape of curves indicating the maxima at even younger age [108].

Comparing the ultimate values of rat and human skin in *in vitro* experiments one finds almost complete agreement. There is an increase during maturation for skin thickness, ultimate load, tensile strength and modulus of elasticity during maturation, a maximum at early adulthood and a slow but continuous decrease of these parameters during aging or senescence. Ultimate strain is in both species much less influenced by maturation and aging. These results give definite confidence that results obtained in rat skin can be extrapolated to human skin.

Further Analysis of Stress-Strain Curves

A more in-depth analysis of stress strain curves in rats showed that they differed depending on age not only in the ultimate values but also in the shape, especially in the lower part. Since all attempts failed to calculate the stress-strain curve by a simple mathematical formula tangents being drawn at the lower part of the curve were used to calculate moduli of elasticity at low extension degrees.

In contrast to the ultimate modulus of elasticity, these values, related to extension degrees between 5% and 20%, decreased sharply during early maturation, then re-

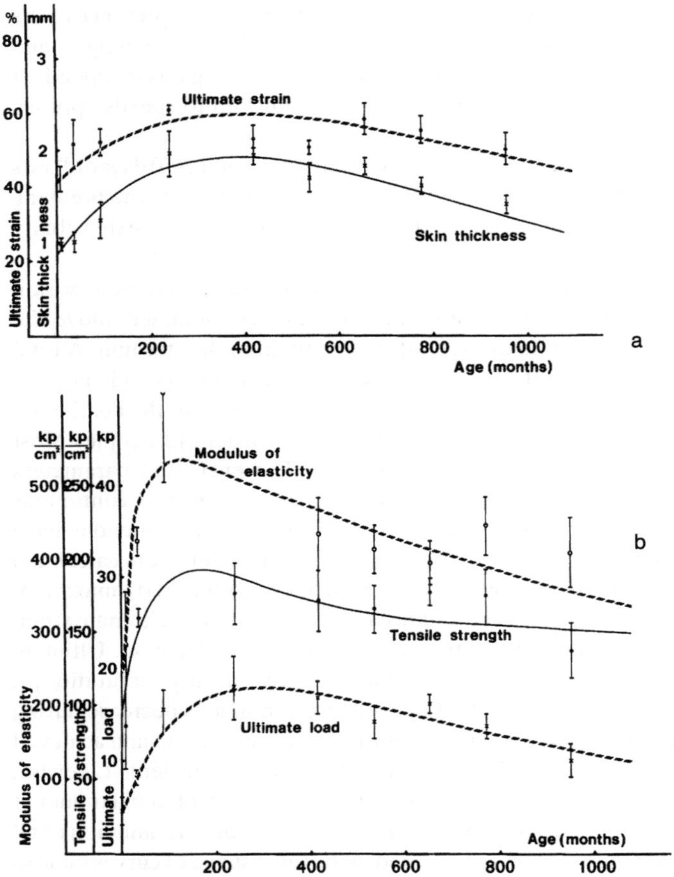

Fig. 3. Mechanical properties of human skin *in vitro* depending on age: **a** skin thickness and ultimate strain; **b** ultimate load, tensile strength, and modulus of elasticity

mained fairly constant, and decreased only slightly further during senescence [118]. At low stress values elongation decreased during early maturation and remained constant until senescence.

Only in perpendicular samples and only at medium and high stress values was a decrease of the elongation values found [98, 112]. The directional variations and the age dependence at the lower part of the stress-strain curves was analyzed in further studies [27, 98, 100, 102, 103, 112]. Whereas at medium and high extension degrees the load and the stress values for longitudinal samples were higher than for perpendicular direction, the reverse was true for extensions below 40%. In this case the perpendicular samples showed the higher stress values (Fig. 4). Therefore, a crossing of the stress-strain curves was noted. Consequently, at low stress values up to 0.2 N/mm^2 elongation in the longitudinal direction was higher than perpendicular to the body axis [103] (Fig. 5). In both directions elongation decreased during early maturation. Afterwards a slight increase was noted reaching a maximum at 4 months and a slight decrease thereafter. From 0.5 N/mm^2 upwards only the perpendicular samples followed the same age dependence, i.e., a decrease of elongation during early maturation, an increase during late maturation, and a decrease during senescence. Longitudinal values showed only the decrease during early maturation and almost constant values during late maturation and senescence. Therefore, from 0.5 N/mm^2 upwards the curves crossed at least once. If the age dependence of load and stress values at various extension degrees was evaluated [100, 102, 106] an increase during early maturation up to 1 month was noted followed by a slight decrease. At extension degrees up to 30% the perpendicular samples showed higher stress values at all age intervals. From 40% extension onwards the crossing phenomenon was again noticed. In both directions stress values rose during early maturation; however, whereas in longitudinal samples the values remained almost constant with age, in perpendicular samples a decrease during late maturation and again an increase during senescence were realized. Therefore at the extension degrees between 30% and 70% the perpendicular stress values were higher in young animals and lower in old rats.

Similar evidence was achieved when the hysteresis experiments [92, 101] and relaxation experiments in rats [105, 106] were evaluated for stress and modulus of elasticity at low extension degrees. In these cases the values showed a steady increase during aging without a decrease during senescence.

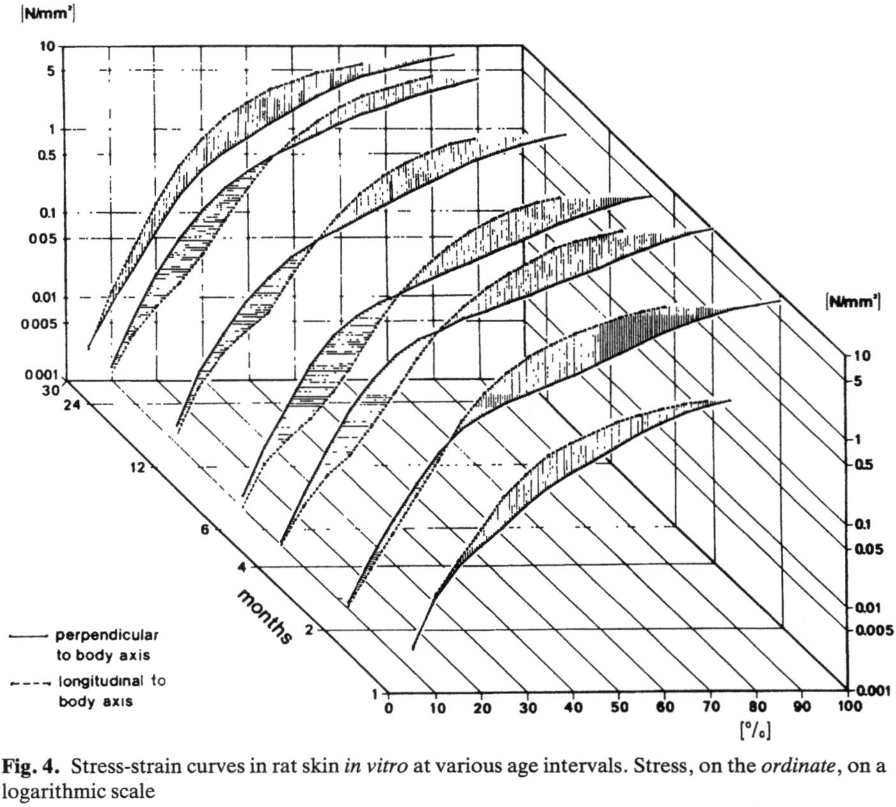

Fig. 4. Stress-strain curves in rat skin *in vitro* at various age intervals. Stress, on the *ordinate*, on a logarithmic scale

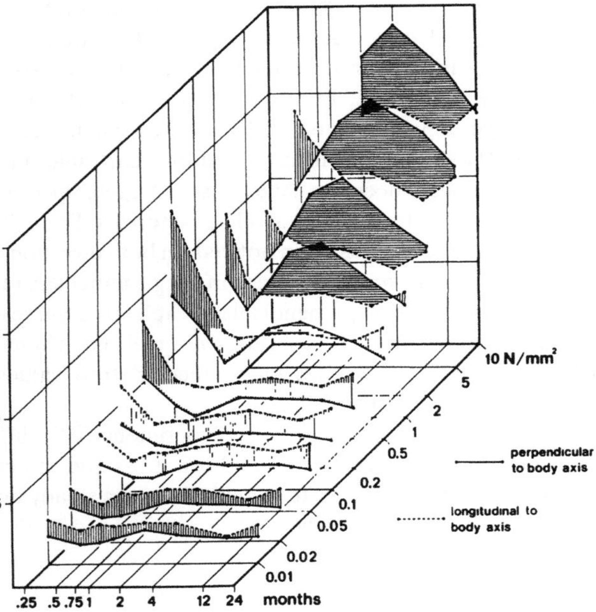

Fig. 5. Elongation of rat skin *in vitro* at various stress values depending on age

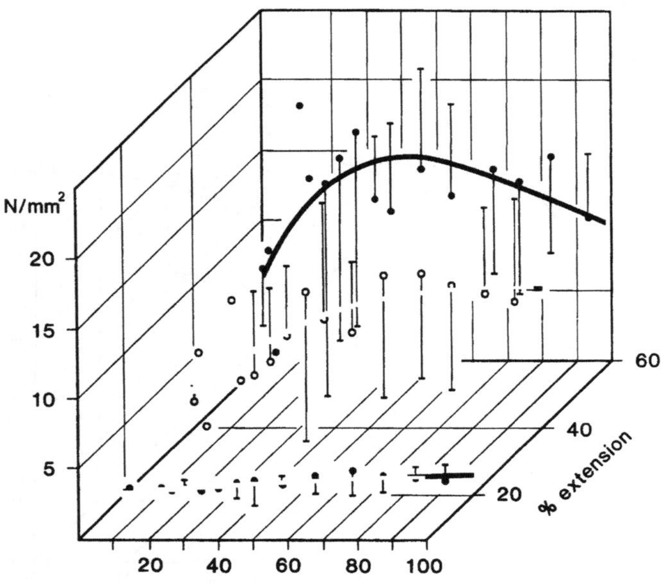

Fig. 6. Age dependence of stress at various extension degrees in human skin. Data from initial tension values of relaxation experiment

Likewise, in human skin strips stress and modulus of elasticity at low extension degrees rose during childhood and continued to rise during maturation and senescence in contrast to the ultimate values and values at high extension degrees, which showed a clear-cut maximum at adulthood and a decrease during senescence [109] (Fig. 6).

Viscosity and Secondary Elasticity

Parameters indicating viscosity or plasticity and secondary elasticity have been analyzed *in vitro* both in animals and in human skin by several experiments such as hysteresis, relaxation, mechanical recovery, creep, and repeated strain.

Hysteresis Experiments

The same method has been used for rat skin [87, 88, 92, 112] and for human skin samples [109]. Using the Instron® instrument, the samples were stretched up to a given extension degree (e.g., 20%) with an extension rate of 20 mm/min. When the given extension was achieved the crosshead was immediately moved back to the starting position with the same velocity. As Fig. 7 shows the upwards and the downwards curves were different, forming the hysteresis loop. The area below the upwards curve measured by planimetry indicated the energy input, whereas the area between the curves indicated energy dissipation. Immediately afterwards, the experiment was repeated up to an extension degree of 30%, than to 40% and 50% and finally up to 60%. In several cases the hysteresis loop could be recorded even at higher extension degrees. As a characteristic number the ratio between energy dissipation and energy input was calculated. In rat skin this ratio had a maximum at 30%–40% extension (Fig. 8). At low extension degrees there was an increase with age, at high extension degrees a decrease was noted.

In human skin the ratio was the highest at 20% extension. In both species the age dependence was similar: at low extension degrees there was a very slight increase with maturation and age whereas at medium and high extension degrees a slight but significant decrease was noted. This indicated that at least at medium and higher extension degrees some decrease of plasticity or viscosity of skin depending on age is noted in both species. Figure 9 shows the age dependence for human skin.

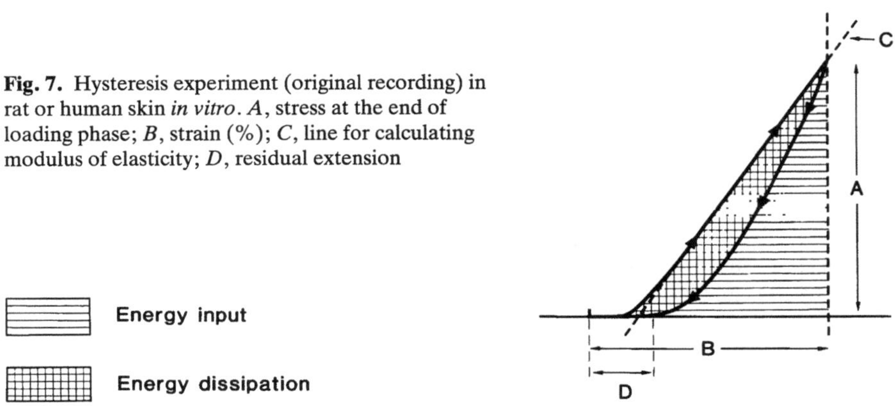

Fig. 7. Hysteresis experiment (original recording) in rat or human skin *in vitro*. *A*, stress at the end of loading phase; *B*, strain (%); *C*, line for calculating modulus of elasticity; *D*, residual extension

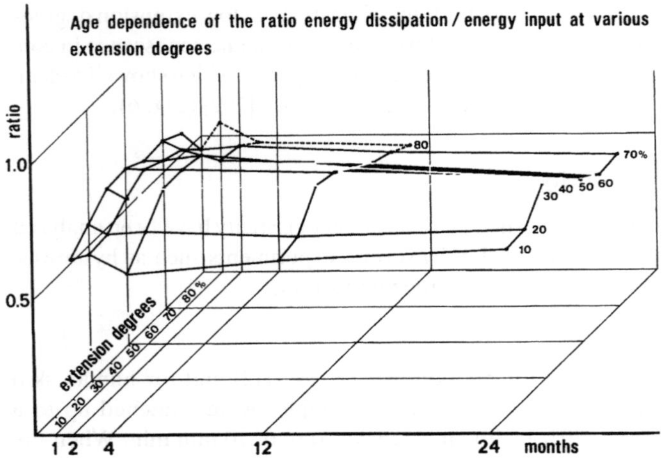

Fig. 8. Hysteresis exeriment in rat skin. Age dependence of energy dissipation/energy input at various extension degrees

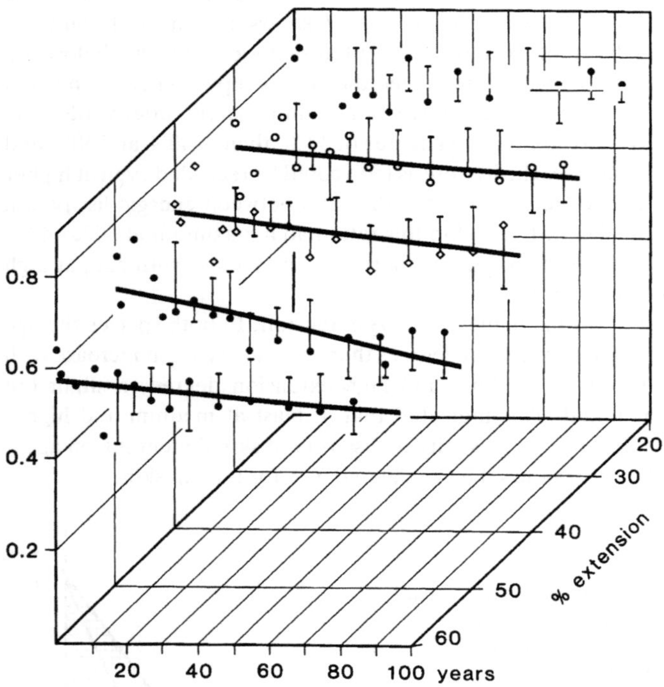

Fig. 9. Age dependence of energy dissipation/energy input of human skin in hysteresis experiments

From the hysteresis curve, as shown in Fig. 7, residual extension as another parameter of plasticity can be calculated. In both animal and human skin a slight age-dependent increase at high extension degrees was noted. Again, an influence of maturation and aging on immediate parameters of plasticity is observed indicating some decrease with aging.

Relaxation Experiments

For relaxation experiments the same method has been used for rat skin and samples from human skin [89, 90, 105, 107, 109]. As Fig. 10 shows, skin strips were extended with the high strain rate of 1.000 mm/min up to 20% extension. This extension was kept constant for 5 min. The chart speed was initially 1.000 mm/min, then 10 mm/min. In this way, the initial tension and the stress values at 0.001, 0.01, 0.1, 1, and 5 min could be measured. Due to relaxation, the stress values dropped roughly with the logarithm of time.

Therefore, for each sample the relaxation was calculated according to the formula:

$$p = A_1 + A_2 \cdot \log t$$

resulting in two constants (A_1 and A_2) for each sample. The ratio between the coefficents A_2 and A_1 has to be considered as the most characteristic parameter of the relaxation experiment. Furthermore, the residual stress after the 5 min relaxation period was measured and calculated as a a percentage of the original stress. After 5 min the sample was returned to 90% of the original strain, for example, from 20% to 18%.

The stress following such unloading was recorded and again calculated as a percentage of the original stress. Immediately after unloading, the mechanical recovery was observed as the spontaneous increase of measured load.

Mechanical recovery was calculated as a percentage of the initial tension and as a percentage of stress after unloading. The relaxation experiment was repeated with increasing degrees of extension of 40%, 60%, 80% and eventually 100% until the specimen broke. In rat skin, a definite decrease of the ratio A_2/A_1 was found at 40% and 60% extension degrees indicating a decrease of plasticity with age. At a 20% extension degree, only in the perpendicular but not in the longitudinal axis was a decrease found (Fig. 11). Almost identical results were obtained in human skin. At 40% and 60% extension degrees a clear decrease of the A_2/A_1 ratio was found depending on age.

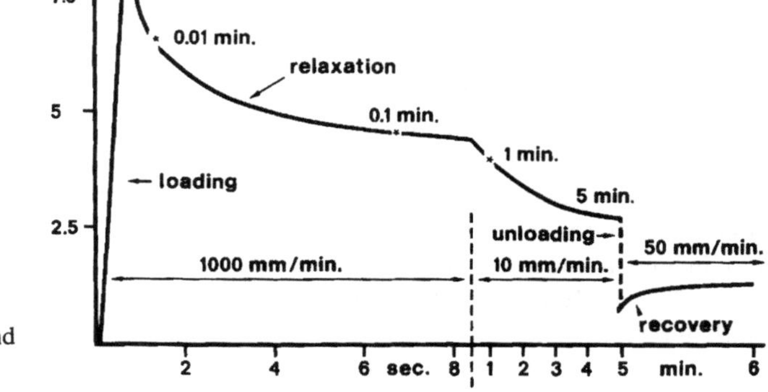

Fig. 10. Relaxation experiment (original recording) in human and rat skin *in vitro*

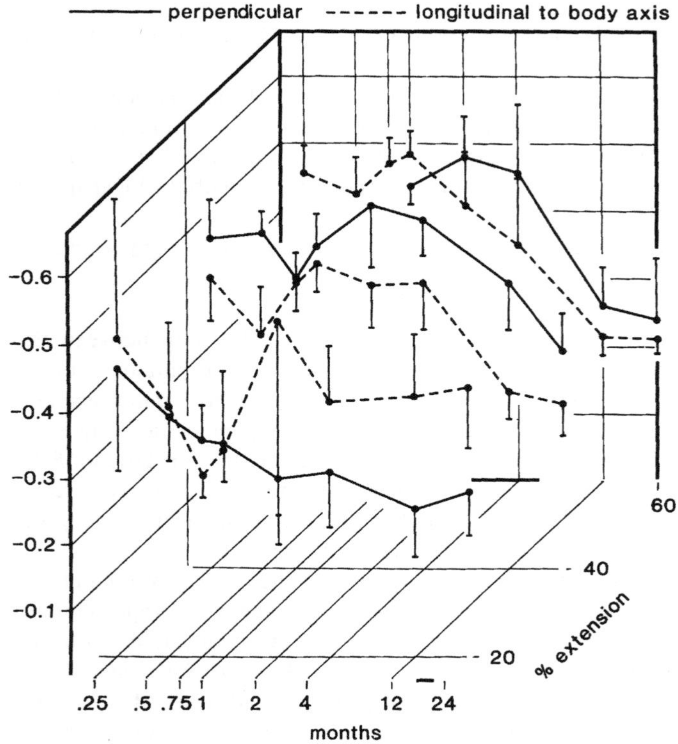

Fig. 11. Ratio between coefficient A_2 and A_1 (from expression $p = A_1 + A_2 \log t$) for consecutive relaxation experiments in rat skin depending on age

Striking similarities between rat and human skin were also found for mechanical recovery which has to be considered as an indicator of secondary elasticity. In both species a decrease of mechanical recovery expressed as percentage of initial tension is noted at 20% extension degree, whereas at 40% and 60% extension this parameter was higher with increasing age (Fig. 12).

Secondary elasticity, which means the behavior of skin after unloading, therefore depends on the degree of initial extension: At low extension degrees it is worse, at medium extension degrees better in old than in young individuals.

Creep Experiments

Again, in creep experiments strips from rat and human skin were studied by the same method [91, 109, 112, 120, 121] using a special apparatus to measure extension under constant load. After loading of skin specimens with 100, 200, or 500 g, a sudden extension occurred which was followed by a slow and almost continuous creep (Fig. 13) being measured as ultimate extension rate. This parameter showed a sharp decrease during maturation but also a continuous decrease during aging in rat skin (Fig. 14). Likewise, also in human skin a continuous decrease with aging was noted at 500 g but not at 200 g load (Fig. 15). Extension after 1 h of constant load was decreased depending on age both in rat and in human skin. The creep experiments indicate that viscosity or plasticity of rat and human skin decrease with maturation and age.

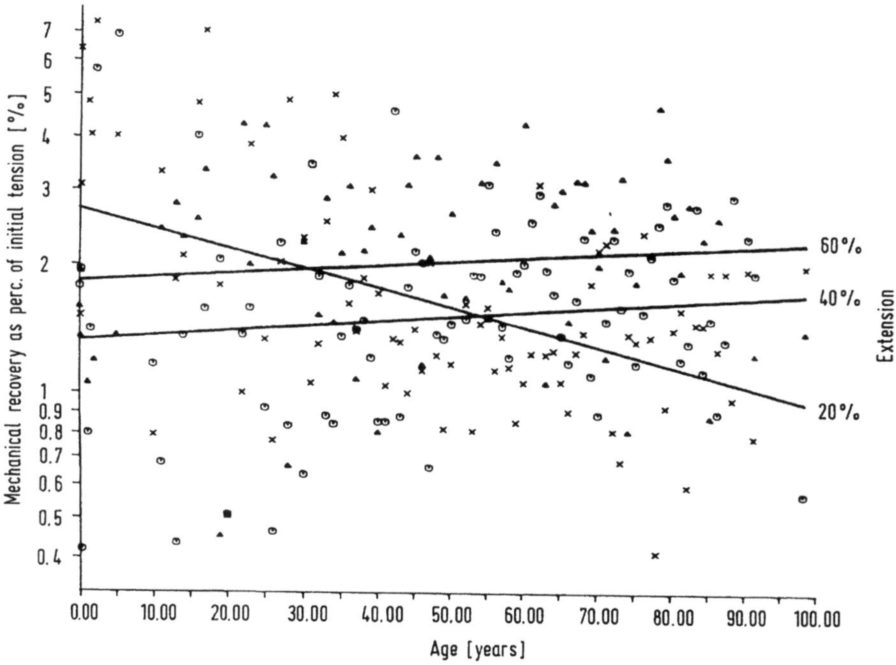

Fig. 12. Mechanical recovery as percentage of initial tension in relaxation experiments in human skin depending on age

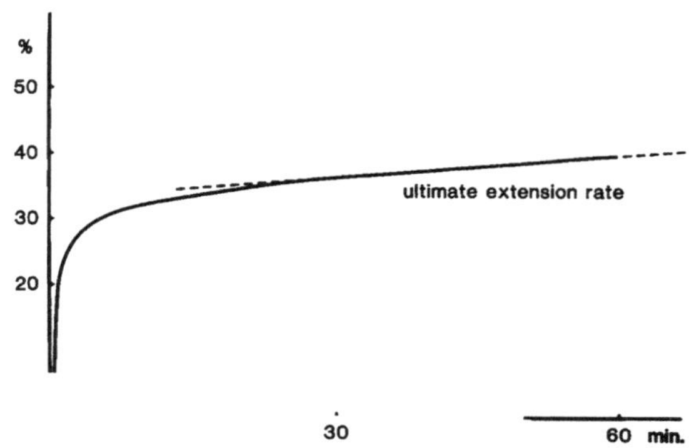

Fig. 13. Creep experiment (original recording) in rat and human skin *in vitro*

Repeated Strain

The studies were performed in a similar way for rat [119] and human [109, 112] skin. Samples were stretched up to 20% with an extension rate of 100 mm/min and unloaded again, followed by further cycles with the same extension rate. The peak of the second cycle was considerably lower than the first one, followed by a further decrease. The number of cycles was calculated until the stress value was only one half that of the first cycle. Immediately afterwards, the degree of extension was increased by a further 10% (Fig. 16).

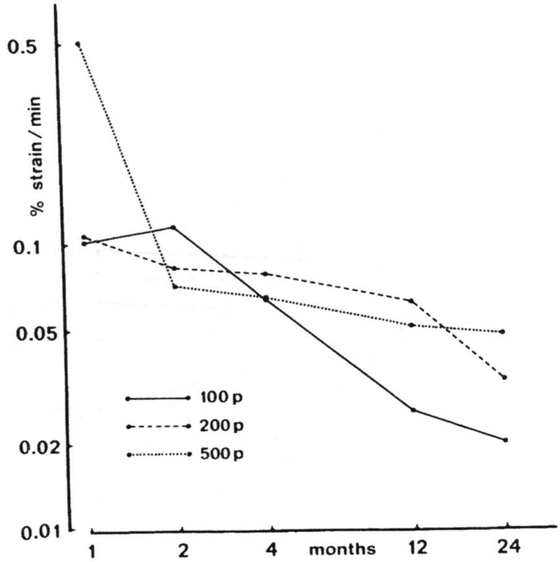

Fig. 14. Influence of age on ultimate extension rate in creep experiments in rat skin

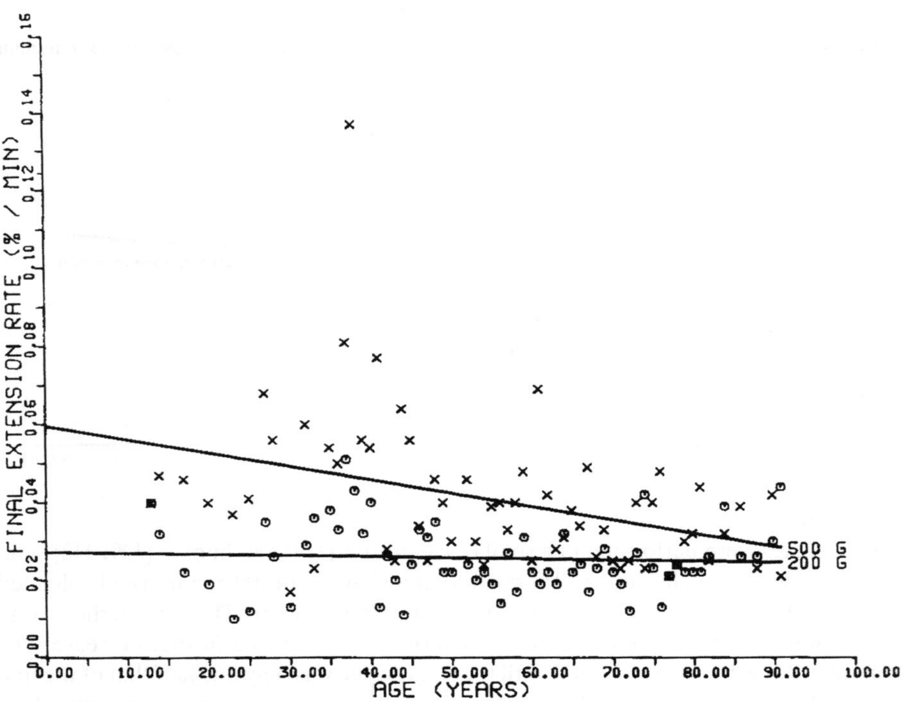

Fig. 15. Creep experiment in human skin; final rate of extension

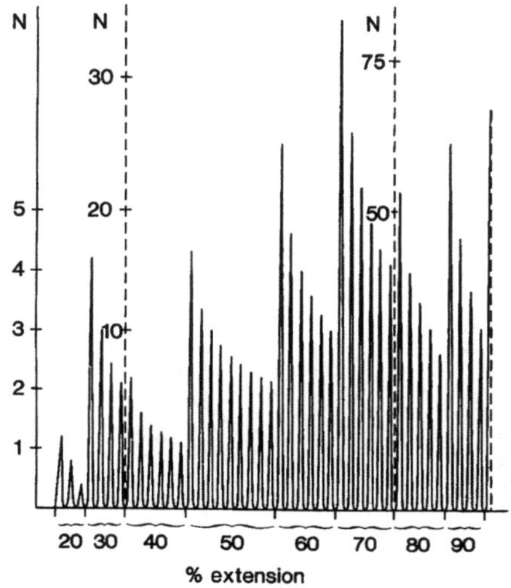

Fig. 16. Experiment (original recording) with repeated strain in human skin *in vitro*

In this way, the number of cycles indicating the half-life of tension due to relaxation was calculated at 30%, 40%, 50%, 60%, 70%, 80%, 90% and eventually 100% extension.

In rats 1 month of age or more, the number of cycles decreased from step 1 to step 3. After a minimum at step 3 or 4, the number of cycles increased as a nearly exponential function of the number of steps. In young rats (2 weeks) this biphasic behavior was absent. The number of cycles at each step was increased depending on maturation. The highest values were found in 20 month old rats. The values of 24 month old rats, however, were relatively decreased. This study also indicated that in rats three periods of life have to be taken in account: early maturation, late maturation, and senescence. Plasticity at medium extension is most pronounced after early maturation.

In human skin initial tension at degrees of extension below 60% rose during maturation and aging, whereas at higher values (above 70%) maxima of stress were found between 20 and 40 years, which shifted to a lower age at higher degrees of extension.

The number of cycles up to a decrease of one half of stress showed a dependence on age and also on the degree of extension. At a low extension of 20% no influence of age was seen. At degrees of extension between 30% and 70% an increase was observed and between 80% and 100% a decrease was found. Values of 80% and 100% extension can only be achieved by stepwise repeated stretching. These data show that resistance increases with age at medium and high degrees of extension; a decrease is noted only at very high extensions (Fig. 17).

The experiment with repeated strain confirms the data from the hysteresis, relaxation, and recovery experiments, that at low degrees of extension, viscosity and plasticity are barely influenced by maturation and age or slightly increased. At medium and higher degrees of extension plasticity decreases with age. The experiment with repeated strain in human skin further indicates that at very high degrees of extension plasticity is agian increased.

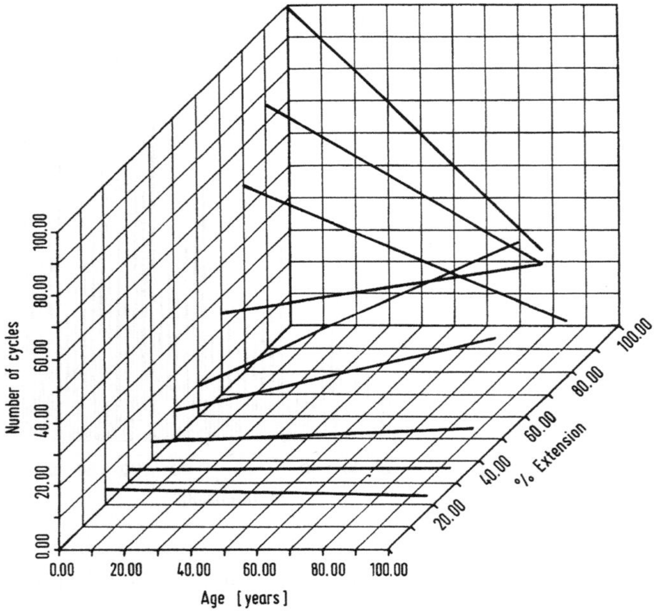

Fig. 17. Repeated strain in human skin. Age dependence of the number of cycles until one half of initial stress at various extension degrees

In vivo Studies in Rat Skin

Comparison Between *in vivo and in vitro* Results

Only experiments in animals allow measurement of the mechanical properties of skin both *in vivo* under anesthesia and *in vitro* after excision of a sample at the same site [95, 96, 100, 115, 117]. The experimental conditions were chosen to be as similar as possible. For the *in vivo* experiments small metal tabs (14 x 14 mm) were glued to the shaved back skin of rats at the same distance used as gauge length for the *in vitro* experiments. Also, the strain rate and the instrumental equipment were identical. In spite of the similar experimental conditions, remarkable differences between the stress – strain curves were found. The stress values reached much lower values with increasing strain *in vivo* than *in vitro*. When the tab distance was varied similar stress-strain curves *in vivo* were achieved with a tab distance of 5 cm as with a gauge length of 3 cm *in vitro*. The contribution of the tissue besides the area between the tabs has to be taken into account, but seems to be of minor importance when compared with the *in vitro* studies [27].

Further experiments showed that the ratio of distance between the tabs to the area below the tabs influences the shape of the stress-strain curves. The differences between the *in vitro* and *in vivo* data can be explained by the experimental conditions: In the *in vitro* experiment the sample is fastened into clamps from both sides, whereas in the *in vivo* experiment only the upper (epidermal) layer is fastened to the tabs. The forces are transmitted to the lower layer (cutis) which can slide over a larger area depending on the size of the tabs. Only under identical conditions (unilateral fixation, same tab distance) were the results the same after *in vivo* testing as after *in vitro* [27].

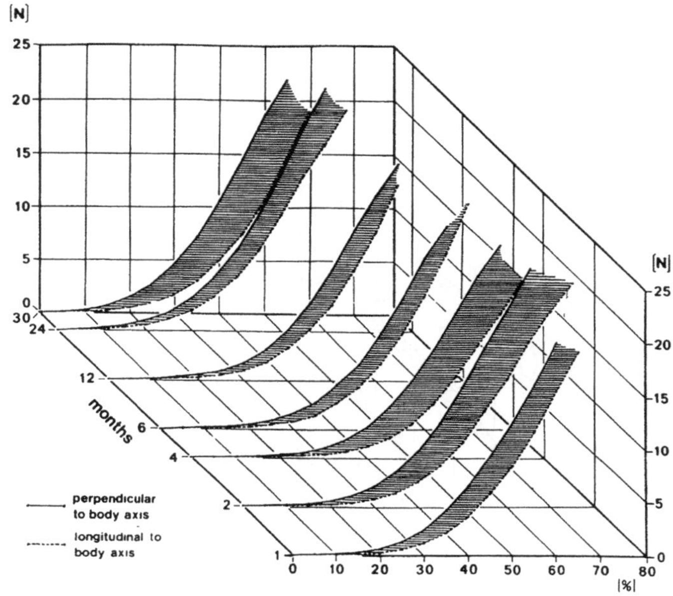

Fig. 18. *In vivo* experiment in rats. Load depends on elongation at various age intervals

Age Dependence of Stress – Strain Curves *in vivo*

Similar to the *in vitro* experiments, *in vivo* a pronounced anisotropy of rat skin was found. *In vitro* ultimate extension was lower perpendicular to the body axis than longitudinal to it in very young rats whereas in adult rats perpendicular ultimate extension was higher. This resulted in a crossing of the curves at an age of about 5 weeks (Fig. 4). The anisotropic differences for ultimate load, tensile strength, and ultimate modulus of elasticity were less pronounced [98, 101, 105, 112]. The anisotropic differences were not only true for ultimate extension but also for medium and high loads below the point of rupture. However, at very low load or stress values another difference was observed *in vitro*. There, in rats of every age elongation was higher in the longitudinal than in the perpendicular direction (Fig. 5). Consequently, at very low extension degrees load or stress were lower in the longitudinal than in the perpendicullar direction [98, 100, 102, 103].

The *in vivo* experiments allowed only moderate loads. Consequently, the anisotropic behavior reflected the situation *in vitro* at low loads or low extension degrees. In all age groups the *in vivo* stress – strain curves were higher in the perpendicular than in the longitudinal direction [27, 102, 112, 116] (Fig. 18).

A detailed analysis of the stress-strain curves *in vivo* revealed that at very low extension degrees again a crossing of the curves occurred which had however, nothing to do with the crossing observed *in vitro* at much higher load and extension degrees (Fig. 19). Nevertheless, for both directions a clear age dependence of the parameters load, stress and modulus of elasticity was found *in vivo*. There was a decrease during maturation, a minimum at adulthood at 4 months, and a steady increase until 30 months (Fig. 20). At this time, load and stress values were as high as in 1 month old rats [27, 100, 102, 103,

112, 116]. Extensibility of rat skin in both directions is the highest at adulthood (4 months). This is in agreement with earlier studies *in vitro* [98, 100, 102, 103, 118].

From this experimental data one has to conclude that *in vivo* results are comparable to *in vitro* data obtained at low extension degrees or low loads but not with the ultimate values.

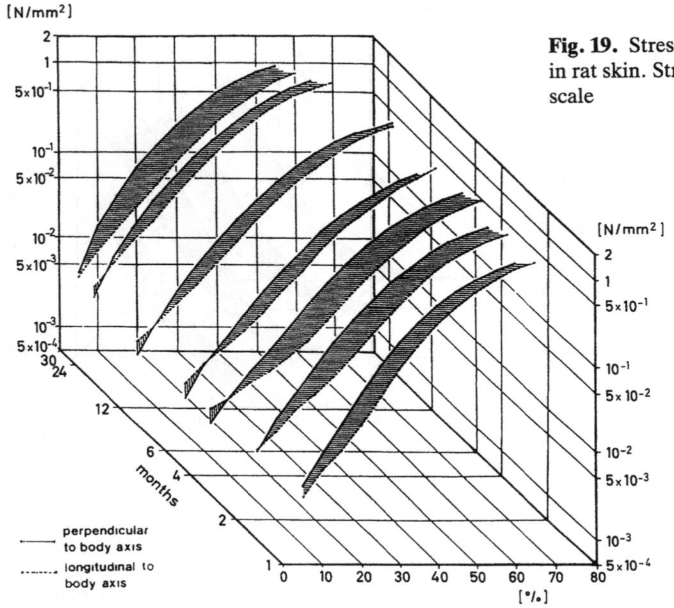

Fig. 19. Stress strain curves *in vivo* in rat skin. Stress on a logarithmic scale

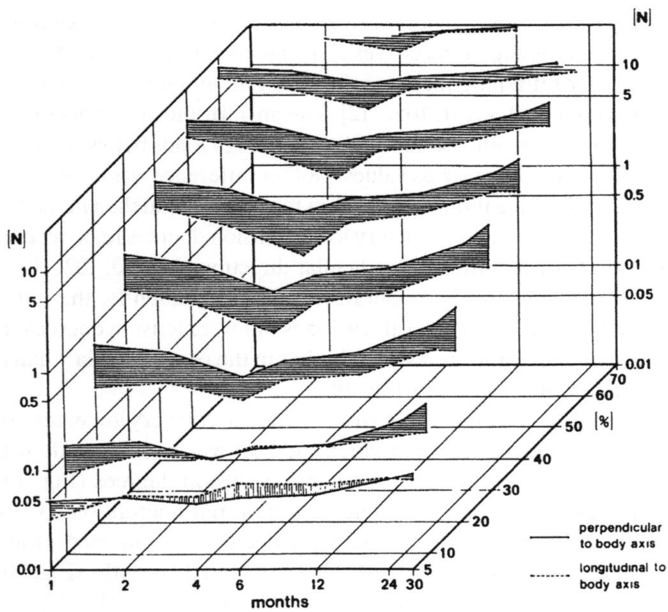

Fig. 20. Load depending on age at various extension degrees. *In vivo* experiment in rats perpendicular and longitudinal to the body axis

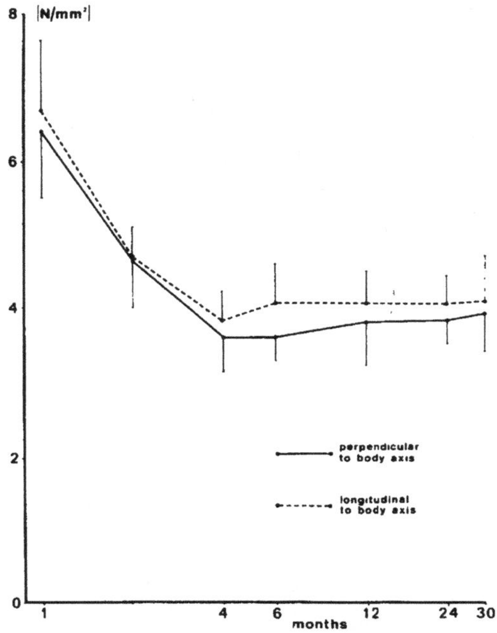

Fig. 21. Modulus of elasticity of the upper part of the stress-strain curves *in vivo* in rat skin depending on logarithm of age

Modulus of elasticity was calculated from the upper, almost linear, part of the stress-strain curve *in vivo*. In contrast to the ultimate values *in vitro* this parameter decreased with maturation, showed a minimum at 4 months, and increased slightly up to 30 months of age in both directions (Fig. 21) [116].

Repeated Strain *in vivo*

A special method has been developed to study the mechanical properties of rat skin after repeated strain *in vivo* and the course of recovery during different time intervals [27, 111–113, 117]. Tabs were fastened on the back skin of rats with a distance of 25 mm either perpendicular or longitudinal to the body axis. With an extension rate of 100 mm/min, the skin was extended 30 times for a 50% strain under anesthesia. Load was recorded and stress calculated by dividing by skin thickness measured from a skin fold obtained with calipers. The 1st, 5th, 10th, 15th, 20th, 25th, and 30th cycles were recorded with a faster paper speed in order to facilitate the evaluation of modulus of elasticity and load and stress values. Modulus of elasticity was calculated from the upper part of the stress-strain curve. As Fig. 22 shows, stress values decrease after repeated loading approximately with the logarithm of number of cycles. The area under the curve of 30 cycles was evaluated by computerized calculation according to Simpson's formula [27, 111, 112]. Stress values and the area under the curve were higher perpendicular than longitudinal to the body axis as found in earlier *in vivo* experiments [102, 116]. For the recovery experiment this was denominated as the first run. The age dependence of the stress values was dependent on the direction vs the body axis (Fig. 23). In longitudinal samples the stress values fell from 1 to 12 months and increased until 24 months.

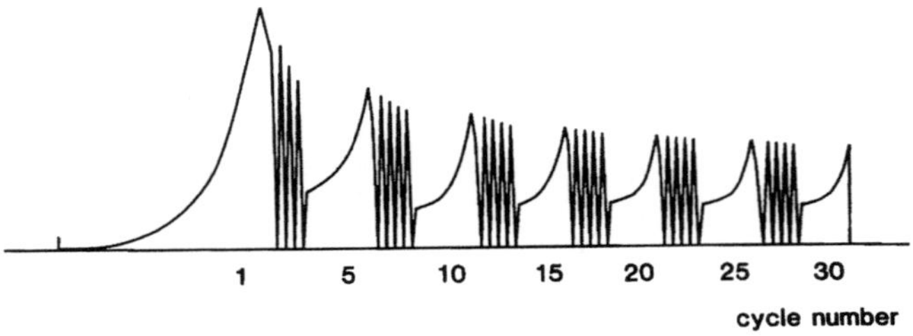

Fig. 22. Original recording of stress – strain curves after repeated strain of rat skin *in vivo*

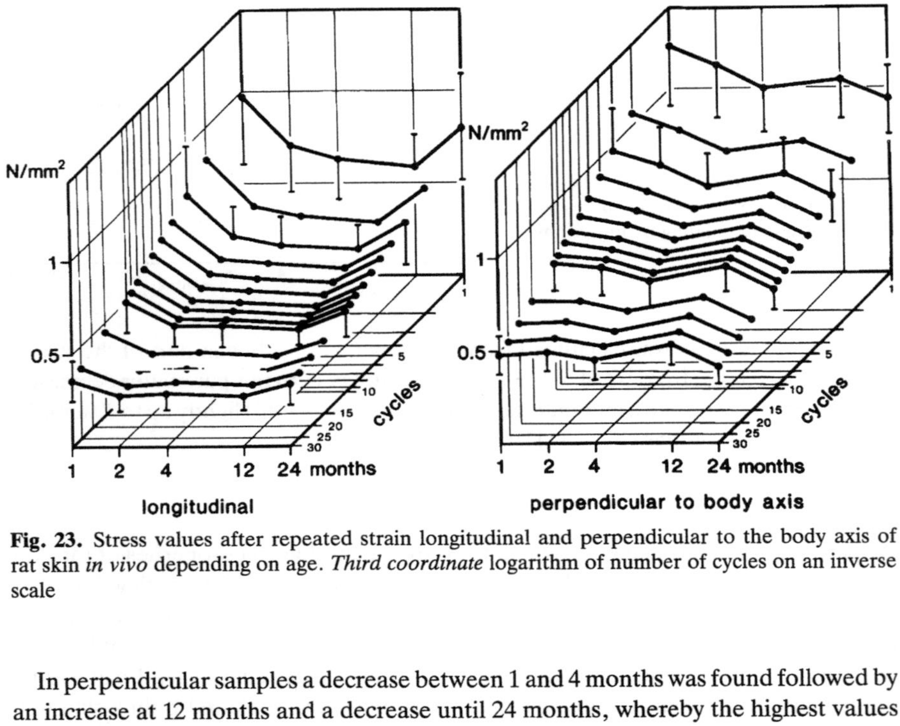

Fig. 23. Stress values after repeated strain longitudinal and perpendicular to the body axis of rat skin *in vivo* depending on age. *Third coordinate* logarithm of number of cycles on an inverse scale

In perpendicular samples a decrease between 1 and 4 months was found followed by an increase at 12 months and a decrease until 24 months, whereby the highest values were at 1 month and the lowest at 24 months. Modulus of elasticity increased in both directions from the first to the fifth cycle. This may be explained by the "conditioning" of connective tissue [58]. Afterwards, a decay is noted which is approximately dependent on the logarithm of cycles. As Fig. 24 shows, age dependence of modulus of elasticity is similar to that of stress values. In both directions a decrease during maturation is found. The behavior during senescence, i.e., between 12 and 24 months, however, is different. In longitudinal samples an increase and in perpendicular samples a decrease are noted. The area under the curve calculated for stress values resembled closely the pattern of initial stress indicating that this value dominates for the area under the curve and that the decay is only of secondary importance. During senescence in the *in vivo* experiments initial load, initial stress, modulus of elasticity and the area

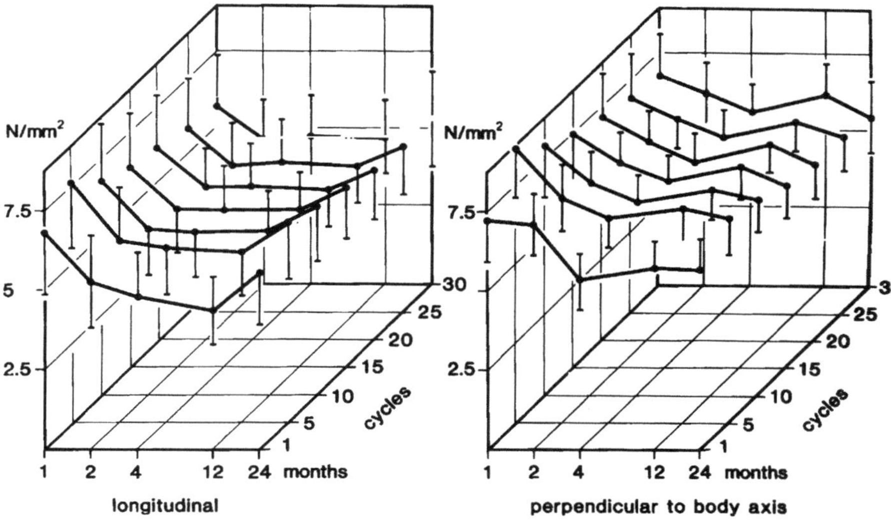

Fig. 24. Modulus of elasticity after repeated strain longitudinal and perpendicular to the body axis of rat skin *in vivo* depending on age

under the curve show the same tendency: a decrease in the perpendicular and an increase in the longitudinal direction. This indicates that the aging of the dermis is different between the longitudinal and the perpendicular direction.

Age Dependence of *in vivo* Recovery After Repeated Strain

This experimental setup was suitable to establish new parameters for living tissue, i.e., the time interval until partial and complete restituto ad integrum by applying a second run of repeated strain after different time intervals between 15 min and 16 h.

After the first run, the animals were taken back to their cages with the attached tabs still in position. They were tested in the same way under anesthesia after different time intervals. The stress values in the second run were definitely lower than in the first run. When calculated as percentage of the first run, the differences diminished with extended time intervals, as Fig. 25 shows. By this method, not only the mechanical recovery, which can also be observed *in vitro*, but also the biological recovery, i.e., the restitutio ad integrum, can be measured. In the first studies, the time until 100% restoration was approximately 16 h. In a second study [111] the age dependence of biological recovery was studied. For this purpose the values of the second run were calculated as a percentage of the first run.

Figure 26 shows the stress at the first cycle of the second run as a percentage of the first run. In both the longitudinal and perpendicular directions the values were less than 50% after 5 min and 1 h, but rose continuously until 16 h, reaching or even exceeding 100% after this time. Apparently, the restoration process for this parameter starts almost immediately and is detectable after 1 h. In both directions, the lowest values were for the youngest animals and the highest for the 12 month old animals.

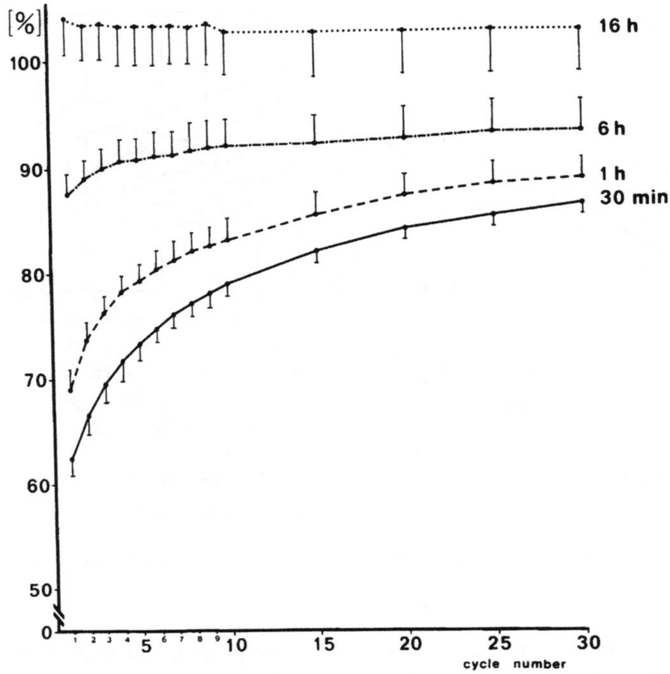

Fig. 25. Repeated strain of rat skin *in vivo*. Stress values of the second run as percentage of the first, perpendicular to the body axis

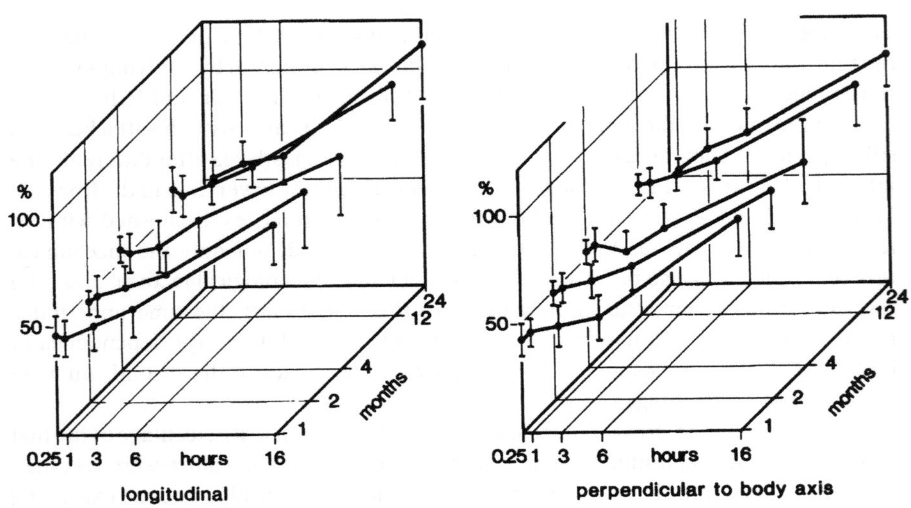

Fig. 26. Stress of the first cycle of the second run as a percentage of the first run, longitudinal and perpendicular to the body axis of rats depending on the time interval between both runs. *Third coordinate*, logarithm of age

When the 30th cycle was evaluated in the same manner, expressing the values of the second run as a percentage of the first run, smaller differences were observed. The values of the second run were between 70% and 80% of the first after 15 min.

However, in most instances these values dropped further, reaching a minimum after

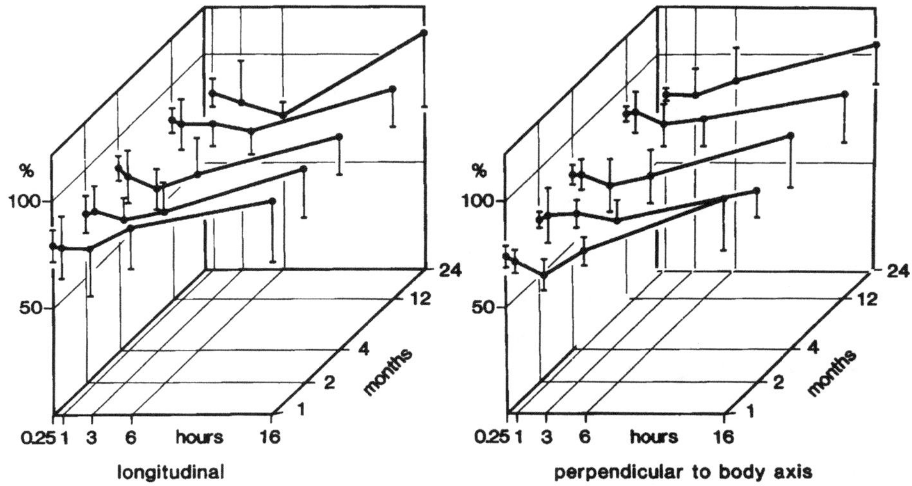

Fig. 27. Stress at the 30th cycle of the second run as percentage of the first run, longitudinal and perpendicular to the body axis of rats depending on the time interval between both runs. *Third coordinate*, logarithm of age

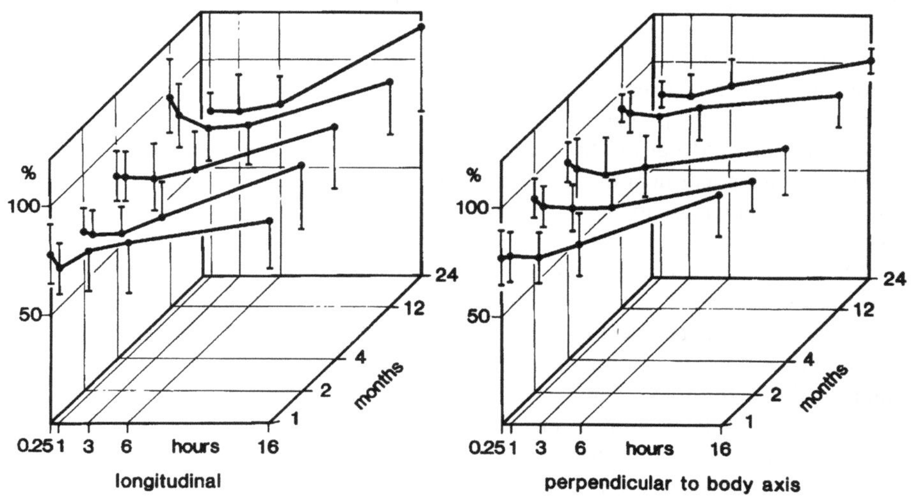

Fig. 28. Modulus of elasticity at the first cycle of the second run in percentage of the first run, longitudinal and perpendicular to the body axis of rats depending on the time interval of both runs. *Third coordinate*, logarithm of age

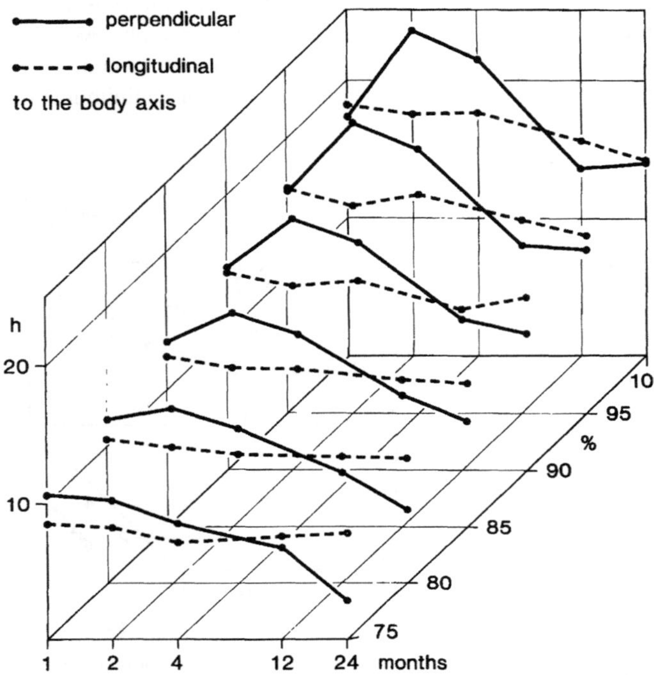

Fig. 29. Amount of time elapsed before reaching various degrees of biological recovery in repeated strain experiments in rat skin longitudinal and perpendicular to the body axis depending on age. *Third coordinate*, percent of the first run

about 3 h, and rose thereafter up to around 100% (Fig. 27). This may indicate that restoration of the skin has at least two components, one which appears immediately and is already apparent after 1 h and a second part in which the damage reaches a maximum later and restoration starts later.

When the modulus of elasticity at the first cycle of the second run was expressed as a percentage of the corresponding value of the first run, the percentage values were much higher than the percentage of tension, indicating that the modulus of elasticity was less affected. Moreover, the changes were the highest in young and the lowest in 12 month old animals in both directions. A minimum after 1 or 3 h was also observed, followed by an increase to almost normal values after 16 h (Fig. 28). Again, these data indicate at least two phases of damage and restoration of the skin.

When the area under the curve was compared, expressing the values of the second run as a percentage of the first run, the values were between 60% and 70% of the first run. In some instances a decline until 3 h was observed, followed by a steady increase. Again, the calculation of the area under the curve indicates that several components of damage and restoration are involved.

In order to recognize more clearly the various phases of recovery the time intervals within various degrees of restoration were achieved have been calculated by graphical evaluation of the restoration curves.

The time necessary to achieve biological recovery (75%–100% of the initial values of the area under the envelope curve) was measured, as shown in Fig. 29. Testing the skin in the longitudinal direction resulted in a shortening of the time to recovery with increased maturation and increased age. This finding is surprising, because it means that biological recovery in rat skin increases with maturation and during aging. Conversely, perpendicular to the body axis we found an increase of biological recovery time at early maturation but a decrease at late maturation and aging. This agrees with the *in vitro* findings that perpendicular to the body axis, rat skin behaves differently during late maturation. This is clearly demonstrated if one compares perpendicular with longitudinal samples. During aging, the recovery times are slightly higher for longitudinal samples, but during maturation, more time is needed to recover after perpendicular than after longitudinal stretching. This means that biological recovery is diminished during maturation in perpendicular samples. However, perpendicular samples had the shortest time for biological recovery during aging.

In both directions the shortest time for recovery was needed at 12 or 24 months indicating that restitutio ad integrum is even better in old than in young animals.

Interpretation of the Presented Experimental Results

Even if highly standardized experimental conditions have been used the mechanical properties of skin turned out to be rather complex. Nevertheless, some conclusions can be drawn.

Comparison of Rat and Human Skin in vitro

The physical properties of rat and human skin *in vitro* are quite similar. The age dependence of ultimate values (ultimate strain, ultimate load, tensile strength and ultimate modulus of clasticity) indicating a pronounced increase during maturation, a maximum at puberty or adulthood, and a slight but definite decrease during senescence is similar in rat and human skin.

The pronounced directional differences found in rat skin (perpendicular or longitudinal to the body axis) were not found in human skin. This is probably due to the experimental conditions because in our experiments human samples were obtained above the sternum, where directional differences related to Langer's lines play a minor role [64].

In animal as well as in human skin the evaluation of the lower part of the stress-strain curves *in vitro*, which is much more difficult to standardize, gives different values than the values before rupture. The age dependence may be just the reverse of the ultimate values.

The methods measuring viscosity or plasticity at short intervals (hysteresis experiments), medium intervals (relaxation experiments), and prolonged intervals (creep experiments) give the same results for rat and human skin: a decrease of plasticity or viscosity with age which is more pronounced at medium or higher extension degrees than at low extensions.

Comparison of Rat Data in vitro and in vivo

Due to the experimental conditions (fastening bilateral *in vitro* and unilateral *in vivo*) the stress-strain curves are different in that higher extension degrees are needed *in vivo* to achieve the same stress values as *in vitro*. Taking into account these conditions the results are comparable.

The results on age dependence *in vivo* reflect the data obtained from the low part of the stress-strain curves *in vitro*. A decrease of stress values at testable elongation degrees and a decrease of modulus of elasticity are found during maturation, achieving a minimum at adulthood followed by an increase during aging.

In vivo Recovery Experiment

New results have been achieved by the *in vivo* recovery experiment. The experiment with repeated strain, causing a definite insult on living tissue, gave surprising insight into the restoration process. (a) at least two phases of the recovery process have to be distinguished; (b) ultimate recovery is better in old than in young animals.

Clinical Relevance of the Presented Data

Ultimate Values

Ultimate values, e.g., mechanical properties at rupture, have relevance to severe injury of the skin. The experimental data show that the skin of children has the highest vulnerability. The best values of ultimate extension, ultimate load, tensile strength, and modulus of elasticity are achieved at puberty or adulthood. During senescence only a slight decrease of these parameters occurs. That means that even in senile patients the resistance of skin to severe trauma is very good and still much better in young children.

Values at Low Extension Degrees

At extension degrees which can occur during normal living conditions a decrease of stress and modulus of elasticity are noted during maturation. After a minimum at adulthood a slight increase is found during senescence. In this respect, skin of old individuals is almost as good as that of adults.

Viscosity or Plasticity

Viscosity or plasticity decrease with maturation and age. This result was found both *in vitro* (hysteresis, relaxation, creep, repeated loading) and *in vivo*. The decrease was more pronounced at higher extension values. This decrease of viscosity may be the cause of the phenomenon which is described as slackness of old skin.

Recovery After Mechanical Insult

The results obtained in rat skin do not yet have corresponding experimental data in human skin. If one may extrapolate animal data to human skin one has to conclude that skin of old individuals has excellent facilities for a restitutio ad integrum after a repeated insult of medium severity.

Comparison of Reported Results with Data from the Literature

In vitro Data from Animals

There is fair agreement between our data and results from animals reported elsewhere. Fry et al. [36] studied the mechanical properties of skin rings from the lower part of the legs of rats. They found an increase of extensibility at early maturation and afterwards a continuous decrease.

Breaking strength showed a steady increase even from 9 to 20 months of age. Mendoza and Milch [57] found, both in male and female rats, significantly higher values of skin tensile strength in old than in young animals. Flandin et al. [35] found in very young rats a biphasic behavior of extensibility.

In vitro Data from Human Skin

With a morphometric procedure used on skin biopsies an age-dependent decrease of skin thickness was found by Branchet et al. [14]. Rollhaeuser [68] studied the mechanical properties of skin strips from human cadavers *in vitro*. He found low values for tensile strength and modulus of elasticity in children below 3 years and a sharp increase of these parameters until 15–30 years which continued up to the group of 50–80 years. Measuring only extensibility at relatively low loads, Jansen and Rottier [44] found no significant changes depending on age. In a later study [45] these authors found a decrease of ultimate extension with age and an age-dependent increase of elasticity modulus at medium extension degrees but no clear-cut changes of tensile strength or ultimate modulus of elasticity. Using tension developed during thermal shrinking as a parameter, Rasmussen et al. [62] found an age-dependent increase. Le Lous et al. [54] measured the relaxation half time of hydrothermal isometric tension at boiling point in skin biopsies of human individuals form birth to 70 years of age and found an increase with maturation and age, however, a decrease during puberty. In a very few post-mortem samples Kenedi et al. [46] found a decrease of extensibility during maturation and age and an increase of tensile strength and modulus of elasticity following maturation.

Ridge and Wright [64] tried to describe the stress-strain curve of skin strips by the equation $E = k \cdot L^{b}$, whereby E is extension, L is load, k is characterized by the dimension of the specimen and b is the degree of curvature of the stress-strain curve, measuring the rate at which the specimen becomes stiffer. This constant increased with maturation and decreased with age.

Generally, the *in vitro* data from the literature are in agreement with our results.

In vivo Data from Animal Skin

Besides our data very few *in vivo* studies in animals are reported in the literature. Baker et al. [8] used uniaxial extension of skin *in vivo* in pigs and found an increase of stiffness between 15 and 30 weeks of age.

In Vivo Data from Human Skin

General Considerations

The data on age dependence of *in vivo* mechanical properties of human skin are rather contradictory. This can be explained by several factors:

1. Since all attempts failed to achieve a constitutive equation for the physical properties of skin *in vitro*, the situation for interpretation of *in vivo* data is even more difficult.
2. The investigators used different methods which makes a comparison between the results rather difficult. According to Leveque [51] four groups measuring the elastic modulus of skin reported values differing for three orders of magnitude. Two of these groups found an increase of elastic modulus with age, the two other ones a decrease.
3. The values were obtained from different stress regions of the stress-strain curves according to the equipment being used [23] or at different extension degrees. Therefore completely contradictory conclusions regarding age dependence were found.
4. The suggestions for standardization of *in vivo* mechanical testing have to be taken seriously [11]. As a consequence, each result has to be discussed in view of the type of method and the experimental conditions being used.
5. Several attempts have been made to correlate rheological parameters of skin with morphological structures and biochemical constituents, such as collagen, elastin, glycosaminoglycans, and water content [82, 83, 86, 89, 108, 125]. Only for *in vitro* experiments has a correlation between tensile strength and collagen content and between decreased viscosity and decreased glycosaminoglycan been found. For the *in vivo* situation such correlations can be extrapolated only by comparison of experimental data from different sources.

Skin Thickness

Using skinfold calipers Leveque et al. [52, 53] found an increase of skin thickness until the age of 20 years in women and until 40 years in men and a considerable decrease thereafter. Shuster et al. [77] described a decrease of skin thickness with age which correlated with the content of skin collagen. Hall et al. [41] found high values in infants which fell until the age of 20 years, remained constant until the age of 60 years, and diminished thereafter significantly. Chappard et al. [20] described a significant negative correlation between skinfold thickness and age. Using different pressures Brozek and Kinzey [15] found no age dependence of skinfolds but a decreased compressibility.

Recently, human skin thickness was studied by ultrasound techniques. Tan et al. [79] found an increase of skin thickness during maturation until 20 years and a linear decrease with age subsequently. Also, Serup [76] and Dena and Takahashi [26] found and age-dependent decrease with this method. In contrast, Escoffier et al. [32] and de Rigal et al. [66] found, with an ultrasound technique, that skin thickness remains constant until the seventh decade of life and diminishes thereafter.

Methods Using Forces Perpendicular to the Skin Surface

Pressure on a Defined Surface Area

Indentometry. The method originally described by Schade [71, 72] using an elastometer or indentometer, has been taken over by various groups. Kirk and Kvorning [47] found lower values of total indentation in elderly than in young individuals. Furthermore, the percentage of primary rebound was lower in the group of older individuals. In a later study Kirk and Chieffi [48] found a continuous age-dependent decrease of immediate indentation and immediate rebound between 18 and 100 years.

Since no younger individuals have been tested no conclusions can be drawn for the maturation period. Using a similar method but an apparatus described by Dikstein and Hartzshtark [29] Robert et al. [67] found that the degree of indentation increased with age in a group of male white collar workers but not in other cohorts. Elasticity expressed in percentage of indentation decreased with age in all groups.

With the same method Lanier et al. [50] found a higher indentation degree in old (64–80 years) than in young (20–26 years) subjects, whereby the differences were not significant and less pronounced at higher loads.

Ballistometry. With the ballistometer, as described by Tosti et al. [81], a sudden drop impact on skin is exerted by a hammer followed by a number of rebounds with decreasing amplitude. The calculated factor for percent rebound energy decreased from 8 to 80 years. Since no mathematical data can be calculated in terms of stress or strain the results obtained with this apparatus cannot be compared with those of other methods.

Elevation of a Defined Surface Area

Suction Methods. A suction cup device has been developed by Grahame and Holt [39] and used to study the influence of aging on the *in vivo* elasticity of human skin. Besides sex differences the authors found an increase of calculated modulus of elasticity in individuals between 19 and 83 years. Using a suction cup method Alexander and Cook [3, 4] described a decrease in the average slope of the curves of skin for male individuals through maturation, a minimum between 15 and 20 years, and an increase with advancing age. Cook et al. [22] tested subjects between 4 and 83 years with a suction cup elastometer. The parameters indicating stiffness decreased whereas hysteresis showed an increasing trend. Cua et al. [24] used a commercially available suction device (cutometer) to study the elastic properties of human skin in relation to age, sex, and anatomical region. The ratio of viscoelastic properties to immediate extension was higher in old than in young individuals, whereas the ratio between immediate retraction to total distension was lower in old than in young test subjects. These differences, however, were significant only for a few anatomical regions. Using a suction cup method, Sato [70] found a decrease of skin extensibility and skin contractility with age. This author underlined the uncertainity of the measurement of skin elastic modulus by this method.

Generally, these methods hardly allow one to express the data in terms of physical parameters.

Levarometry. A special device developed by Dikstein and Hartzshtark [29] has been developed as a modification of an indentometer, exerting pull instead of pressure to the skin. Lanir et al. [50] found higher elevations in old than in young subjects and recommended this method to be more sensitive in assessing than indentometry to aging.

Other Traction Devices. Piérard and Lapiere [59] applied pull through a disk of 20 mm diameter glued to the skin by cyanoacrylate and measured deformations after tractions between 100 and 400 g. An index of deformability was calculated as the ratio between two deformations. The authors found differences in pathological conditions but no changes related to age.

Methods Using Forces Horizontal to the Skin Surface

Extension Methods

Using uniaxial extension Daly and Odland [25] found an increase of the so called inelastic region of the lowest part of the stress-strain curve in old individuals.

An in-plane extensometer was used by Wijn [123] and Wijn et al. [124]. A decrease of elasticity with age at small deformations was found in these studies.

Berardesca et al. [12] used a special extensometer in which the displacement between two tabs was measured at a given low load. An age-dependent increase of the values measuring extension was found.

Torsional Methods

Torsional methods have been used by various groups to study age-related changes. Finlay [34] used a motor-driven disc of 15 mm diameter surrounded by a fixed guard ring. Either trapezoidal rotational displacement is applied and the resulting torque is registered or a given torque is used as input and the angle of twist is measured as output [23]. Furthermore, the relaxation phenomenom can be studied. Finlay [34] found a decrease of low-load extensibility with age and a decrease of relaxation.

Agache et al. [1, 2] using a similar technique, found at high torque a sudden fall of immediate extensibility at the age of 30 years, whereas at low torque a continuous fall of extensibility was noted.

The ratio of delayed to immediate extension increased with aging. Escoffier et al. 32] employed an apparatus called a twistometer using a low and a higher torque. They found a slight decrease of extensibility at senescence and a continuous decrease of elasticity and of the recovery vs extensibility ratio at both given torques. Furthermore, creep relaxation time decreased with age.

By contrast with a similar technique Sanders [69] found that at a given load extensibility increases with age. Furthermore, moduli of elasticity calculated from this experiment decreased with age.

Other Methods

Pliquet et al. [61] and Haferkorn et al. [40] described the age dependence of human skin obtained by a special method using both mechanical and electrical (impedance) parameters. They found a decrease of maturation, then an increase and a maximum between 40 and 50 years, and a decrease thereafter. The data are not comparable or in accordance with other reports in the literature.

Conclusions and Recommendations

From our own studies and from the data reported in the literature the following conclusions can be drawn and recommendations can be made.

Data from *in vitro* and *in vivo* experiments can be compared only if the experimental conditions (unilateral or bilateral fixation) are taken in account. *In vivo* methods have the drawback that the calculation of physical parameters is more difficult than *in vitro*. *In vivo* studies reflect the lower part of the stress-strain curve compared to *in vitro* data. The age-dependence of the lower part of the stress-strain curve is different from the values at or before rupture.

Changes at low extension degrees reflect more closely the age-related visual appearance of skin. Even at the lower part of the stress-strain curve, the results depend on the degree of given extension or load. This can explain contradictory results from different authors. Therefore, regardless of the type of method being used, the studies should be done at various given extension or load degrees. Arbitrary units should be avoided. Instead, extension degrees in percent of initial value and stress and elastic moduli in terms of N/mm^2 should be calculated.

Values indicating viscosity or plasticity such as found in hysteresis, relaxation and creep experiments show a different age dependence than values indicating stiffness or elasticity. Viscoelastic properties not only depend on the degree of given extension or load but also on the time of observation. The age-dependence of short term viscosity (seconds to minutes) and long-term viscosity (minutes to hours) may be different.

Skin has a memory effect. Repeated straining or loading gives different results than do single experiments. Measurements of age dependence are influenced by phenomena such as the conditioning effect. Skin has the possibility to overcome the memory effect after insults in vivo by complete restoration, the so-called restitutio ad integrum. Studies to investigate the age dependence of this phenomenon in human beings are recommended.

References

1. Agache PG, Leveque J-L, de Rigal J, Monneur C (1980) Biomechanical properties of human skin in vivo, and aging. Bioeng Skin 2: 20–30
2. Agache PG, Monneur C, Leveque JL, de Rigal J (1980) Mechanical properties and Young's moduls of human skin in vivo. Arch Dermatol Res 269: 221–232
3. Alexander H, Cook T (1975) Variations with age in the mechanical properties of human skin in vivo. Proceedings of the Strathclyde bioengineering seminar Biomechanics of tissue viability, pp 1–12
4. Alexander H, Cook T (1976) Variations with age in the mechanical properties of human skin in vivo. In: Kenedy RM (ed) Bedsore biomechanics. University Park, Baltimore, pp 109–117
5. Alexander H, Cook T (1977) Accounting for natural tension in the mechanical testing of human skin. J Invest Dermatol 69: 310–314
6. Adhout H, de Rigal J, Popoff B, Bohin D, Leveque JL, Privat J (1985) Influence of PUVA treatment on the thickness and elastic properties of skin. Bioeng Skin 1: 245
7. Aubert L, Anthoine P, de Rigal J, Leveque JL (1985) An in vivo assessment of the biomechanical properties of human skin modifications under the influence of cosmetic products. Int J Cosmet Sci 7: 51–59

8. Baker MR, Bader DL, Hopewell JW (1988) An apparatus for testing of mechanical properties of skin in vivo: its application to the assessment of normal and irradiated pig skin. Bioeng Skin 4: 87–103
9. Ballou SP, Mackiewicz A, Lysikiewicz A, Neumann, MR (1990) Direct quantitation of skin elasticity in systemic sclerosis. J Rheumatol 17: 790–794
10. Barbenel JC, Evans JH (1977) The time-dependent mechanical properties of skin. J Invest Dermatol 69: 318–320
11. Barbenel JC, Payne PA (1981) In vivo mechanical testing of dermal properties. Bioeng Skin 3: 8–38
12. Berardesca E, Borroni G, Gabba P, Borlone R, Rabbiosi G (1986) Evidence for elastic changes in aged skin revealed in an in vivo extensometric study at low loads. Bioeng Skin 2: 261–270
13. Brakkee AJM, Jagtman BA, Kuiper JP, Wijn PFF (1981) Clinical investigations of the mechanical properties of human skin in vivo for small deformations. Bioeng Skin 3: 105
14. Branchet MC, Boisnic S, Robert AM, Frances C (1990) Skin thickness changes in normal aging skin. Gerontology 36: 28–35
15. Brozek J, Kinzey W (1969) Age changes in skinfold compressibility. J Gerontol 15: 45–51
16. Burlin TE, Hutton WC, Ranu HS (1977) A method of in vivo measurement of the elastic properties of skin in radiotherapy patients. J Invest Dermatol 69: 321–323
17. Burlin TE (1980) Towards a standard for in vivo testing of the skin subject to uniaxial extension. Bioeng Skin 2: 37–40
18. Burlin TE (1981) Towards a standard for in vitro testing of the skin subject to uniaxial extension. Bioeng Skin 3: 75–77
19. Burlin TE (1981) Towards a standard for in vivo testing of the skin subject to biaxial extension. Bioeng Skin 3: 47–49
20. Chappard D, Alexandre C, Robert JM, Riffat G (1991) Relationships between bone and skin atrophies during aging. Acta Anat 141: 239–244
21. Cook TH, Alexander H, Cohen M (1977) Experimental method for determining the 2-dimensional mechanical properties of living human skin. Med Biol Eng Comput 15: 381–390
22. Cook TH, Darr DJ, Grove GL (1981) Skin's mechanical properties changes as a function of age. Bioeng Skin 3: 109–114
23. Cook TH (1989) Mechanical properties of human skin with aging. In: Balin AK, Kligman (eds) Aging and the skin. Raven, New York, pp 205–225
24. Cua AB, Wilhelm KP, Maibach HI (1990) Elastic properties of human skin: relation to age, sex and anatomical region. Arch Dermatol Res 282: 283–288
25. Daly HC, Odland GF (1979) Age-related changes in the mechanical properties of human skin. J Invest Dermatol 73: 84–87
26. Denda M, Takahashi M (1990) Measurement of facial skin thickness by ultrasound method. J Soc Cosmet Chem Jpn 23: 316
27. Denkel K (1983) Vergleich rheologischer Parameter "in vivo" und "in vitro" an der Rückenhaut der Ratte. Frankfurt
28. Dikstein S (1979) In vivo mechanical properties of the skin measured by Indentometry and Levarometry. Bioeng Skin 2: 23–24
29. Dikstein S, Hartzshtark A (1981) In vivo measurement of some elastic properties of human skin. In: Marks R, Payne PA (eds) Bioengineering and the skin. Proceedings of the European Society for Dermatological Research symposium, Cardiff, 1979. MTP Press Lancaster, p 45–53
30. Dikstein S, Hartzshtark A (1982) The performance of a medicocosmetic consultation unit. Ärztl Kosmetol 12: 280–286
31. Elsner P, Wilhelm D, Maibach HI (1990) Mechanical properties of human forearm and vulvar skin. Br J Dermatol 122: 607–614
32. Escoffier C, de Rigal J, Rochefort A, Vasselet R, Leveque, JL, Agache PG (1989) Age-related mechanical properties of human skin: an in vivo study. J Invest Dermatol 93: 353–357
33. Finlay B (1970) Dynamic mechanical testing of human skin "in vivo". J Biomech 3: 557–568
34. Finlay B (1971) The torsional characteristics of human skin in vivo. Biomed Eng 6: 567–572

35. Flandin F, Buffevant C, Herbage D, Bazin S (1978) Age related changes in the mechanical properties of rat skin and the biochemical properties of its collagens. Proceedings of the 6th colloqium of the Federation of European Connective Tissue Clubs. Biochemistry of normal and pathological connective tissues. Int Colloq CNRS (RCP n°.08.0533): 86–88
36. Fry P, Harkness MLR, Harkness RD (1964) Mechanical properties of the collagenous framework of skin in rats of different ages. J Physiol 206: 1425–1429
37. Gibson T, Stark H, Evans JH (1969) Directional variation in extensibility of human skin in vivo. J Biomech 2: 201–204
38. Grahame R (1969) Elasticity of human skin in vivo. Ann Phys Med 10: 130–136
39. Grahame R, Holt PJL (1969) The influence of ageing on the in vivo elasticity of human skin. Gerontologia 15: 121–139
40. Haferkorn M, Weiss A, Barth J, Pliquett F (1979) Untersuchungen zum passiv-elektrischen und mechanischen Verhalten der Haut in Abhängigkeit vom Alter. Dermatol Monatsschr 165: 97–103
41. Hall DA, Blackett AD, Zajac AR et al. (1981) Changes in skinfold thickness with increasing age. Age Ageing 10: 19–23
42. Holzmann H, Korting GW, Kobelt D, Vogel HG (1971) Prüfung der mechanischen Eigenschaften von menschlicher Haut in Abhängigkeit von Alter und Geschlecht. Arch Klin Exp Dermatol 239: 355–367
43. Jagtman BA, Wijn PFF, Brakkee AJM, Kuiper JP (1982) Clinical investigations of the mechanical properties of human skin in vivo for small deformations. Bioeng Skin 4: 32–40
44. Jansen LH, Rottier, PB (1957) Elasticity of human skin related to age. Dermatologica 115: 106–111
45. Jansen LH, Rottier PB (1958) Some mechanical properties of human abdominal skin measured on excised strips. Dermatologica 117: 65–83
46. Kenedi RM, Gibson T, Daly CH (1965) Bio-engineering studies of the human skin: II. Biomechanics and related bio-engineering topics. Oxford, pp 147–158
47. Kirk JE, Kvorning SA (1949) Quantitative measurements of the elastic properties of the skin and subcutaneous tissues in young and old individuals. J Gerontol 4: 273–284
48. Kirk JE, Chieffi M (1962) Variation with age in elasticity of skin and subcutaneous tissue in human individuals. J Gerontol 17: 373–380
49. Lanir Y, Dikstein S, Hartzshtark A, Manny V (1990) In-vivo indentation of human skin. J Biomech Eng 112: 63–69
50. Lanir Y, Manny V, Zlotogorski A, Shafran A, Dikstein S (1992) The influence of ageing on the in-vivo mechanics of the skin. Skin Pharmacol in press
51. Leveque JL (1987) In vivo methods for measuring the viscoelastic properties of the skin. Bioeng Skin 3: 375–382
52. Leveque JL, Corcuff P, de Rigal J, Agache P (1984) In vivo studies of the evolution of physical properties of the human skin with age. Int J Dermatol 23: 322–329
53. Leveque JL, de Rigal J, Agache PG, Monneur C (1980) Influence of ageing on the in vivo extensibility of human skin at a low stress. Arch. Dermatol Res 269: 127–135
54. Le Lous M, Cohen-Solal L, Allain JC, Bonaventure J, Maroteaux P (1985) Age related evolution of stable collagen reticulation in human skin. Connect Tissue Res 13: 145–155
55. Manschot JFM, Brakkee AJM (1987) Characterisation of in vivo mechanical skin properties independent of measuring configuration. Bioeng Skin 3: 1–10
56. Manschot JFM, Brakkee AJ M(1987) Seasonal variations in the mechanical properties of the human skin. Bioeng Skin 3: 25–33
57. Mendoza SA, Milch RA. (1964) Age variations of nominal tensile strength of Wistar rat skins. Gerontologia 10: 42–46
58. Nemetscheck T, Riedl H, Jonak R, Nemetschek-Gansler H, Bordas J, Koch MHJ, Schilling V (1980) Die Viskoelastizität parallelsträngigen Bindegewebes und ihre Bedeutung für die Funktion. Virchows Arch [A] 386: 125–151
59. Piérard GE, Lapiere CM (1977) Physiopathological variations in the mechanical properties of skin. Arch Dermatol Res. 260: 231–239
60. Piérard GE (1980) Investigating rheological properties of skin by applying a vertical pull. Bioeng Skin 2: 31–33

61. Pliquett F, Haferkorn M, Weiss A (1978) Altersbedingte Veränderungen der passiv elektrischen und mechanischen Eigenschaften der menschlichen Haut. Z Altersforsch 33: 523–528
62. Rasmussen DM, Wakim KG, Winkelmann RK (1964) Effect of aging on human dermis: Studies of thermal shrinkage and tension. In: Montagna W (ed) Advances in biology of skin: VI, Aging Pergamon, Oxford pp 151–162
63. Ridge MD, Wright V (1966) The directional effects of skin. A bioengineering study of skin with particular reference to Langer's lines. J. Invest Dermatol 46: 341–346
64. Ridge MD, Wright V (1966) The ageing of skin. A bio-engineering approach. Gerontologia 12: 174–192
65. De Rigal J, Leveque JL (1985) In vivo measurement of the stratum corneum elasticity. Bioeng Skin 1: 13–23
66. De Rigal J, Escoffier C, Querleux B, Faivre B, Agache P, Leveque JL (1989) Assessment of aging of the human skin by in vivo ultrasonic imaging. J Invest Dermatol 93: 621–625
67. Robert C, Blanc M, Lesty C, Dikstein S, Robert L (1988) Study of skin ageing as a function of social and professional conditions: modification of the rheological parameters measured with a noninvasive method – Indentometry. Gerontology 34: 284–290
68. Rollhäuser H (1950) Die Zugfestigkeit der menschlichen Haut. Gegenbaurs Morph Jahrb 90: 249–261
69. Sanders R (1973) Torsional elasticity of human skin in vivo. Pflügers Arch 342: 255–260
70. Sato S (1982) On the skin extensibility and contractility with regard to aging. Jpn J Geriat 19: 376–380
71. Schade H (1912) Untersuchungen zur Organfunction des Bindegewebes: I. Mitteilung: Die Elasticitätsfunction des Bindegewebes und die intravitale Messung ihrer Störungen. Z Exp Pathol Ther 11: 369–399
72. Schade H (1926) Gewebselastometrie zu klinischem und allgemeinärztlichem Gebrauch. Münch Med Wochenschr 53: 2241–2246
73. Schmidt-La Baume F (1927) Elastometrie in der Dermatologie. Arch Dermatol Syph 153: 564–573
74. Schmidt-La Baume F (1927) Über Dermoelastometrie. Arch Dermatol 153: 765–771
75. Schmidt-La Baume F (1928) Über Dermoelastometrie. Arch Dermatol Syph 156: 383–423
76. Serup J (1984) Quantification of acrosclerosis: measurement of skin thickness and skin-phalanx distance in females with 15 MHZ pulsed ultrasound. Acta Derm Venerol (Stockh) 64: 35–40
77. Shuster S, Black MM, McVitie E (1975) The influence of age and sex on skin thickness, skin collagen and density. J Dermatol 93: 639–643
78. Suominen H, Heikkinen E, Moisio H, Viljamaa K (1978) Physical and chemical properties of skin in habitually trained and sedentary men. Br J Dermatol 99: 147–154
79. Tan CY, Statham B, Marks R, Payne PA (1982) Skin thickness measurement by pulsed ultrasound: its reproducibility, validation and variability. Br J Dermatol 106: 657–667
80. Thacker JG, Lachetta FA, Allaire PE, Edgerton MT, Rodeheaver GT, Edlich RF (1977) In vivo extensometer for measurement of the biomechanical properties of human skin. Rev Sci Instrum 48: 181–185
81. Tosti A, Compagno G, Fazzini ML, Villardita S (1977) A ballistometer for the study of the plastoelastic properties of skin. J Invest Dermatol 69: 315–317
82. Viidik A (1973) Rheology of skin with special reference to age-related parameters and their possible correlation to structure. Front Matrix Biol 1: 157–189
83. Viidik A (1976) Aging in skin-assessments in vivo and in vitro. Akt Gerontol 6: 11–14
84. Vogel HG (1970) Beeinflussung der mechanischen Eigenschaften der Haut von Ratten durch Hormone. Arzneimittelforschung 20: 1849–1857
85. Vogel HG (1972) Influence of age, treatment with corticolsteroids and strain rate on mechanical properties of rat skin. Biochim Biophys Acta 286: 79–83
86. Vogel HG (1974) Correlation between tensile strength and collagen content in rat skin. Effect of age and cortisol treatment. Connect Tissue Res 2: 177–182
87. Vogel HG (1976) Einfluß von Alter und Corticosteroid-Behandlung auf die mechanischen Parameter der Haut von Ratten bei zyklischer Beanspruchung (Mechanical parameters in rat skin following repeated load. Influence of age and corticosteroid treatment). GIT Lab Med 20: 113–121

88. Vogel HG (1976) Measurement of some viscoelastic properties of rat skin following repeated load. Connect Tissue Res 4: 163–168
89. Vogel HG (1976) Altersabhängige Veränderungen der mechanischen und biochemischen Eigenschaften der Cutis bei Ratten. Akt Gerontol 6: 477–487
90. Vogel HG (1976) Tensile strength, relaxation and mechanical recovery in rat skin as influenced by maturation and age. J Med 7: 177–188
91. Vogel HG. (1977) Strain of rat skin at constant load (creep experiments). Influence of age and desmotropic agents. Gerontology 23: 77–86
92. Vogel HG (1978) Age dependence of mechanical parameters in rat skin following repeated strain. Akt Gerontol 8: 601–618
93. Vogel HG (1978) Influence of maturation and age on mechanical and biochemical parameters of connective tissue of various organs in the rat. Connect Tissue Res 6: 161–166
94. Vogel HG (1980) Experimental approaches to maturation and ageing of skin. Cosmet Toil 95: 20–29
95. Vogel HG (1981) Attempts to compare in vivo and in vitro measurement of mechanical properties in rat skin. Bioeng Skin 3: 39–46
96. Vogel HG (1981) Comments on the paper by BARBENEL and PAYNE: "In vivo mechanical testing of dermal properties". Bioeng Skin 3: 53–56
97. Vogel HG (1981) Influence of desmotropic agents on the directional variations of mechanical properties in rat skin. Bioeng Skin 3: 85–97
98. Vogel HG (1981) Directional variations of mechanical parameters in rat skin depending on maturation and age. J Invest Dermatol 76: 493–497
99. Vogel HG (1981) Mechanical properties of rat skin at high and low loads. Influence of age and desmotropic drugs. In: Marks R, Payne PA (eds) Bioengineering and the skin. Proceedings of the European Society for Dermatological Research symposium, Cardiff, MTP Press, Lancaster, pp 79–101
100. Vogel HG (1982) Mechanical properties of rat skin as compared by in vivo and in vitro measurement. Bioeng Skin 3: 198–209
101. Vogel HG (1983) Age dependence of viscoelastic properties in rat skin. Directional variations in stress-strain and hysteresis experiments. Bioeng Skin 4: 136–155
102. Vogel HG (1983) Effects of age on the biomechanical and biochemical properties of rat and human skin. 1983 IFSCC/SCC joint conference on skin, San Francisco
103. Vogel HG (1983) Effects of age on the biomechanical and biochemical properties of rat and human skin. J Soc Cosmet Chem 34: 453–463
104. Vogel HG (1985) Reifung und Alterung der Haut. Experimentelle Grundlagen. Parfüm Kosmet 66: 219–225
105. Vogel HG (1985) Age dependence of viscoelastic properties in rat skin; Directional variations in relaxation experiments. Bioeng Skin 1: 157–174
106. Vogel HG (1985) Repeated relaxation and determination of the isorheological point in skin strips of rats as influenced by maturation and ageing. Bioeng Skin 1: 321–335
107. Vogel HG (1986) In vitro test systems for evaluation of the physical properties of the skin. In: Marks R, Plewig G (eds) Skin models; models to study function and disease of skin. Springer Berlin Heidelberg New York, pp 412–419
108. Vogel HG (1987) Age dependence of mechanical and biochemical properties of human skin: I. Stress-strain experiments, skin thickness and biochemical analysis. Bioeng Skin 3: 67–91
109. Vogel HG (1987) Age dependence of mechanical and biochemical properties of human skin: II. Hysteresis, relaxation, creep and repeated strain experiments. Bioeng Skin 3: 141–176
110. Vogel HG (1988) Further studies on directional variations and the "Step-Phenomenon" in rat skin depending on age. Bioeng Skin 4: 297–309
111. Vogel HG (1988) Restitution of mechanical properties of rat skin after repeated strain. Influence of maturation and ageing. Bioeng Skin 4: 343–359
112. Vogel HG (1989) Mechanical properties of rat skin with aging. In: Balin AK, Kligmann AM (eds) Aging and the skin. Raven, New York, pp 227–275
113. Vogel HG (1990) Restitutio ad integrum der mechanischen Eigenschaften von Rattenhaut nach wiederholter Dehnung. Einfluß von Reifung und Alterung. Z Gerontol 23: 126–127

114. Vogel HG (1991) Biomechanik des Bindegewebes. In Platt D (ed) Biologie des Alterns. Ein Handbuch. De Gruyter, Berlin, pp 111–122
115. Vogel HG, Denkel K (1982) Methodological studies on biomechanics of rat skin comparing in vivo and in vitro results. Bioeng Skin 4: 71–79
116. Vogel HG, Denkel K (1985) Influence of maturation and age, and of desmotropic compounds on the mechanical properties of rat skin in vivo. Bioeng Skin 1: 35–54
117. Vogel HG, Denkel K (1985) In vivo recovery of mechanical properties in rat skin after repeated strain. Arch Dermatol Res 277: 484–488
118. Vogel HG, Hilgner W (1977) Analysis of the low part of stress-strain curves in rat skin. Influence of age and desmotropic drugs. Arch Dermatol Res 258: 141–150
119. Vogel HG, Hilgner W. (1978) Viscoelastic behaviour of rat skin after repeated and stepwise increased strain. Bioeng Skin 1: 22–33
120. Vogel HG, Hilgner W (1979) The "Step Phenomenon" as observed in animal skin. J Biomech 12: 75–81
121. Vogel HG, Hilgner W (1979) Influence of age and of desmotropic drugs on the step phenomenon observed in rat skin. Arch Dermatol Res 264: 225–241
122. Vogel HG, Kobelt D, Korting GW., Holzmann H (1970) Prüfung der Festigkeitseigenschaften von Rattenhaut in Abhängigkeit von Lebensalter und Geschlecht. Arch Klin Exp Dermatol 239: 296–306
123. Wijn PFF (1980) The alinear viscoelastic properties of human skin in vivo for small deformations. PhD thesis, University of Nijmwegen
124. Wijn PFF, Manschot JFM, Brakkee AJM (1983) The angular distribution function of the elastin fibers in the skin as derived from in vivo measurements. Bioeng Skin 4: 124–135
125. Wilkes GL, Brown IA, Wildnauer RH. (1973) The biomechanical properties of skin. Crit Rev Bioeng 1: 453–495

The Effect of Aging on the Barrier Function of Human Skin Evaluated by In Vivo Transepidermal Water Loss Measurements

K. P. Wilhelm[1,2] and H. I. Maibach[2]

Introduction

Measurements of transepidermal water loss (TEWL) are used in many laboratories for characterization of skin barrier function in vivo, in clinical research, and as a supplementary tool in clinical examination for objective evaluation of certain diseases, e.g., allergic and irritant contact dermatitis, psoriasis, atopy, ichthyosis [1–6].

It is generally accepted that TEWL is higher in preterm infants than in term infants although sweat glands are nonfunctioning [7–9]. During the first 2–4 weeks of life the skin barrier gradually matures and with increasing chronologic age, TEWL gradually becomes comparable to adult levels. At the other end of the age spectrum, i.e., from adulthood through senescence, the age dependence of TEWL is controversially discussed.

Stratum Corneum as a Physical Barrier

It is now established that the stratum corneum (SC), the outermost skin layer at the environment-individual interface, is the principle permeability barrier to TEWL and to percutaneous absorption of topically applied compunds [10–12]. SC is typically 6–20 μm thick, except for the palms and soles, where thickness is approximately 400–600 μm [13, 14].

As a part of the epidermis, SC is constantly renewed from the granular layer and the outermost corneocytes are gradually desquamated from the surface. The internal structure of SC is well organized and has often been schematically described by a "brick-wall model" [12, 15]. Terminally differentiated, keratin-filled corneocytes of polyhedral shape, arranged as interdigitating vertical columns, are represented by the "bricks" while the intercellular lipoidal material in a multilamellar bilayer arrangement represents the "mortar". Lipid metabolism within the SC has been documented and TEWL seems to play a role in the regulation of lipid synthesis via regulation of HMG-CoA-reductase activity [16, 17].

Though today there is circumstantial evidence that SC is not homogeneous throughout its thickness [18, 19], initial claims that the true barrier layer resides at the base of the SC [19–21] have been shown to be an inappropriate interpretation of

---

[1] Department of Dermatology, Medical University of Lübeck, Lübeck, Germany
[2] Department of Dermatology, Universtity of California-San Francisco, San Francisco, CA, USA

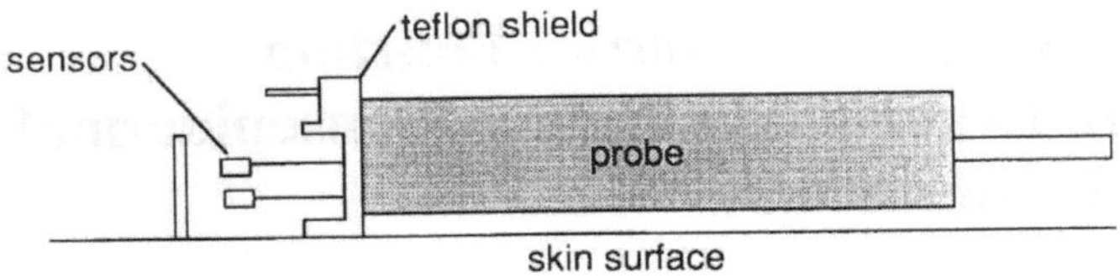

Fig. 1. Measurement probe with the open unventilated chamber. Two hygrosensors coupled with a fast thermistor at a constant distance between each other are vertically held against the skin surface. Thus water evaporation is obtained by water vapor pressure gradient calculation

experiments in which SC was removed, layer by layer, by adhesive tape stripping. More appropriate studies have shown the contrary, that the barrier properties are more evenly distributed across the entire thickness of the membrane [22, 23]

Transepidermal water loss Measurements To Examine Skin Barrier Properties

Today measurement of TEWL is a generally accepted parameter for the evaluation of skin barrier function [7, 24–27]. The relationship between TEWL and percutaneous absorption has been clearly demonstrated in preterm infants [7] and in respect to anatomic variability [25].

Different methodology has been used for assessing TEWL as reviewed by Wilson and Maibach [28] and by Grice [29]. Today, the majority of clinical studies are performed with the open unventilated chamber technique (Fig. 1) and instrumental calculation of the water evaporation gradient developing from the skin surface to atmospheric humidity [30]. The instrument measures relative air humidity, water vapor partial pressure, and evaporation rate. The probe contains two sensors vertically placed at a known distance from the skin surface. Each sensor is coupled to a fast thermistor and both are enclosed in a cylindrically shaped Teflon capsule. For measurements the probe is held against the skin surface, orienting the sensors perpendicularly to the water vapor pressure gradient. To perform accurate and reliable measurements, several sources of variation need to be taken into account, as reviewed by Pinnagoda et al. [31]. Most important are constant ambient temperature and relative humidity, minimizing air convection and recording skin temperature as the variable with the most significant influence on TEWL.

Skin temperature should always be reported since TEWL increases exponentially with skin temperature [32, 33]. Some investigators therefore prefer a correction of absolute TEWL to a standard skin temperature, conventionally 30°C [32, 33] while others do not [31].

Transepidermal Water Loss of Aging Skin

While there is no doubt that the permeability barrier matures within the first 2–4 weeks of life, no consent has yet been established about the skin permeability barrier and baseline TEWL at the opposite end of the age spectrum, i.e., from adulthood through senescence (Table 1).

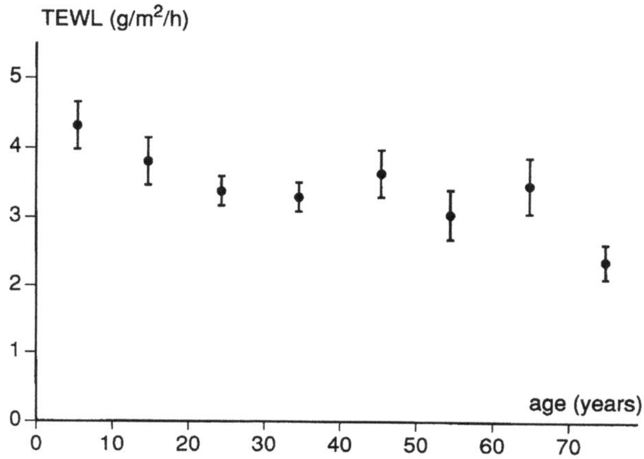

Fig. 2. Baseline transepidermal water loss (TEWL) on the volar forearm decreases during the first 20 years of life (n = 145). A second decrease is noted after the age of 70 years. (Modified from [34])

The majority of published studies, however, note a significant decrease of TEWL with age, especially after the age of 60–70 years. A study performed by Leveque [34] on 145 healthy volunteers reports a significant decrease of TEWL on the forearm during the first 20 years of life and a second decrease after the age of 70 years as compared with adulthood levels (Fig. 2). Wilhelm et al. [35] demonstrated that TEWL was significantly lower in an aged group (70.5 + 13.8 years) than in young individuals (26.7 ± 2.8 years) (Fig. 3). In the same study no significant differences in skin capacitance as a measure for SC hydration were demonstrated, however (Fig. 4). There are also reports that failed to demonstrate any significant correlation between age and TEWL [24, 36, −38]. The critical reader might wonder why results can be so conflicting even though the method of measurement and group size are very similar. While no information about the age of the study group was provided by Grice and Bettley [38], Tupker et al. [24] studied individuals age 20–48 years representing mid-adulthood levels. A correlation between age and TEWL could not be expected in their study because TEWL does apparently not decrease before the age of 60–70 years [34]. While studying individuals age 60 years and older Roskos and Guy [36] and Rougier et al. [37] still failed to demonstrate significant age-related changes in TEWL, possibly because of high ambient temperature (23°C ± 2°C) in the first study or high relative humidity (70%) in the second study. Both groups, however, demonstrated an increase in the skin permeability barrier in aged individuals by reduced percutaneous penetration of topically applied compounds [37, 39]. Roskos and Guy [36] also examined the water barrier in young and old individuals under "stressed" conditions by first preventing TEWL for 24 h by occluding the skin and then monitoring the recovery of TEWL to baseline values. The authors hypothesized that occlusion might enhance the "signal-

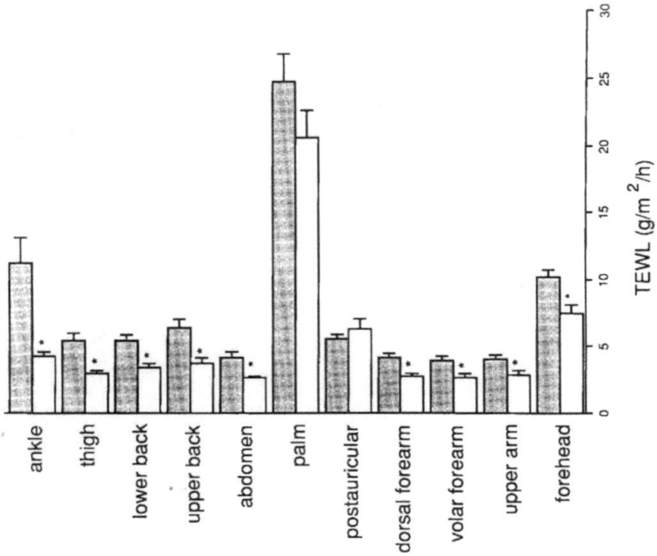

Fig. 3. Age differences in TEWL rates at different anatomical locations. Young group, *hatched bars*; aged group, *open bars*. Shown are means ± 1 S.E.M ($n = 14–15$); *statistically significant difference between the two groups ($p \leq 0.05$). (Modified from [35])

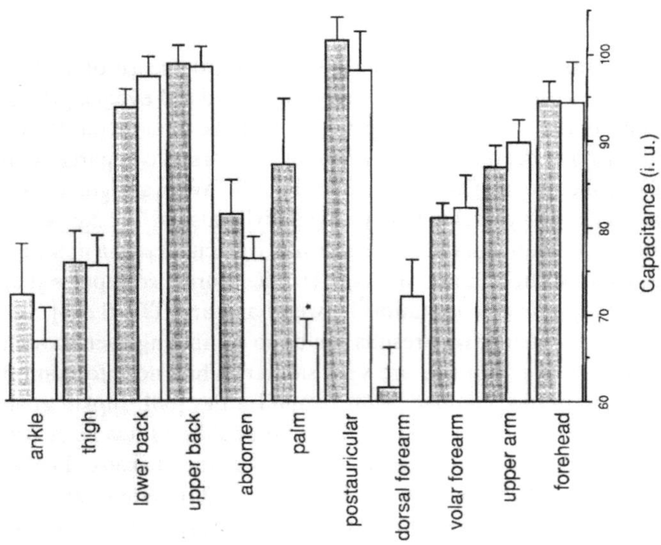

Fig. 4. Age differences in stratum corneum hydration at different anatomical locations as evaluated by capacitance measurements. Young group, *hatched bars*, aged group *open bars*, *i. u.*, instrumental units; means ± 1 S.E.M.; n = 14–15; *statistically significant differences between the age groups ($p \leq 0.05$). Since these age difference appear site-specific, it is possible that the responsible mechanism(s) are local rather than systemic. (Modified from [35])

to-noise" ratio associated with TEWL measurements. Indeed, with this "stress test" the authors demonstrated a relatively slower relaxation of TEWL in the aged group. Their results confirmed earlier work by Tagami [40], who used conductance measurements in a"water sorption-desorption test" to distinguish between young and old skin. Whether this procedure of hydrating the SC first, either by occluding the skin or by applying water to it, and then measuring TEWL really reflects water permeability barrier properties remains open for discussion.

Table 1. Age dependence of transepidermal water loss (TEWL)

Author (reference)	Group size (*n*)	Result	Anatomic site
Baker [41]	87	Lower water loss in individuals older than 70 years	–
Grice and Bettley [38]	39	TEWL tended to decrease with increasing age; however corelation was not statistically significant (age range of the group was not indicated)	Abdomen
Jemec et al. [59]	21	Significant negative correlation between TEWL and age (22–71 years)	Onychial
Kligman [42]	21	Lower TEWL in 66–81 year old individuals than in 19–26 years olds	Leg and forearm
Leveque [34]	145	Decreased TEWL after 60 years of age	Forearm
Roskos et al. [36, 39]	33	No correlation between baseline TEWL and age (range: 19–85 years); however four out of six radiolabeled drugs showed significantly decreased percutaneous penetration in aged individuals	Forearm
Rougier et al. [37]	23	No difference in TEWL between age groups (20–30 vs 65–80 years); the percutaneous penetration of benzoic acid, however, was significantly reduced in aged individuals	Upper arm
Tagami [40]	22	TEWL decreased in the age group (19–22 vs 61–85 years)	Pretibial
Tupker et al. [24]	43	TEWL showed no correlation with age (age range: 20–48 years)	Forearm
Wilhelm et al. [35]	29	Significant decrease with age on most anatomical regions (mean age 26.7 vs 70.5 years)	Eleven different regions

Summarized are the results of some recently published studies (without intention of completeness) on the effect of aging on in vivo TEWL measurements in humans.

Discussion

The clinical aspect of dry skin encountered in the majority of subjects age 65 or older has not been associated with a perturbed barrier to water permeability as evaluated by TEWL measurements [34]. In contrast, the majority of studies demonstrated lower TEWL in individuals age 60–70 and older [34, 35, 40–44]. An explanation for reduced TEWL in the aged is not obvious. Skin physiology and biochemistry changes in many regards with increasing age [45]. It is not to be expected that the barrier function is excluded from this modification. Reduced sweating associated with the aging process [46] is probably not contributing to the observed decrease in TEWL, and sweating does not significantly influence baseline TEWL [47]. It has been shown that there is an inverse relationship between corneocyte size and TEWL [48]. However, in the case of skin senescence, there seems to be no clear correlation between these parameters [49].

Although the thickness of the SC is not altered by age, its renewal time is greatly prolonged; in young adults, SC transit time, as estimated by the dansyl chloride staining method, is about 20 days, whereas in older adults it is more than 30 days [50]. But the relevance of the increased SC renewal time in aged skin is not yet known.

Decreased density and efficiency of the skin microvasculature [51] resulting in decreased skin temperature might explain reduced TEWL in elderly individuals, although Wilhelm et al. [35] corrected their TEWL measurements to a standard skin reference temperature of 30°C and still noted lower TEWL values in the elderly.

A significant correlation between TEWL and percutaneous absorption of diverse drugs has been demonstrated by several studies [25, 37, 52]. It appears that the decreased TEWL in aged individuals reflects also a less permeable membrane to topically applied compounds [37, 38, 51, 53]. Rougier et al. [37] report a decreased percutaneous absorption of [14 C] benzoic acid in older subjects (65–80 years). Roskos et al. [39] confirm a decreased penetration for four out of six radioisotope-labeled substances in older individuals. Only the percutaneous penetration of the two most lipophilic compounds considered was not significantly different in their experiments. This was in agreement with earlier studies by Christophers and Kligman [53] and Tagami [51] who concluded that the barrier function of human skin in vivo increases with increasing chronologic age. Furthermore, the recent study by Cua et al. confirms a decreased irritant response after application of sodium lauryl sulfate in older individuals [44].

In summary, the majority of studies including TEWL measurements and/or percutaneous penetration experiments support a further increasing skin barrier function with increasing chronologic age. Age-associated changes in the SC as the principle permeability barrier are most probably responsible for this effect.

Physicochemical Interpretation

The most simple way of modeling both the process of percutaneous absorption and TEWL is to assume that Fick's first law of diffusion is applicable, although the SC is not an inert membrane. The form of the equation often quoted ist:

$$\frac{\mathrm{d}Q}{\mathrm{d}t} = \frac{\mathrm{D}Kpc}{h}$$

where $\mathrm{d}Q/\mathrm{d}t$ is the rate of skin penetration (TEWL); D is the effective diffusion coefficient of drug (water) in SC; Kp is the partition coefficient of drug (water) between membrane and solution; c is the concentration gradient of drug (water); h is the effective thickness of the skin barrier.

For water diffusing through the SC in the opposite direction $\mathrm{d}Q/\mathrm{d}t$ is measurable at the skin surface as TEWL. Thus, all factors relevant to $\mathrm{d}Q/\mathrm{d}t$ apply to TEWL. SC thickness is not altered by age [13, 50] and may therefore not account for the increased in vivo barrier. One may also assume that c is constant, although epidermal atrophy and a reduced tissue hydration in the aged might decrease the concentration gradient for water [54].

Recent in vitro observations suggest that a lower lipid content leads to an increased penetration of tritiated water and of [14 C] salicylic acid [55]. A lowered lipid content might not only reduce the diffusion coefficient but also Kp, as recently demonstrated by Surber et al. [56]. They showed that delipidization of isolated human SC significantly reduced *Kp*, especially for hydrophilic compounds. Interestingly, Roskos found an overall diminution of SC epidermal lipid content with increasing age in humans in vivo by means of attenuated total reflectance infrared spectroscopy (ATR–IR) [57]. A decreased epidermal lipid content in the elderly would reduce the partitioning of water (*Kp*) in SC and hence explain the reduced TEWL.

In addition, no significant difference in SC water content between young and old individuals was demonstrated by capacitance or conductance measurements [35, 40]. Using more sensitive ATR-IR spectroscopy instrumentation, however, it has been demonstrated that the SC of elderly is drier than the young adult equivalent [58]. And by use of a water sorption-desorption test Tagami confirmed a lower water binding capacity of old SC [40]. A reduced presence of water in the SC of old subjects [58] would imply that the environment of aged skin is less attractive to hydrophilic molecules and to water resulting in a decreased *Kp*, hence decreased dQ/dt.

Acknowledgement. Supported by a grant from the Deutsche Forschungsgemeinschaft (DFG Wi 879/3–1). The authors appreciate the collaboration with Dr. A. B. Cua who generated much of the experimental data considered for this chapter.

References

1. Thune P (1989) Evaluation of the hydration and the water-holding capacity in atopic skin and so-called dry skin. Acta Derm Venereol (Stockh) Suppl 144: 133–135
2. Frost P, Weinstein GD, Bothwell JW, Wildnauer R (1968) Ichthyosiform dermatoses; III. Studies of transepidermal water loss. Arch Dermatol 98: 230–233
3. Silverman RA, Lender J, Elmets CA (1989) Effects of occlusive and semiocclusive dressings on the return of barrier function to transepidermal water loss in standardized human wounds. J Am Acad Dermatol 20: 755–760
4. Grice K, Sattar H, Baker H (1973) The cutaneous barrier to salts and water in psoriasis and in normal skin. Br J Dermatol 88: 459–463
5. Serup J, Staberg B (1987) Differentiation of allergic and irritant reactions by transepidermal water loss. Contact Dermatitis 16: 129–132
6. Van der Valk PJM, Nater JP, Bleumink E (1984) Skin irritancy of surfactants as assessed by water vapor loss measurements. J Invest Dermatol 82: 291–293
7. Rutter N (1988) The immature skin. Br Med Bull 44: 957–970
8. Hammerlund K, Sedin G, Stromberg B (1983) Transepidermal water loss in newborn infants. Acta Paediatr Scand 72: 721–728
9. Wilson DR, Maibach HI (1982) An in vivo comparison of skin barrier function. In: Maibach HI, Boisits EK (eds) Neonatal skin, structure and function. Dekker, Basel pp101–110
10. Blank IH, Scheuplein RJ (1969) Transport into and within the skin. Br J Dermatol 81: 4–10
11. Scheuplein RJ (1976) Percutaneous absorption after twenty-five years: or "old wine in new wineskins". J Invest Dermatol 67: 31–38
12. Elias PM (1981) Epidermal lipids, membranes, and keratinization. Int J Dermatol 20: 1–19
13. Holbrook KA, Odland GF (1974) Regional differences in the thickness (cell layers) of the human stratum corneum: an ultrastructural analysis. J Invest Dermatol 62: 415–422
14. Plewig G, Scheuber E, Reuter B, Waidelich T (1983) Thickness of corneocytes. In: Marks R, Plewig G, (eds) Stratum corneum. Springer Berlin, Heidelberg, New York, pp 171–174
15. Michaels AS, Chandrasekaran SK, Shaw JE (1975) Drug permeation through human skin, theory and in vitro experimental measurement. Journal of the American Institute of Chemical Engineers 21: 985–996

16. Grubauer G, Elias PM, Feingold KR (1989) Transepidermal water loss: the signal for recovery of barrier structure and function. J Lipid Res 30: 323–333
17. Proksch E, Elias PM, Feingold KR (1990) Regulation of 3-hydroxy-3-methylglutaryl-co-enzyme A reductase activity in murine epidermis. Modulation of enzyme content and activation state by barrier requirements. J Clin Invest 85: 874–882
18. Bommannan D, Potts RO, Guy RH (1990) Examination of stratum corneum barrier function in vivo by infrared spectroscopy. J Invest Dermatol 95: 403–408
19. Eriksson G, Lamke L (1971) Regeneration of human epidermal surface and water barrier function after stripping. Acta Derm Venereol (Stockh) 51: 169–178
20. Bowser PA, White RJ (1985) Isolation, barrier properties and lipid analysis of stratum compactum, a discrete region of the stratum corneum. Br J Dermatol 112: 1–14
21. Blank IH (1953) Further observations on factors which influence the water content of the stratum corneum. J Invest Dermatol 21: 259–271
22. Blank IH, Gould E (1962) Location and reformation of the epithelial barrier to water vapor. Arch Dermatol 78: 702–714
23. Blank H, Gould E (1962) Study of mechanisms which impede the penetration of synthetic anionic surfactants into skin. J Invest Dermatol 37: 311–315
24. Tupker RA, Coenraads PJ, Pinnagoda J, Nater JP (1989) Baseline transepidermal water loss (TEWL) as a prediction of susceptibility to sodium lauryl sulphate. Contact Dermatitis 20: 265–269
25. Lotte C, Rougier A, Wilson DR, Maibach HI (1987) In vivo relationship between transepidermal water loss and percutaneous penetration of some organic compounds in man: effect of anatomic site. Arch Dermatol Res 279: 351–356
26. Onken HD, Moyer CA (1963) The water barrier in human epidermis. Arch Dermatol 87: 90–96
27. Murahata RI, Crowe DM, Roheim JR (1986) The use of transepidermal water loss to measure and predict the irritation response to surfactants. Int J Cosmet Sci 8: 225–231
28. Wilson DR, Maibach HI (1989) Transepidermal water loss: a review. In: Leveque JL (ed) Cutaneous investigation in health and disease. Noninvasive methods and instrumentation. New York, pp 113–134
29. Grice KA (1980) Transepidermal water loss. In: Jarret A (ed) The physiology and pathophysiology of the skin, vol 6. Academic, London, pp 2115–2127
30. Nilsson GE (1977) Measurement of water exchange through skin. Med Biol Eng Comput 15: 209–218
31. Pinnagoda J, Tupker RA, Agner T, Serup J (1990) Guidelines for transepidermal water loss (TEWL) measurement. Contact Dermatitis 22: 164–178
32. Mathias CGT, Wilson DM, Maibach HI (1981) Transepidermal water loss as a function of skin surface temperature. J Invest Dermatol 77: 219–220
33. Grice K, Sattar H, Sharrett M, Baker H (1978) Skin temperature and transepidermal water loss. J Invest Dermatol 57: 108–110
34. Leveque JL (1989) Measurement of transepidermal water loss. In: Leveque JL (ad) Cutaneous investigation in health and diseas. Noninvasive methods and instrumentation. New York, pp 135–152
35. Wilhelm KP, Cua AB, Maibach HI (1991) Skin aging: Effect on transepidermal water loss, stratum corneum hydration, skin surface pH, and casual sebum content. Arch Dermatol 127: 1806–1809
36. Roskos KV, Guy RH (1989) Assessment of skin barrier function using transepidermal water loss-effect of age. Pharm Res 6: 949–953
37. Rougier A, Lotte C, Corcuff P, Maibach HI (1988) Relationship between skin permeability and corneocyte size according to anatomic site, age, and sex in man. J Soc Cosmet Chem 39: 15–26
38. Grice KA, Bettley FR (1967) Skin water loss and accidental hypothermia in psoriasis, ichthyosis and erythrodermia. BMJ 4: 195–201
39. Roskos KV, Maibach HI, Guy RH (1989) The effect of aging on percutaneous absorption in man. J Pharmacokinet Biopharm 17: 617–630
40. Tagami H (1988) Aging and the hydration state of the skin. In: Kligmann AM, Takase Y (eds), Cutaneous aging. University of Tokyo Press, Tokyo, pp 99–109

41. Baker H (1971) Deperdition d'eau par voie trans-epidermique. Ann Dermatol Syph 98: 289–296
42. Kligman AM (1979) Perspectives and problems in cutaneous gerontology. J Invest Dermatol 73.39-46
43. Thune P, Nilsen T, Gustavson T, Lövig Dahl H (1988) The water barrier function of the skin in relation to the water content of stratum crneum, pH and skin lipids. Acta Derm Venerol (Stockh) 68: 277–283
44. Cua AB, Wilhelm KP, Maibach HI (1990) Cutaneous sodium lauryl sulfate irritation potential: age and regional variability. Br J Dermatol 123: 607–613
45. Gilchrest BA (1989) Skin aging and photoaging: an overview. J Am Acad Dermatol 21: 610–613
46. Sato K, Timm DE (1988) Effect of aging on pharmacological sweating in man. In: Kligman AM, Takase Y (eds) Cutaneous aging. University of Tokyo Press, Tokyo, pp 111–126
47. Pinnagoda J, Tupker RA, Coenraads PJ, Nater JB (1989) Transepidemal water loss with and without sweat gland inactivation. Contact Dermatitis 21: 16–22
48. Marks R, Nicholls S, King CS (1981) Studies on isolated corneocytes. Int J Cosmet Sci 3: 251–258
49. Leveque JL, Corcuff P, de Rigal J, Agache P (1984) In viov studies of the evolution of physical properties of the human skin with age. Int J Dermatol 23: 322–329
50. Grove GL, Kligman AM (1983) Age-Associated changes in human epidermal cell renewal. J Gerontol 38: 137–142
51. Tagami H (1971/1972) Functional characteristics of age skin: 1. Percutaeous absorption. Acta Dermatol Kyoto Eng. Ed 66/67: 19–21
52. Dupuis D, Rougier A, Lotte C, Wilson DR, Maibach HI (1986) In vivo relationship between percutaneous absorption and transepidermal water loss according to anatomic site in man. J Soc Cosmet Chem 37: 351–357
53. Christophers E, Kligman AM (1965) Percutaneous absorption in aged skin. In: Montagna W (ed) Advanced in biology of skin: Pergamon, Oxford, pp 163–175
54. Miyake I (1988) Histological aging of facial skin. In: Kligman AM, Takase, Y (ed) Cutanous aging. University of Toky Press, Tokyo, pp 571–588
55. Elias PM, Cooper ER, Korc A, Brown BE (1981) Percutaneous transport in relation to stratum corneum structure and lipid composition. J Invest Dermatol 76: 297–301
56. Surber C, Wilhelm KP, Hori M, Maibach HI, Guy RH (1990) Optimzation of topical therapy: partitioning of drugs into stratum corneum. Pharm Res 7: 1320–1324
57. Roskos KV (1989) The effect of skin aging on the percutaneous penetration of chemical through human skin. Dissertation, University of California, San Francisco
58. Potts RO, Buras EM (1985) In vivo changes in the dynamic viscosity of human straum corneum as a function of age and ambient moisture. J Soc Cosmet Chem 36: 169–176
59. Jemec G, Agner T, Serup J (1989) Transonychial water loss. Relation to sex, age and nailplate thickness. Br J Dermatol 121: 443–446

In Vivo Study on Age-Related Elastic Properties of Human Skin

K. P. WILHELM[1,2], A. B. CUA[2], and H. I. MAIBACH[2]

Introduction

The skin performs numerous functions vital to the maintenance of homeostasis. Faced with a variety of extrinsic factors, such as physical trauma from the sun, wind, temperature changes, microorganisms, and the dynamic movements of the body, as well as the intrinsic aging processes, its integrity is well preserved by a complex interaction of the three layers: epidermis, dermis, and subcutaneous tissue.

The epidermis, particularly the stratum corneum layer, provides a barrier to permeability. It is tough and resilient due to the presence of fibrous keratin. Evidence for stratum corneum elasticity has been described [10, 13]; intraepidermal elasticity has also been associated with the presence of sweat [26]. The relatively thick dermis together with the subcutaneous fat gives the skin its toughness and elasticity, an important mechanical property primarily attributable to the intra- and intermolecular cross-links of collagen, elastic, and reticulin fibers embedded in ground substance [22, 32]. The extensibility of skin, however, shows directional variation characterized as anisotropy [15, 35].

Studies on the mechanical properties of skin began with Dupuytren and Langer [17, 22]. There is continuing interest particularly in the evaluation of the aging process [1, 5, 20, 34, 37], and other clinical conditions such as edema and atrophy [3, 9, 36], connective tissue disorders [6, 8, 23, 27], and psoriasis [28]. Various instruments have been employed, as reviewed recently [19] (Table 1):

1. Methods utilizing devices working perpendicular to the skin surface: indentation, elevation, suction, ballistometry
2. Methods measuring the skin's properties in its own plane: stretching, torsion and wave propagation.

Unfortunately, no uniform nomenclature to describe the phenomena observed in skin elasticity experiments has been agreed upon. Table 2 lists important terms regarding elasticity as a glossary.

Although different methodologies have been employed most studies noted increased extensibility but decreased elasticity with increasing chronologic age. However, results on the effect of aging on the elastic properties of skin in vivo as measured with the various techniques have been contradictory, as summarized in Table 3.

[1] Department of Dermatology, Medical University of Lübeck, Lübeck, Germany
[2] Department of Dermatology, University of California-San Francisco, San Francisco, CA, USA

Table 1. Methods for in vivo skin elasticity measurements

Devices operating perpendicular to the skin surface

Suction: skin deformation after application of a negative pressure is measured.
Elevation/traction: Skin is pulled by a mechanical force and the displacement of the skin surface is measured.
Indentation: compression of the skin by a mechanical force and measurement of the displacement of the skin surface.
Ballistometry: measurement of the drop impact of a body onto a stationary surface (the skin).

Methods working in the plane of the skin (horizontal to the surface)

Stretching: displacement of a small tab glued onto the skin in response to a sinusoidal driving force is recorded by a gas bearing electrodynanometer. In an alternative approach two metallic tabs are glued onto the skin surface and moved by a small motor. The force needed to elongate or compress the skin is recorded.
Torsion: rotation of a disc glued onto the skin surface is measured as response to a given force (torque).
Wave propagation: mechanical waves travelling longitudinally to the skin surface generated by piezoelectric components are recorded by piezoelectric sensors. Their amplitude, phase, and velocity can be determined and related to the elastic properties of the tissue.

Overview of various methods to study in vivo elasticity in human skin (withouts intention of completeness. Modified from [18].

Table 2. Nomenclature used in the elasticity literature

Parameter	Explanation
Elasticity	Measure of the ability of the skin to return to its original position after deformation by elastic retraction.
Extension (extensibility, tensile distension)	Deformation of the skin when a force (suction, torque) is first applied to the skin.
Elongation, elevation	Corresponds to extension, in the case of suction devices.
Stretchability	Equals extension for methods operating in the skin's own plane.
Immediate distension	Initial part of the distension governed by elastic fibers.
Delayed distension	Applies to the viscoelastic part of skin deformation.
Resilient distension	Applies to repeated extension-retraction cycles and describes the skin's residual deformation measured at the end of the last cycle.
Retraction	Describes the repositioning of the skin after the extension force (suction, torque) is discontinued. Like the extension process it can be divided into immediate, late, and total retraction.
Hysteresis	When skin elasticity measurements are repeated for several cycles the skin extensibility increases from cycle to cycle and it takes longer for the skin to retract to its inital position. Hysteresis is measured as the difference in maximum extensibility between the first cycle and the last cycle.
Coefficient of restitution	Amount of energy returned by the tissue in ballistometric studies.

Explanation of various terms used in the pertinent literature (see also Fig. 2).

Table 3. Aging and skin elasticity

Author (reference)	Method	Result
Agache et al. [1]	Torsion	Diminished elasticity and stretchability after the age of 30, associated with an increase in the visco elastic component.
Alexander and Cook [2]	Suction	Extension ratio decreased through maturation, reached a minimum between the ages of 15 and 25, and then increased with further advancing age.
Berardesca et al. [5]	Stretching	Extensibility increased with age (male volunteers only).
Elsner et al. [14]	Suction	Elasticity was decreased in the aged group; significant difference between volar forearm and vulvar skin.
Escoffier et al. [15]	Torsion	Extensibility was constant up to the seventh decade; – elasticity highest in very young individuals and progressively decreased with aging.
Leveque et al. [20]	Torsion	Exentsibility decreased with age; females hat lower extensibility than males.
Sato [25]	Suction	Extensibility and contractility decreased with age.
Tosti et al. [30]	Ballistometry	Coefficient of restitution was highest in very young people and a progressive decrease occurred with aging; differences among 12 anatomic sites were prominent.
Cua et al. [11]	Suction	Measurements were performed on 11 anataomic regions; biologic elasticity decreased while the viscoelastic portion of the extension process increased on most test sites.

Summarized are the results of some recently published studies (without intention of completeness) on the effect of aging on in vivo skin elasticity in humans.

This study utilizes noninvasive, in vivo, suction device for measuring skin elasticity and to evaluate potential age- and sex-dependent differences in viscoelastic properties of the skin and its regional variability, an aspect not previously thoroughly examined.

Experimental Methods

Subjects

A total of 33 volunteers participated in the study after giving written informed consent. The study was approved by the University of California-San Francisco Committee on Human Research. The population was divided into four groups: (1) group A, eight young females (age 25.8 ± 3.0; mean ± sd); (2) group B, nine elderly female (74.7 ± 5.7); (3) group C, eight young males (age 28.3 ± 1.2); and (4) group D, eight elderly males (age 75.1 ± 4.8). All participants were Caucasians with no signs of apparent skin disease. Subjects were instructed not to treat their skin with cosmetics or moisturizers 24 h prior to the measurements.

Measurements were performed on 11 anatomic regions: forehead (center), post-auricular region, upper arm (inner middle third), volar and dorsal forearm (center between wrist and elbow), palm (thenar aspect), abdomen (3 cm above umbilicus), thigh (anterior, upper third), ankle (medial malleoli), upper back (scapula), and lower back (at level of L1). Except for measurements of the abdomen during which volunteers were recumbent, all measurements were taken with volunteers seated.

Elasticity Measurements

Skin elasticity was measured with a recently designed commercially available instrument (Cutometer SEM 474, Courage and Khazaka, Cologne, West Germany). This instrument measures the elastic properties of skin based on the principle of suction/elongation. The device (Fig. 1) consists of a hand-held probe with a central suction head (2 mm in diameter) fitted to a spring, which ensures that the head is applied to the skin at constant pressure. Due to the small test area (approximately 3 mm^2), the skin elongation contribution from the dermosubepidermal junction – a drawback of previous, much larger, suction devices – is negligible [14]. The probe is attached to the main unit linked to an IBM PC/AT or compatible computer and is entirely controlled by the computer. The main unit consists of a vacuum pump which generates vacuum or load from 50 to 500 mbar, a pressor sensor, an electrical circuit controlling the pump, and an analog to digital data conversion (Fig. 1). Measurements of skin deformation by application of vaccum perpendicular to the skin surface are registered by an optical measuring unit with an accuracy of 0.01 mm and a frequency of 100 Hz.

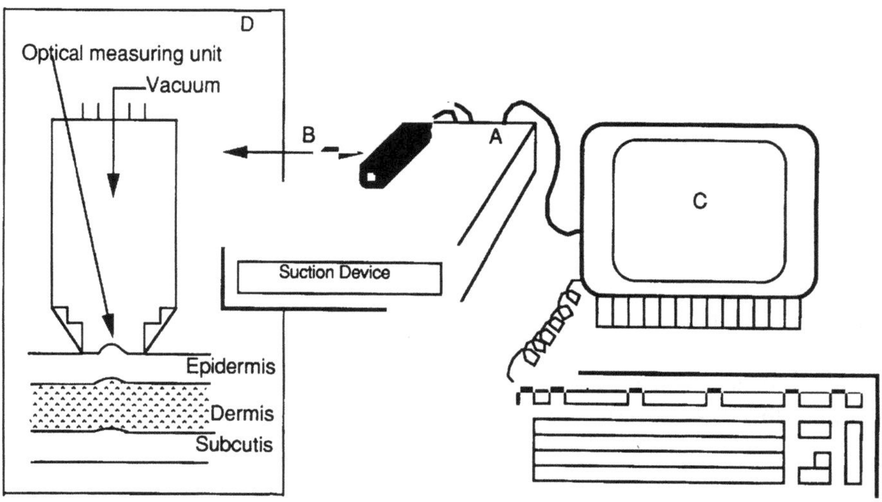

Fig. 1. Elasticity measurement apparatus. The main unit of the suction device consists of a vacuum pump, pressor sensor, electrical circuit controlling pump, and an analog to digital data conversion (*A*): Through two rubber tubes the probe (*B*) is attached to the main unit and is linked to an IBM PC/AT or compatible computer. A magnification of the probe, applied perpendicularly to the skin surface, is shown (*D*). (Adapted from [11])

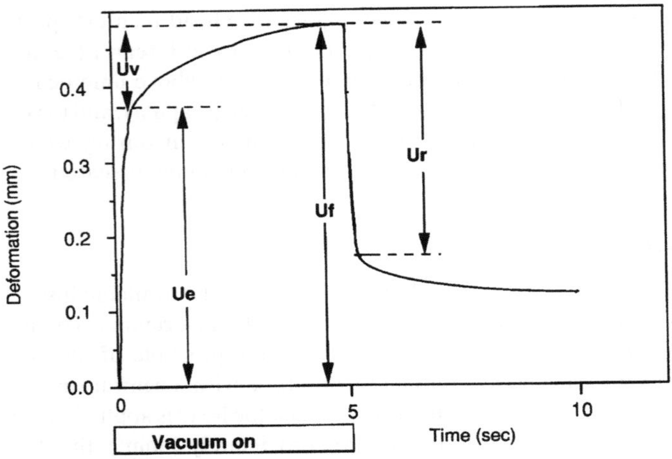

Fig. 2. Typical skin deformation plotted as a function of time. The parameters are: immediate distension (*Ue*), delayed distension (*Uv*), immediate retraction (*Ur*), and final distension (*Uf*). (Modified from 11])

The time/strain mode was used with a 5 s application of three different loads: 100, 200, and 500 mbar, followed by a 5 s relaxation period. Skin deformation was plotted as a function of time. A typical time/strain recording is illustrated in Fig. 2. The following parameters were recorded: immediate distension (Ue), measured at 0.48 s; delayed distension (Uv); immediate retraction (Ur); and final distension (Uf) [1,20]. The deformation curve consists of an initial purely elastic component, followed by a viscoelastic, and a final purely viscous part [14].

All parameters are a function of skin thickness and can thus not be simply compared between subjects and regions. However, for the time being, in vivo skin thickness measurements are not without difficulty. Fortunately, certain biologically relevant ratios of these parameters are independent of skin thickness and can be compared between subjects and anatomical regions [1, 14, 15, 23]. For each group, two relative parameters independent of skin thickness were calculated: Firstly, the viscoelastic to elastic ratio (Uv/Ue). Increasing values of Uv/Ue indicate an increasing viscoelastic portion of the deformation process (which is controlled by the collagen fibers) and a relative decrease of the elastic part. Secondly, Ur/Uf (biologic elasticity) was calculated, which measures the ability of skin to regain its initial position after deformation. A value of 1 would indicate 100% elasticity. Decreasing elasticity will result in smaller ratios. Variations in the mechanical properties of the skin were analyzed with respect to age, sex, and region.

Differences were tested for their statistical significance using Student's test for unpaired data and analysis of variance for regional variation [38]. A p value less than or equal to 0.05 was considered statistically significant.

Results

Typical extension/retraction curves for young versus old skin are shown in Fig. 3. Note that the final distension (Uf) is higher in the aged individual while the immediate retraction (Ur) did not increase to the same extent. Thus, the calculation of the biologic elasti-

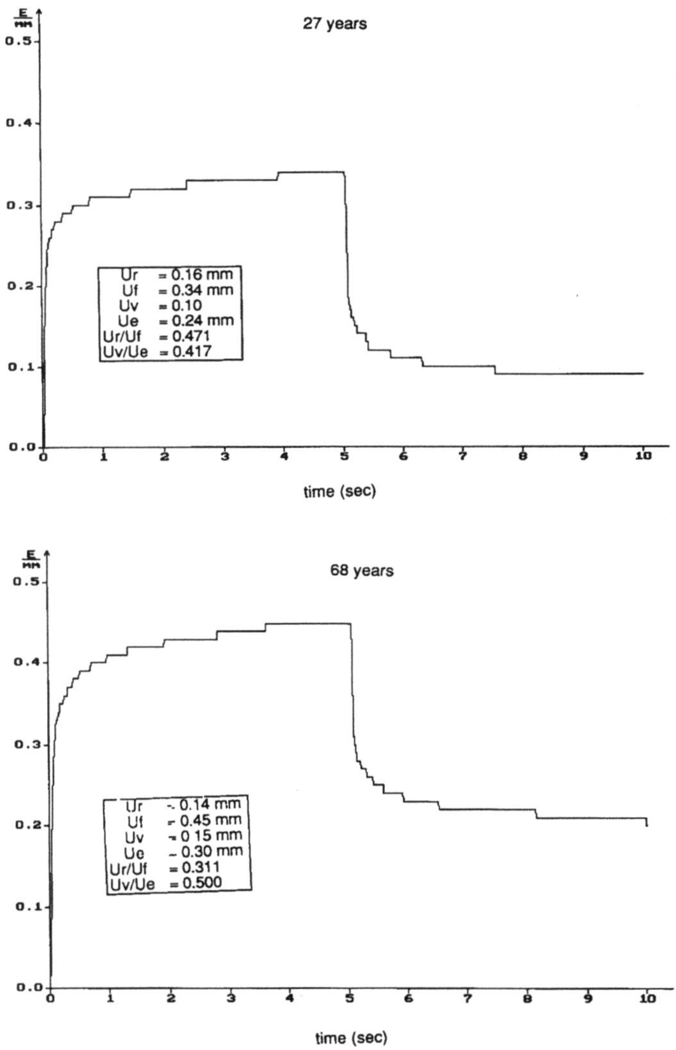

Fig. 3. Typical deformation curves (500 mbar) in young (*top*) and old (*bottom*) skin. Note that the total distension (*Uf*) is increased in the aged individual while the immediate retraction (*Ur*) is smaller. It can also be seen that the residual deformation after the end of the cycle is higher in the aged. *Uv*, delayed distension; Ue, immediate distension

city yields significantly lower numbrs in the aged person (0.311 vs 0.471; old vs young). Similarly, but less pronounced in this example, are the effects in the extension phase, in which the viscoelastic portion increased slightly over the elastic part. The uncorrected results of skin elasticity measurements with respect to anatomic region and age for a load of 200 mbar are summarized in Table 4. All parameters tended to be increased in the elderly at most anatomic regions. Since the increase in extensibility with increasing age is at least partly due to atrophy of the skin in this group, we also calculated the parameters that describe the elasticity of the skin independent of skin thickness. Here we found that the viscoelastic to elastic ratio (Uv/Ue) was increased with increasing loads and tended to be higher in the aged group for almost all anatomic sites. Age differences were specially apparent when medium loads were applied (Table 5, Fig. 4). The ratios as a function of load for the dorsal and volar forearm are illustrated in Fig. 5.

The biologic elasticity (Ur/Uf) increased with increasing loads in both age groups. It was generally lower in the aged group at all anatomic sites (Table 6, Fig. 6). The ratios as a function of load for the dorsal and volar forearm are illustrated in Fig. 7.

However, regardless of the load applied, no significant differences (data not shown) were noted between the sexes for either ratio for most body regions.

Table 4. Parameters of skin elasticity measurements at load 200 mbar (modified from) [11]

	Ue		Uv		Ur		Uf	
Region	Young	Old	Young	Old	Young	Old	Young	Old
Forehead	0.28±0.05	0.43±0.06*	0.12±0.02	0.23±0.05*	0.29±0.06	0.38±0.07	0.40±0.07	0.66±0.10*
Post auricular	0.57±0.10	0.94±0.17*	0.23±0.03	0.42±0.06*	0.63±0.12	0.93±0.20	0.80±0.13	1.36±0.19*
Upper arm	0.33±0.08	0.61±0.08*	0.10±0.02	0.27±0.03*	0.39±0.09	0.73±0.09*	0.43±0.09	0.87±0.10*
Volar forearm	0.14±0.02	0.47±0.08*	0.05±0.01	0.24±0.04*	0.16±0.02	0.56±0.11*	0.19±0.03	0.72±0.11*
Dorsal forearm	0.11±0.02	0.19±0.04	0.03±0.01	0.11±0.03*	0.11±0.02	0.20±0.06	0.15±0.02	0.31±0.07*
Palm	0.06±0.01	0.08±0.01*	0.03±0.00	0.04±0.01*	0.05±0.01	0.06±0.01	0.09±0.01	0.12±0.02
Abdomen	0.68±0.14	0.30±0.05*	0.17±0.02	0.15±0.04	0.77±0.15	0.39±0.08*	0.85±0.15	0.45±0.08*
Tigh	0.16±0.02	0.30±0.04*	0.04±0.00	0.12±0.02*	0.17±0.02	0.32±0.06*	0.20±0.02	0.37±0.05*
Ankle	0.09±0.01	0.25±0.01*	0.03±0.01	0.02±0.00	0.09±0.02	0.04±0.01*	0.13±0.02	0.07±0.01*
Upper back	0.24±0.02	0.27±0.04	0.09±0.01	0.18±0.04*	0.29±0.03	0.32±0.06	0.33±0.03	0.44±0.07
Lower back	0.23±0.04	0.35±0.06	0.07±0.01	0.17±0.03*	0.26±0.04	0.40±0.07	0.30±0.04	0.51±0.08*

Ue, immediate distension; Uv, delayed distension; Ur, immediate retraction; and Uf, final deformation.
* statistically significant difference ($p \leq 0.05$) between the age groups (Student's t-test).
A 5 s application of load (200 mbar) was applied followed by a 5 s relaxation period.
Generally, parameters were noted to be increased in the aged group at all anatomic regions except for the abdomen and ankle.
mean ± S.E.M; n = 13–16 volunteers.

Discussion

In our present youth-oriented society with a growing population of elderly, much attention has been focused on cutaneous aging. In this study, using a simple, noninvasive, suction device, we compared in vivo skin elasticity between two age groups. Although comparison between the age groups with respect to skin thickness is not provided for our data correlate well with earlier studies on the dorsal forearm by Leveque et al [20]. Correcting their data for skin thickness, the authors reported variations of the intrinsic

Table 5. Viscoelastic proportion of the total distension (Uv/Ue) at different loads (modified from [11]

Region	Load (mbar)	**Young**	**Old**
	500	0.56 ± 0.07	0.61 ± 0.07
Forehead	200	0.51 ± 0.06	0.52 ± 0.07
	100	0.50 ± 0.08	0.59 ± 0.08
	500	0.49 ± 0.07	0.46 ± 0.07
Postauricular	200	0.47 ± 0.05	0.56 ± 0.06
	100	0.49 ± 0.03	0.60 ± 0.05
	500	0.43 ± 0.05	0.42 ± 0.05
Upper arm	200	0.33 ± 0.03	0.48 ± 0.04*
	100	0.26 ± 0.02	0.38 ± 0.05*
	500	0.59 ± 0.02	0.55 ± 0.05
Volar forearm	200	0.36 ± 0.02	0.53 ± 0.04*
	100	0.31 ± 0.04	0.39 ± 0.04
	500	0.46 ± 0.04	0.64 ± 0.05*
Dorsal forearm	200	0.34 ± 0.06	0.50 ± 0.06
	100	0.30 ± 0.04	0.35 ± 0.04
	500	0.49 ± 0.05	0.53 ± 0.04
Palm	200	0.41 ± 0.03	0.46 ± 0.05
	100	0.60 ± 0.13	0.63 ± 0.11
	500	0.27 ± 0.04	0.49 ± 0.07*
Abdomen	200	0.30 ± 0.03	0.47 ± 0.04*
	100	0.26 ± 0.02	0.33 ± 0.04
	500	0.34 ± 0.02	0.44 ± 0.03
Thigh	200	0.26 ± 0.04	0.44 ± 0.03
	100	0.40 ± 0.08	0.41 ± 0.06
	500	0.42 ± 0.04	0.52 ± 0.05
Ankle	200	0.34 ± 0.04	0.39 ± 0.04
	100	0.44 ± 0.03	0.52 ± 0.05
	500	0.50 ± 0.03	0.65 ± 0.06*
Upper back	200	0.37 ± 0.03	0.61 ± 0.04*
	100	0.32 ± 0.03	0.41 ± 0.04
	500	0.38 ± 0.03	0.54 ± 0.06*
Lower back	200	0.33 ± 0.04	0.49 ± 0.07
	100	0.35 ± 0.11	0.38 ± 0.09

* Statistically significant difference ($p \leq 0.05$) between the age groups.
Means ± S.E.M.; n = 13–16 volunteers.
Uv/Ue increased with increasing loads and tended to be higher in the aged group. Age differences were especially apparent when high loads were applied.

skin extensibility in relation to age with a minimum at age 45 for men, when skin thickness reached a maximum; for women, results were approximately similar 10 years earlier [20].

To compare between subjects and anatomic regions, we calculated two relative parameters of skin elasticity independent of skin thickness: the viscoelastic to elastic ratio of the total extension process (Uv/Ue) and Ur/Uf, as a measure of the biologic elasticity of the skin. The viscoelastic properties are thought to be dependent on alterations in the equilibrium of the "ground substance" of the dermis [12]; the content of glycosamino-

Table 6. Elasticity (Ur/Uf) at different loads (modified from [11]

Region	Load (mbar)	**Young**	**Old**
Forehead	500	0.72 ± 0.04	0.66 ± 0.05
	200	0.68 ± 0.05	0.61 ± 0.06
	100	0.64 ± 0.04	0.53 ± 0.06
Postauricular	500	0.76 ± 0.04	0.65 ± 0.06
	200	0.73 ± 0.03	0.66 ± 0.06
	100	0.65 ± 0.05	0.60 ± 0.05
Upper arm	500	0.92 ± 0.01	0.84 ± 0.04
	200	0.90 ± 0.01	0.83 ± 0.02*
	100	0.85 ± 0.02	0.78 ± 0.03
Volar forearm	500	0.88 ± 0.02	0.77 ± 0.03*
	200	0.81 ± 0.03	0.75 ± 0.03
	100	0.72 ± 0.04	0.67 ± 0.03
Dorsal forearm	500	0.77 ± 0.05	0.64 ± 0.04*
	200	0.72 ± 0.05	0.58 ± 0.04*
	100	0.74 ± 0.04	0.48 ± 0.04*
Palm	500	0.66 ± 0.03	0.53 ± 0.02*
	200	0.60 ± 0.03	0.45 ± 0.02*
	100	0.53 ± 0.03	0.45 ± 0.02*
Abdomen	500	0.91 ± 0.02	0.87 ± 0.03
	200	0.91 ± 0.01	0.83 ± 0.03*
	100	0.87 ± 0.02	0.77 ± 0.03*
Thigh	500	0.92± 0.01	0.88 ± 0.03
	200	0.83 ± 0.04	0.85 ± 0.02
	100	0.82 ± 0.02	0.79 ± 0.03
Ankle	500	0.78 ± 0.02	0.62 ± 0.02*
	200	0.71 ± 0.04	0.59 ± 0.03*
	100	0.65 ± 0.04	0.52 ± 0.03*
Upper back	500	0.91 ± 0.02	0.81 ± 0.02*
	200	0.78 ± 0.06	0.71 ± 0.04
	100	0.75 ± 0.04	0.66 ± 0.03
Lower back	500	0.90 ± 0.02	0.86 ± 0.04
	200	0.88 ± 0.01	0.76 ± 0.05*
	100	0.8 ± 0.03	0.73 ± 0.04

* Statistically significant difference ($p \leq 0.05$) between the age groups.
Means ± S.E.M.; n = 13–16 volunteers.
Ur/Uf tended to increase with increasing load in both age groups and was generally lower in the aged than in the young group.

glycans or soluble collagen may be related to viscosity, decreasing with maturation and age [33]. Ur/Uf is correlated with the function of the elastic fiber network [14]. The increased Uv/Ue and decreased Ur/Uf values with aging observed in this study are in agreement with earlier reports [1, 14, 20, 24]. There is, however, variability dependent on the load or pressure. No significant differences between young and old skin were observed on the forehead and postauricular region, although values show a general tendency for increased Uv/Ue and decreased Ur/Uf with aging, similar to the other body regions. Note that in comparing visibly apparent aged skin of the face character-

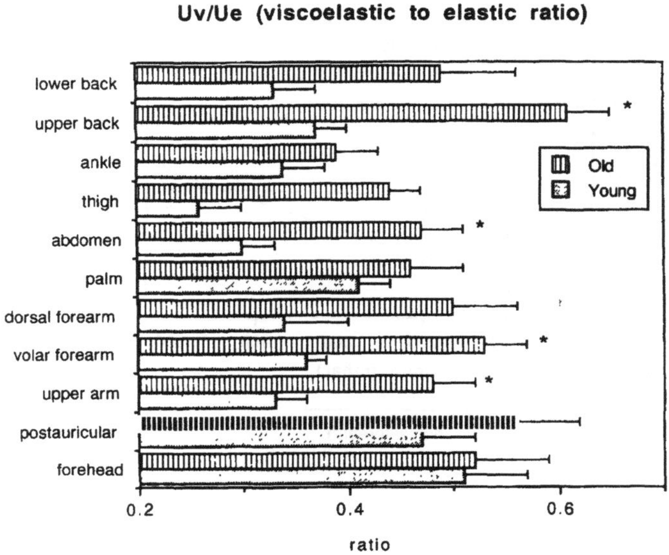

Fig. 4. Viscoelastic to elastic ratio (Uv/Ue) after 200 mbar load for 5 s followed by a 5 s relaxation period at 11 different anatomic sites. Means ± SEM; $n = 13–16$ volunteers; *asterisk*, statistically significantly different ($p \leq 0.05$)

ized as having fine and coarse wrinkling and sagging, with young skin, the difference in the measurements are not dramatic. This may be due to the fact that our "young" group consisted of young adults who already underwent significant photoaging of the elastic fiber network in the face.

As aforementioned, the overall mechanical properties of the skin depend mainly on the dermal and hypodermal collagen and elastic fiber network embedded in a viscous ground matrix, with some contribution from the epidermis. Pierard [22] clearly elucidated this complex interaction in his analogic model for a normal dermis, consisting of a variable number of elements in parallel representing different networks of fibers in the dermis, their properties varying according with three successive phases of extension of the tissue. Elements represent single collagen fibers, thick collagen bundles, elastic fibers, and the interfascicular substances such as proteoglycans. Diseases such as cutis laxa, corticosteroid-induced atrophy, pseudoxanthoma elasticum, Ehlers-Danlos syndrome, and scleromyxedema were characterized employing both the ability of the skin to be elongated (skin extensibility) and its biologic elasticity [22].

Age-related changes in the collagen fiber network are variable but the average collagen fiber bundle is reportedly smaller with increasing age and the total amount of collagen is reduced [29]. Earlier studies suggested that glycosaminoglycan/proteoglycan complexes, which are responsible for hydration of the dermis through their water-binding capacity, may be altered in cutaneous aging; concentration of uronic acid increased with age in sun-exposed areas whereas a decrease was suggested in sun-protected skin [18]. Thus, it was conceived that reduced proteoglycan/hyaluronic acid concentrations could lead to loss of dermal hydration contributing to the aged appearance of skin [31].

Recently, Fazio et al. presented several lines of evidences suggesting that changes in the mechanical properties of the skin accompanying cutaneous aging result from

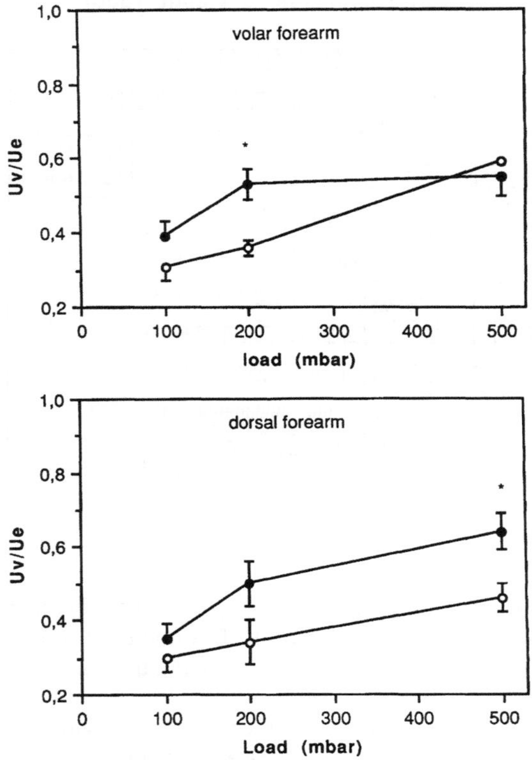

Fig. 5. Influence of load on viscoelastic to elastic ratio (Uv/Ue) on the volar and dorsal forearm in young (*open circles*) and aged (*closed circles*) volunteers. Means ± S.E.M.; $n = 13-16$ volunteers; *asterisk*, statistically significantly different ($p \leq 0.05$)

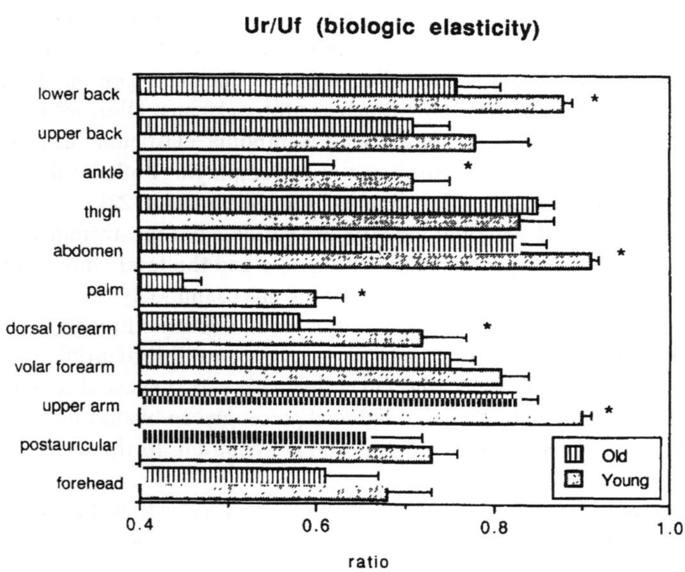

Fig. 6. Biologic elasticity (Ur/Uf) after 200 mbar load for 5 s followed by a 5 s relaxation period at 11 different anatomic sites. Means ± SEM; $n = 13-16$ volunteers; *asterisk*, statistically significantly different ($p \leq 0.05$)

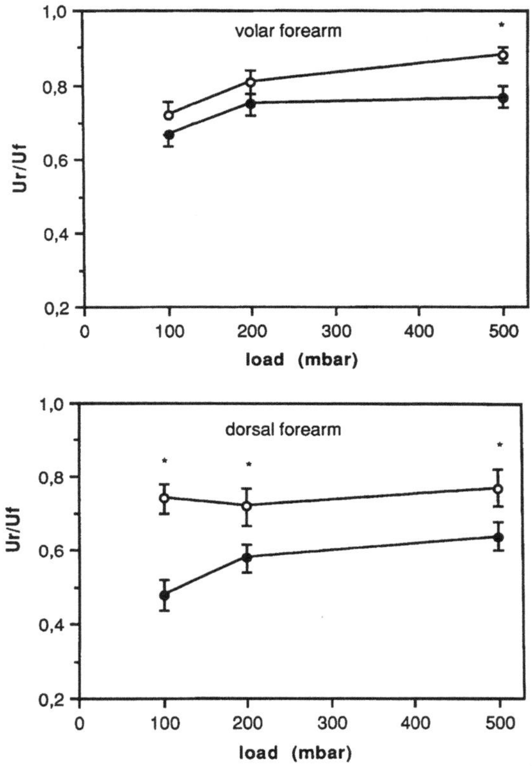

Fig. 7. Influence of load on Ur/Uf on the volar and dorsal forearm in young (*open circles*) and aged (*closed circles*) volunteers: Means +S.E.M.; $n = 13-16$ volunteers; *asterisk*, statistically significantly different ($p \leq 0.05$)

altered elastic fibers [16]. Histopathologic and electron microscopy studies showed that elastic fibers were composed of at least two distinct proteins: elastin and the microfibrillar component, oxytalan and elaunic fibers [16]. Oxytalan fibers have more abundant microfibrils with some elastin while elaunic fibers have a greater proportion of elastin to microfibrils. Balin et al. [4] summarized the changes in elastic fibers with innate aging as: (a) disappearance of subepidermal oxytalan fibers and abnormalities in elaunin and elastic fibers in 30–50 year olds, (b) absence of oxytalan fibers in the papillary dermis, progressive abnormalities in elaunin and elastic fibers, cystic spaces within the elastin matrix in 50–70 year olds, and (c) larger cystic spaces in elastin matrix, presence of lacunae separating microfibrils, thinner elastic core, and clumping of dense microfibrillar areas in individuals age 70 and older. These findings are congruent with those obtained by Bouissou et al. [7]. The consequences of these elastic fiber changes explain mechanical alterations in the skin manifesting as looseness and sagging, poor and delayed recoil following stretching, and fine wrinkling [16].

Lastly, instrinsic aging must be distinguished from photoaging whose mechanisms are biologically, biochemically, and molecularly distinct from each other. Sun damage to elastic fibers is characterized by coarse wrinkling and furrowing, loose and lethery skin largely due to solar elastosis, and reduced elasticity [16]. Histopathologically, a narrow zone of densely packed collagen underlies the dermoepidermal junction and the microfibrillar and elastin network is disrupted by the appearance of fine, amorphous, granular, elastotic materials and accumulation of glycosaminoglycans [7, 31]. In sun-exposed skin, changes due to sun and innate aging are superimposed. Organization of the elastic fiber network is disrupted beyond the extent seen with innate aging alone [29].

In conclusion, precluding invasive techniques such as the biopsy, mechanical properties of the skin can be evaluated using simple bioengineering methods such as the suction device used in this study. The described procedure provides a simple quantitative assessment of elastic properties of the skin. Its use may help in future investigations of connective tissue disorders and in the evaluation of therapeutic approaches or documentation of efficacy of vehicles, cosmetics, and of active compunds.

Acknowledgements The authors thank Courage and Khazaka (Cologne, Federal Republic of Germany) and Aca Derm, Menlo Park, CA. for providing the suction device.

References

1. Agache P, Monneur C, Leveque JL, de Rigal J (1980) Mechanical properties and Young's modulus of human skin in vivo. Arch Dermatol Res 269: 221–232
2. Alexander H, Cook T (1977) Variations with age in the mechanical properties of human skin in vivo. In: Kenedi RM et al. (eds), Bedsore biomechanics. William, London, pp 109–118
3. Baker MR, Bader DL, Hopewell JW (1988) An apparatus for testing of mechanical properties of skin in vivo: its application to the assessment of normal and irradiated pig skin. Bioeng Skin 4: 87–103
4. Balin AK, Pratt LA (1989) Physiological consequences of human skin aging. Cutis 43: 431–436
5. Beradesca E, Borroni G, Gabba P, Borlone R, Rabbiosi G (1985) Evidence for elastic changes in aged skin revealed in an in vivo extensometric study at low loads. Bioeng. Skin 2: 261–270
6. Bjerring P (1985) Skin elasticity measured by dynamic admittance. A new technique for mechanical measurements in patients with scleroderma. Acta Derm Venereol Suppl (Stockh) 120: 83–87
7. Bouissou H, Pieraggi M, Julian M, Savit T (1988) The elastic tissue of the skin: a comparison of spontaneous and actinic (solar) aging. Int J Dermatol 27 5: 327–335
8. Bramont C, Vasselet R, Rochefort A, Agache P (1988) Mechanical properties of the skin in Marfan's syndrome and Ehlers-Danlos syndrome. Bioeng Skin 4: 217–227
9. Burlin TE, Hutton WC, Eng C, Ranu HS (1977) A method of in vivo measurement of the elastic properties of skin in radiotherapy patients. J Invest Dermatol 69: 321–323
10. Christensen MS, Hargens CW, Nacht S, Gans EH (1977) Viscoelastic properties of intact human skin: instrumentation, hydration effects, and the contribution of the stratum corneum. J Invest Dermatol 69: 282–286
11. Cua AB, Wilhelm KP, Maibach HI (1990) Elastic properties of human skin: relation to age, sex and anatomical region. Arch Dermatol Res 282: 283–288
12. Daly CH, Odland GF (1979) Age-related changes in the mechanical properties of human skin. J Invest Dermatol 73: 84–87
13. de Rigal J, Leveque JL (1985) In vivo measurement of the stratum corneum elasticity. Bioeng Skin 1: 13–23
14. Elsner P, Wilhelm D, Maibach HI (1990) Mechanical properties of human vulvar skin. Br J Dermatol 122: 607–614
15. Escoffier C, de Rigal J, Rochefort A, Vasselet R, Leveque JD, Agache P (1989) Age related mechanical properties of human skin. An in vivo study. J Invest Dermatol 93: 353–357.

16. Fazio MJ, Olsen DR, Uitto JJ (1989) Skin aging: lessons from cutis laxa and elastoderma. Cutis 43: 437–444
17. Jagtman BA (1983) Clinical investigation of skin elasticity. An in vivo study of patients with varicose veins and certain connective tissue disorders. Thesis, Nijmegen pp 16–32
18. Johnston KJ, Oikarinen A, Lowne NJ (1985) Ultraviolet-induced connective tissue changes in the skin: models for actinic damage and cutaneous aging. In: Maibach HI, Lowe NT (eds) Models in dermatology, vol 1. Karger, New York, pp 69–76
19. Leveque JL (1987) In vivo methods for measuring the viscoelastic properties of the skin. Bioeng Skin 3: 375–382
20. Leveque JL, de Rigal J, Agache PG, Monneur C (1980) Influence of ageing on the in vivo extensibility of human skin at a low stress. Arch Dermatol Res 269: 127–135
21. Pearce RH, Grimmer J (1972) Age and the chemical constitution of normal human dermis. J Invest Dermatol 58 6: 347–361
22. Piérard GE (1989) A critical approach to in vivo mechanical testing of the skin. In Leveque TL (ed) Cutaneous investigation in health and disease. Dekker, New York, pp 215–240
23. Piérard GE (1989) Histological and rheological grading of cutaneous sclerosis in scleroderma. Dermatologica 179: 18–20
24. Piérard GE, Lapiere CM (1977) Physiopathological variations in the mechanical properties of skin. Arch Dermatol Res 260: 231–239
25. Sato S (1988) A suction method for measuring dermal extensibility and contractility. In: Kligman AM, Takase Y (eds) Cutaneous aging. University of Tokyo Press, Tokyo pp 501–508
26. Serban G, Edelberg R, Garcia M, Hambridge A (1986) Intraepidermal sweat levels and the viscoelastic properties of human skin. Bioeng Skin 2 2: 134
27. Serup J (1986) Localized scleroderma (Morphea): in vivo measurement of skin elasticity. Acta Derm Venereol Suppl (Stockh) 122: 18–23
28. Serup J, Northeved A (1985) Skin elasticity in psoriasis. J Dermatol 12: 318–324
29. Smith LS (1989) Histopathologic characteristics and ultrastructure of aging skin. Cutis 43: 414–424
30. Tosti A, Compagno G, Fazzini ML; Villardita S (1977) A ballistometer for the study of the plastoelastic properties of skin. J Invest Dermatol 69: 315–317
31. Uitto JJ, Fazio MJ, Olsen DR (1989) Molecular mechanisms of cutaneous aging. J Am Acad Dermatol 21: 614–622
32. Uitto J, Oikarinen A, Thody AJ (1986) Mechanical and physical functions of the skin. In: Thody AT (ed) Scientific basis of dermatology. A physiological approach. Churchill Livingstone Edinburgh, pp 7–25
33. Vogel HG (1985) Age dependence of viscoelastic properties in rat skin; directional variations in relaxation experiments. Bioeng Skin 1 2: 157–173
34. Vogel HG (1987) Age dependence of mechanical and biochemical properties of human skin: II. Stress-strain experiments, skin thickness and biochemical analysis. Bioeng Skin 3: 67–91
35. Vogel HG (1981) Directional variations of mechanical parameters in rat skin depending on maturation and age. J Invest Dermatol 76: 493–497
36. Vogel HG (1974) Correlation between tensile strength and treatment. Connect Tissue Res 2: 177–182
37. Vogel HG, Denkel K (1985) Influence of maturation and age, and of desmotropic compounds on the mechanical properties of rat skin in vivo. Bioeng Skin 1: 35–54
38. Zar JH (1974) Biostatistical analysis. Prentice-Hall, Englewood Cliffs

Ultrasound – An Update on Methodology and Application with Special References to Inflammatory Reactions

T. AGNER AND J. SERUP*

Introduction

Vasodilation and edema are the main features of inflammatory skin reactions. The clinical correlates are erythema, skin thickening, papules, and vesicles. In the past most research was directed toward assessment of the vascular reactions, and the edema formation was overlooked. Recently, high frequency ultrasound has become established as an accurate technique to measure skin thickness and skin thickening non-invasively. With this technique much research on the edema component of inflammatory skin reactions can be initiated.

Ultrasound scanning of normal skin and of a number of pathological conditions were recently outlined [1]. Our experiences are based on research and development of a technique and the necessary equipment over the last 10 years. Today, we use the Dermascan A for A-mode scanning (Fig. 1), and the Dermascan C for A, B, C, M-mode scanning (Fig. 2). Both machines are manufactured by Cortex Technology Aps (Hadsund, Denmark) from prototypes developed in our clinic.

One-dimensional ultrasound A-scan is used for quantification of skin thickness. No preconditioning of the subjects is necessary before measurement. In practice the measurement is easily performed. The probe head is held gently toward the skin, and the echoes are displayed on the screen (Fig. 3, upper half). The interval (ns) between the echo from the stratum corneum and the echo from the interface between the dermis and subcutaneous fat is a measure of the thickness of the skin (i.e., epidermis and dermis). The distance in millimeters can be calculated from the sound velocity in the tissue, known to be around 1580 m/s in skin. In most parts of the body a differentiation between epidermis and dermis is difficult; an exception is the palm. With ultrasound B-mode scanning a cross-sectional image of the skin and the tela subcutanea is obtained. With C-mode scanning a number of parallel images are obtained, and a skin lesion is evaluated in three dimensions. Twenty MHz transducers are generally preferred. With this frequency both the axial resolution and the scanning depth are acceptable for the assessment of most dermatological lesions. With high freqeuency, i.e., 50 MHz, the epidermis might be studied more in detail. However, with this frequency level the scanning depth is limited.

The dermis is in most body regions highly echogenic (Fig. 3). It is the regularly ordered fiber network which reflects ultrasound. Disturbances of the fiber network and its regular organization are normally followed by a decrease in reflectance. Thus, the

* Department of Dermatology A, Bispebjerg Hospital, 2400 Copenhagen, Denmark

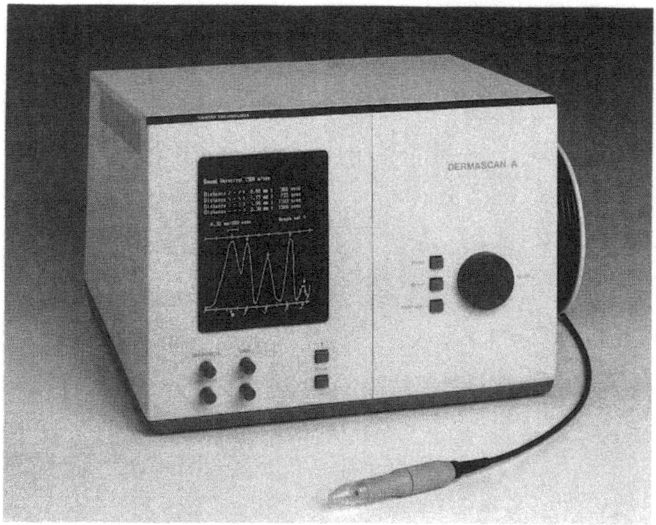

Fig. 1. Dermascan-A skin thickness measurer (20 MHz A-mode scanner).

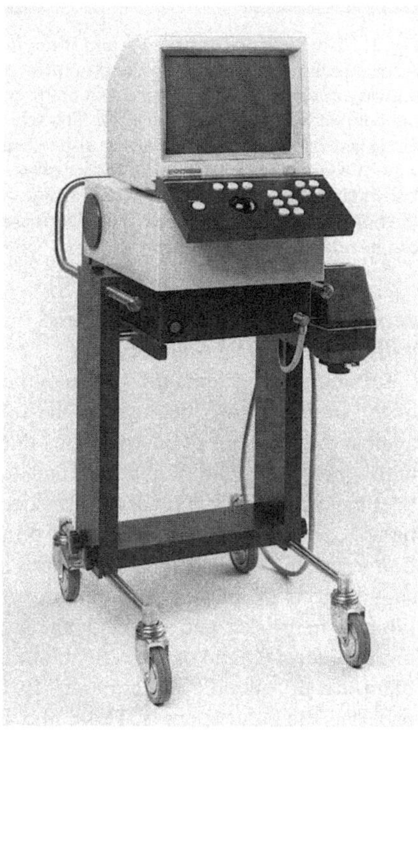

Fig. 2. Dermascan-C for A, B, C, M-mode scanning of the skin, tela subcutanea, and muscle fascia

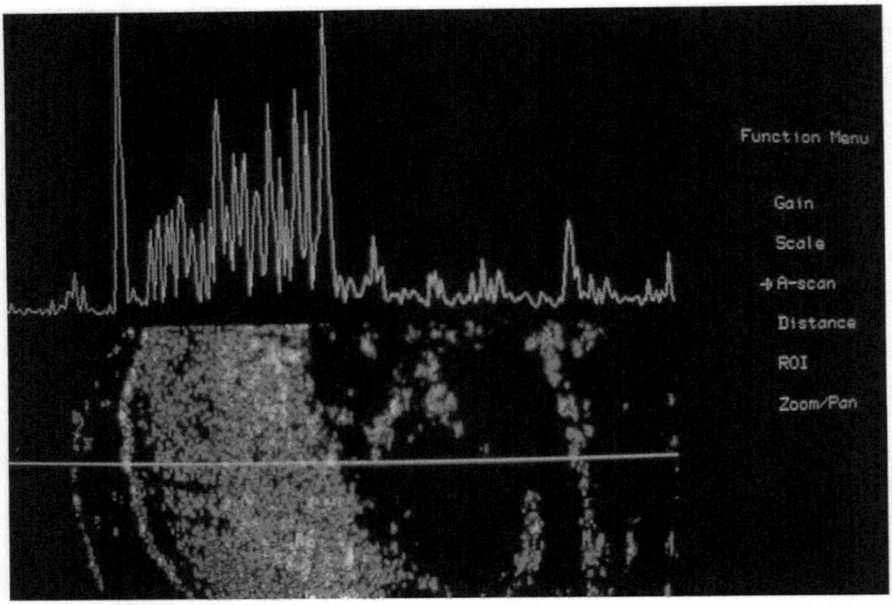

Fig. 3. A-mode scan (*upper half*) and B-mode san (*lower half*) of a + + allergic patch test reaction. A strong echo is reflected from the skin surface, followed by an echolucent zone in the outer dermis, seen as a *black band*. The internal part of the dermis shows quite strong reflections, originating from the connective tissue fiber network. The tela subcutanea is *black* and low reflectant. The muscle fascia is seen to the *right*. For in vivo distance measurement the A-scanner is used. The more precise way to measure skin thickness is to outline the cross-sectional area of the dermis block and, knowing the lateral extension of the scan (22.4 mm), the average thickness is easily calculated. With the built-in computer facilities of the Dermascan-C, the echographic structure of the dermis block can be analyzed.

dermis structure function as a kind of natural contrast medium in which different pathologies may be outlined.

Inflammatory edema formation in the skin will depend on the character and degree of the initial process, its level in the skin, and the mechanical resistance of the skin against the pressure of edema. The adult skin is mechanically a two-layered structure with a more soft and pliable papillar dermis and a more tense reticular dermis. This becomes more prominent as the skin becomes older. In aged skin a characteristic "age-band" corresponding to the papillar dermis is seen [2]. This alteration may explain the fine wrinkling of aged skin. It is in this space of decreased mechanical resistance that suggillations propagate. Inflammatory edema has the same tendency to propagate laterally in the skin and especially to distend the papillar dermis. On ultrasound images a subepidermal band of low reflectance is seen (Fig. 3, 4, 5). This phenomenon and this band are nonspecific in character. In contact dermatitis, atopic dermatitis, and in psoriasis the band appears. There may also be edema formation and distension of the reticular dermis, however, except for occasional vertical cracks through the dermis in advanced edema, such as allergic patch test reactions, ultrasound imaging of inflammatory edema of the deeper parts of the dermis reveals no special pattern.

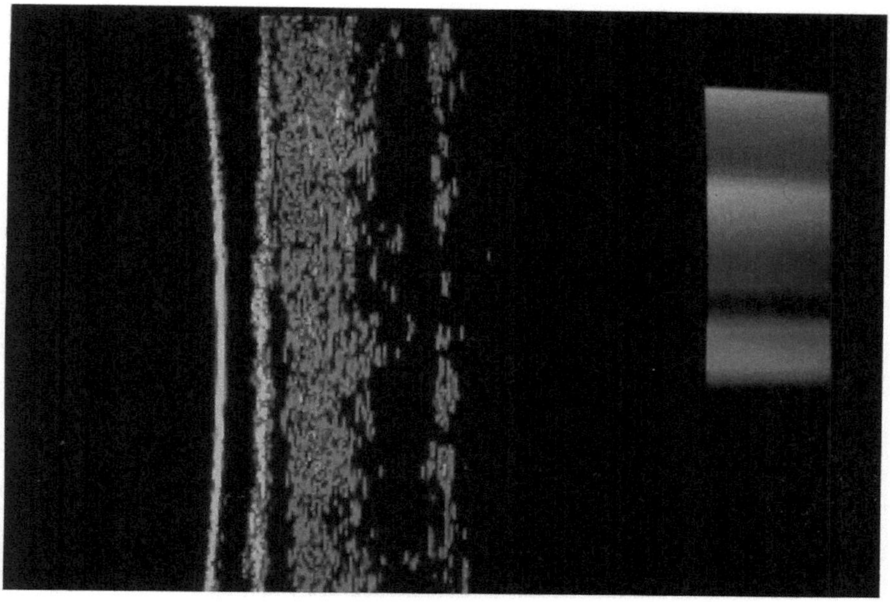

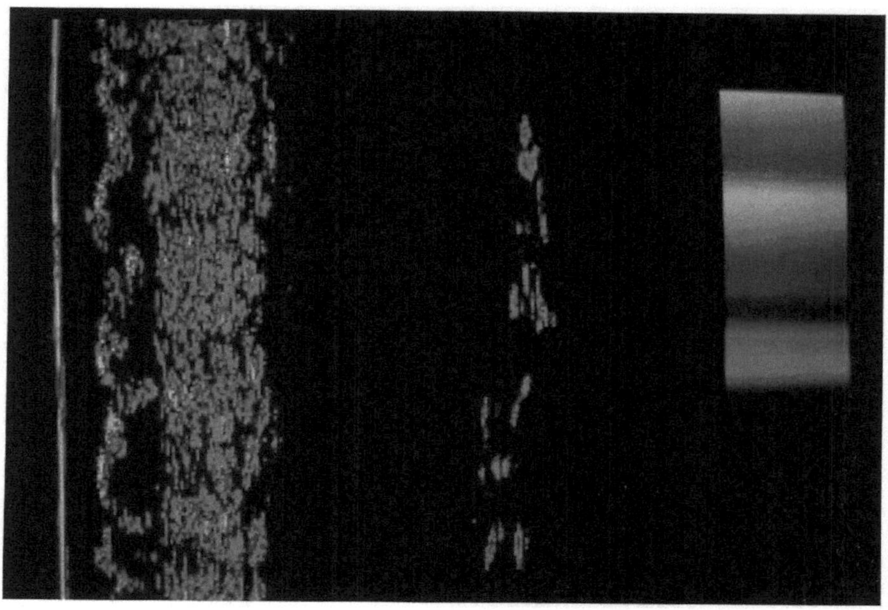

Figs. 4 a–b. Atopic dermatitis. **a** Slightly involved skin with an echolucent band appearing in the *lower half* of the image corresponding to the papillar dermis. To the *left* a membrane holding the coupling medium (water) of the probe is seen. To the *right* the tela subcutanea and the muscle fascia are seen. *Blue* represents a strong ultrasound reflection; *yellow* and *red*, a reflection of moderate strength, and *green* and *light blue*, a weak reflection. **b** Skin heavily afflicted with dermatitis and clinically with lichenification, which is seen as a regular folding of the epidermal surface. The inflammatory band underneath corresponds to the papillar dermis. In contrast the reticular dermis is straight.

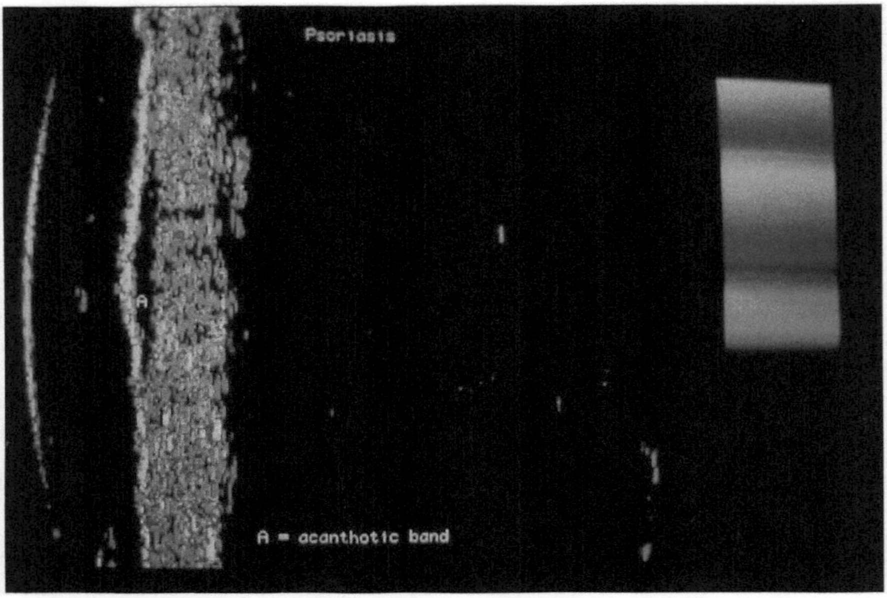

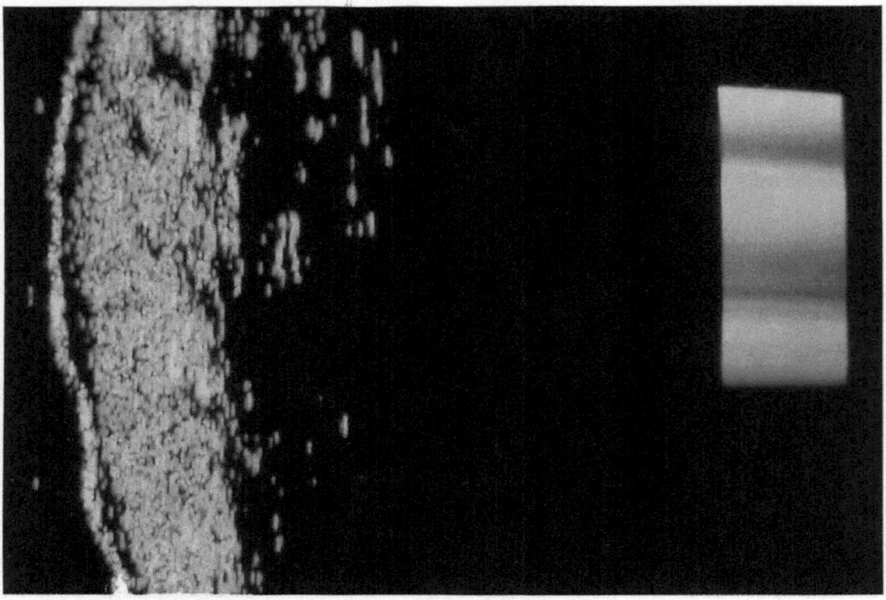

Figs. 5 a–c. Psoriasis vulgaris with subepidermal echolucent band. **a** A patient with a mild affection. **b** A patient with a more severe affection. **c** A patient with pustular psoriasis with the same type of echographic findings, however, in this case more focal.

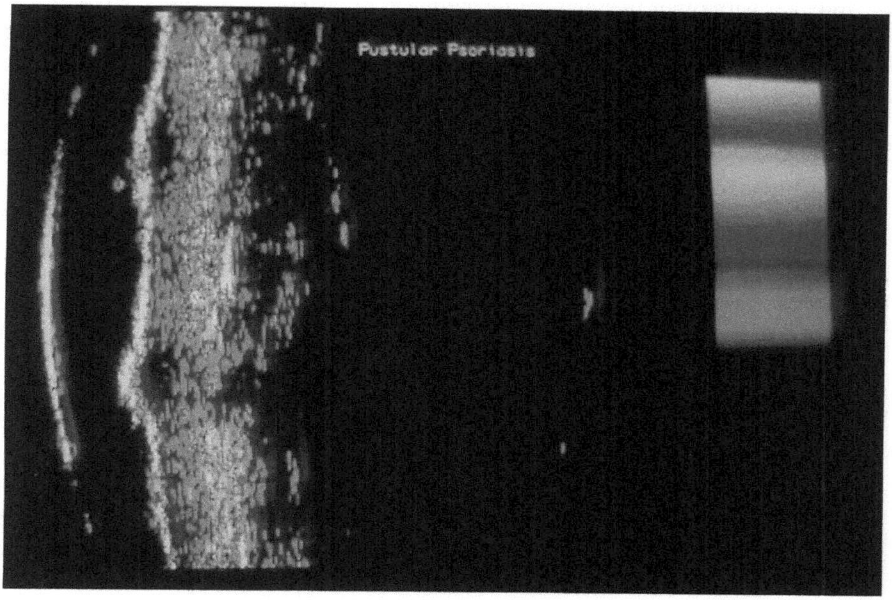

Fig. 5c

A-scan for Quantification of Edema

When the skin is exposed to injury, either chemical or physical, an inflammatory response occurs, including edema formation. The strength of the inflammatory response appears as an increase in skin thickness and can thus be parametrically quantified by ultrasound A-scan. The edema formation leads to a zone with very few and low echoes, while the interface between dermis and subcutis still gives rise to a distinct echo.

Several studies have proved the usefulness of ultrasound A-scan for objective measurement and parametric quantification of edema formation when applied to inflammatory reactions [2–4].

Studying allergic patch test reactions, ultrasound was found suitable for quantification of both doubtful as well as positive patch test reactions [3]. Good separation between (+), +, and + + reactions was obtained by measurements of the absolute difference in skin thickness [3]. Brazier and Shaw [5], however, in 1986 studied 34 positive allergic patch test reactions and found that they could not differentiate (+) and + reactions from the normal skin. In that study, the Cutech dermal depth detector was used, and the authors state that a main drawback with this instrument is difficult in reading the cathode ray oscilloscope. This might explain the authors misfortune in differentiating between different grades of reactions. In another study of both allergic and irritant patch tests [4], using nickel sulfate, nickel chloride, and sodium lauryl sulfat (SLS), the edema was found to be greater in allergic than in irritant reactions that were similar in strength according to the clinical reading [4].

Together with other bioengineering methods, ultrasound was used to study the influence of different irritants on the skin [5]. SLS, nonanoic acid, and hydrochloric acid were applied to the skin, and a different time phase for the maximum inflammatory response of the skin was found [5]. the usefulness of ultrasound was also proved in a study considering the purity of different quality grades of SLS [7]. The inflammatory responses were examined by measurements of edema formation [7], and the products could be graded with regard to irritancy.

Quantification of the DMSO (dimethylsulfoxide) response used for determination of the sensitivity of the skin, is also possible by ultrasound [8], thus improving the objectivity of the test.

The reproducibility of ultrasound A-scan measurements on both normal and inflamed skin was recently investigated [9]. The coefficient of variation was 2.2% and 2.4% for measurement on normal and on SLS exposed skin, respectively [9].

In a recent study the sensitivity of ultrasound A-scan for quantification of SLS induced skin damage was compared to other bioengineering methods, i.e., measurement of transepidermal water loss (TEWL), laser Doppler flowmetry and colorimetry. The sensitivity of ultrasound in this study was found to be consistently better than that of colorimetry and almost as high as measurement of TEWL [10]. Compared to other bioengineering methods used for quantification of inflammation, ultrasound has the advantage that no preconditioning of the subjects is necessary before measurement. Modest changes in ambient temperature, relative humidity, air convection, and emotional status will not influence edema, which is a structural parameter. The main drawback of the method is that a certain amount of experience is needed from the examiner before a high reproducibility of measurements can be obtained.

Inflammatory Edema – A-mode Scanning versus B, C-mode Scanning

The interface between the dermis and the tela subcutanea is far from flat. Variation of the biology itself limits precise thickness measurements. However, if three or more sites are examined and averaged, the reproducibility of ultrasound A-mode skin thickness measurement is high, the coefficient of variation being 2%–4% [11]. As mentioned, some training in A-mode scanning and interface interpretation is needed.

With B, C-mode scanning the A-mode scan line can be chosen guided by the cross-sectional image, and there is no risk of misinterpretation of interfaces. However, measurements based on selection of scan lines from an image carries the risk of observer bias. Problems of scan line selection may be overcome if the contour of the edematous process or tissue block is outlined by the ROI (region of interest) function and the cross-sectional area calculated. From the area a mean thickening based on a maximum of 224 A-mode lines covering a 22.4 mm lateral scanning field can be calculated by the use of the Dermascan C-mode scanner. Today this is probably the more accurate way of measuring skin thickness, since biologic variation in the dermis/subcutaneous fat interface is overcome.

In choosing of a method the cost of equipment is a factor. It is our experience that, with proper training, averaged, triple site, A-mode ultrasound measurement of inflammatory edema is highly accurate, and this more cheap method will suffice in the vast majority of studies, when quantification of inflammatory edema is the intention.

Inflammatory Edema Ultrasound vs Histology

Ultrasound does not have the resolution of histology; inflammatory cells can not be visualized. Nonetheless, during the preparation of biopsy samples water is extracted from the samples and replaced by lipophilic media and later paraffin. Thus, processing is highly intrusive to the interstitial water and to tissue edema, which is only visible under these conditions if it has caused major and more persistent alterations of tissue organization and structure. This is normally not the case in acute edema. Ultrasound does not affect interstitial water or change the true in vivo dimensions. Thus, with respect to interstitial water and edema, ultrasound examination is purely nonintrusive.

A punch biopsy typically 4 mm in diameter will only sample an area of topical alteration from, for example, a positive patch test reaction. With ultrasound a number of sites of an inflammatory process may be examined. With the C-mode scanner a tissue block 22.4 mm x 22.4 mm laterally is imaged, and the process may be evaluated systematically without leaving a scar.

Other Applications of Ultrasound in Dermatology

Increased skin thickness due to increased connective tissue was studied at an early stage in the development of dermatological ultrasonography. In systemic sclerosis and in localized scleroderma the skin thickening may be up to three times the thickness of unaffected skin [12, 13]. Ultrasound is useful to monitor the development of scleroderma and the effects of therapy. The same anatomic site may be followed over years, and several sites may be studied. In localized scleroderma the sclerosis spontaneously turns into thinning and pigmentation resembling Pacini-Pierini atrophy. This stage of thinning can be assessed by ultrasound. Also, corticosteroid atrophy and atrophy following radiotherapy may be evaluated [14].

Skin tumors are a natural field of ultrasound examination. Due to its noninvasiveness ultrasound should have a potential as a preoperative diagnostic technique, which may improve both the strategy and quality of surgery. Tumors such as basal cell carcinoma, malignant melanoma, seborrheic keratoses and Kaposis sarcoma have been evaluated by ultrasound. In melanoma and dysplastic nevi much research has to be done before the value of ultrasound examination can be determined. In tumor evaluation ultrasound cannot replace histology.

Another area which has quite recently been the subject of ultrasound A-scan studies is the nail plate. The structure of the human nail plate was described using a 20 MHz ultrasound scanner [15], and two cmpartments were identified: a superficial dry compartment with an ultrasound velocity of 3103 m/s, and a deep humid compartment with an ultrasound velocity at 2125 m/s [15]. No significant correlation was found between nailplate thickness and measurement of transonychial water loss [16]. The nail is, from a scientific point of view, a relatively neglected area. Perhaps the possibility to elucidate the internal nail structure by noninvasive methods will help to correct this matter.

Ultrasound Examination as a Basis for Advanced Image Analysis of the Skin

The numbers of scientific papers in the field of dermatology dealing with digital imaging and various techniques of recording including ultrasound are increasing exponentially [17]. Recently advanced software technology for the analysis of images became available. The Dermascan C already has built-in facilities for image analysis. Based on examination of Figures 3–5, much information is to be expected from a more detailed analysis of the echographic structure of the dermis. Seidenary et al. recently described how allergic patch test reactions can be quantified with such a technique [18, 19]. Although just introduced, it is already obvious that advanced image analysis based on ultrasound examination is a powerful future tool for the objective assessment of inflammatory lesions of the skin.

References

1. Serup J (1992) Ten years of experience with high frequency ultrasound examination of the skin: development and refinement of technique and equipment. In: Ultrasound Altmeyer P, Hoffmann K, el Gammal S (eds), Ultrasound in dermatology. Springer, Berlin, Heidelberg New York, pp 41–54
2. de Rigal J, Escoffier C, Querleux B, Faivre B, Agache P, Leveque JL (1989) Assessment of ageing of the human skin in vivo. J Invest Dermatol 93: 621–625
3. Serup J (1984) Diameter, thickness, area and volume of skin-prick histamine weals, Allergy 39: 359–364
4. Serup J, Staberg B, Klemp P (1984) Quantification of cutaneous edema in patch test reactions by measurement of skin thickness with high-frequency pulsed ultrasound. Contact Dermatitis 10: 88–93
5. Brazier S, Shaw S (1986) High-frequency ultrasound measurement of patch test reactions. Contact Dermatitis 15: 199–201
6. Serup J, Staberg B (1987) Ultrasound for assessment of allergic patch test reactions. Contact Dermatitis 17: 80–84
7. Agner T, Serup J (1989) Skin reaction to irritants assessed by non-invasive bioengineering methods. Contact Dermatitis 20: 352–359
8. Agner T, Serup J (1989) Different skin irritation abilities of different qualities of sodium lauryl sulphate. Contact Dermatitis 21: 184–189
9. Agner T, Serup J (1989) Quantification of the DMSO-response – a test for assessment of sensitive skin. Clin Exp Dermatol 14: 214–217
10. Agner T, Serup J (1990) Sodium lauryl sulphate for irritant patch testing – a dose-response study using bioengineering methods for determination of skin irritation. J Invest Dermatol 95: 543–547
11. Agner T, Serup J (1990) Individual and instrumental variations in irritant patch-test reactions – clinical evaluation and quantification by bioengineering methods. Clin Exp Dermatol 15: 29–33
12. Serup J (1984) Quantification of acrosclerosis: measurement of skin thickness and skin-phalanx distance in females with 15 MHz pulsed ultrasound. Acta Derm Venereol (Stockh) 64: 35–40
13. Serup J (1984) Localized scleroderma (morphoea): thickness of sclerotic plaques as measured by 15 MHz pulsed ultrasound. Acta Derm Venereol (Stockh) 64: 214–219
14. Serup J, Holm IP, Stender IM; Pichard J (1987) Skin atrophy and telangiectasia after topical corticosteroids as measured noninvasively with high frequency ultrasound, evaporimetry and laser Doppler flowmetry. Methodological aspects including evaluations of regional differences. Bioeng Skin 3: 43–58

15. Jemec GBE, Serup J (1989) Ultrasound structure of the human nail plate. Arch Dermatol 125: 643–646
16. Jemec GBE, Agner T, Serup J (1989) Transonychial water loss: relation to sex, age and nail plate thickness. Br J Dermatol 121: 443–446
17. Perednia DA (1991) What dermatologists should know about digital imaging. J Am Acad Dermatol 25: 89–108
18. Seidenary S, di Nardo A, Pepe P, Gianetti A (1991) Ultrasound B-scanning with image analysis for assessment of allergic patch test reactions. Contact Dermatitis 24: 216–222
19. Seidenary S, di Nardo A (1992) Cutaneous reactivity to allergens at 24-h increases from the antecubical fossa to the wrist: an echographic evaluation by means of a new image analysis system. Contact Dermatitis 26: 171–176.

Biophysical Techniques for the Evaluation of Skin Protective Creams

P. J. Frosch, A. Kurte, and B. Pilz*

Introduction

Irritant contact dermatitis is a major problem in occupational dermatology. While acute severe irritant reactions due to caustic chemicals have become relatively rare, an equally serious danger arises from moderate and low level irritants producing a cumulative insult type contact dermatitis after weeks or months of exposure. Chronic irritant contact dermatitis is very frequent in hairdressers, health care personnel, food handlers, construction workers, and employees of the metal industry [7]. While gloves and other protective garments are regularly worn when severely irritating substances such as concentrated acids or alkalis are handled, this is usually not the case with low level irritants. In many professions it is impossible to wear gloves because of the loss of dexterity. Furthermore, many workers develop a dyshidrotic eczema due to the continuous occlusion when wearing gloves.

This is the basis for the development of so called "barrier creams" against chemical irritants. The term "skin protective creams" seems to be more appropriate since most creams do not provide a real barrier, at least not comparable to the stratum corneum which is a superb shield against noxious environmental agents. The literature in the field of skin protective creams (SPCs) is extremely confusing. There are a few enthusiastic reports but the majority come to the conclusion that the effect in practice is questionable or nonexistent. The subject has been reviewed by Ummenhofer [21] two monographs provide further information [5, 19].

Standardized techniques exist for the evaluation of various dermatological therapeutics (e.g., corticosteroids, topical antibiotics, and sunscreens). These models have proven extremely useful in comparing various commercial products and in developing new more effective drugs [14]. In contrast no generally accepted model for the quantification of SPC efficacy exists. In reviewing the literature we were surprised that most authors used a single and rather high concentration of the irritant; furthermore most of the previous investigators applied the irritant under occlusion for several hours. Even most glove materials cannot resist the penetration of low molecular weight chemicals [6, 16, 18]. Therefore one cannot be surprised that in these investigations most SPCs failed to show any protective effect [2–4, 12, 13, 15, 22].

Based on the literature and on our own experience in the field of cutaneous irritancy we developed therefore two new test models: a guinea pig method and a technique

* Department of Dermatology, Städtische Kliniken Dortmund and University of Witten/Herdecke, Beurhausstraße 40, 4600 Dortmund, Germany

using human subjects. The common pertinent features are (a) repetitive daily exposure of the irritant at a low dose, (b) total irritant exposure for 2 weeks, (c) use of various standard irritants (sodium lauryl sulfate, sodium hydroxide, toluene). As the clinical scoring of erythema will always have a subjective component, we wanted to apply modern noninvasive biophysical techniques in order to measure the degree of inflammation caused by the irritant. Our experiments have been published in detail elsewhere [8–10]. This contribution will summarize the findings and concentrate on the value of the applied biophysical methods.

The Repetitive Irritation Test in the Guinea Pig

Materials and Methods

Young albino guinea pigs weighing 300 to 400 g are used. The skin of the back is clipped and shaved over an area of approximately 7 x 10 cm. The SPC to be evaluated is applied to the skin in a measured amount with a polyethylene glove-covered index finger (ointment 0.03 ml/cm^2). After 2h the irritant is applied with a gauze pad saturated by a solution of the irritant. For the detergent sodium lauryl sulfate (SLS) at a concentration of 5% in water is applied to the skin for 30 min. The alkali sodium hydroxide (NaOH) is used at a concentration of 0.5% (w/v) and the application time is 2 min. The organic solvent toluene (T) is dissolved in ethanol at 20% and applied daily for 2 min as well.

On day 5, after 4 days of exposure, the resulting irritant reaction is evaluated using several parameters. Another exposure follows immediately after the assessment. After an exposure–free interval of 2 days over the weekend the daily exposure to the SPC and the irritant is continued in the second week from Monday until Thursday. Final readings and measurements of irritation are taken on Friday (12th day of experiment and after nine exposures).

Evaluation of the Irritant Response

Three parameters were selected to evaluate the irritant response:

1. *Clinical scoring:* The intensity of the reaction is scored as follows: 0, none; 1+, slight; 2+, moderate; 3+, severe with epidermal defects.
2. *Blood flow volume:* BFV is measured on the basis of the laser–Doppler velocimetry using a Periflux apparatus (Perimed KB, Stockholm). Details of the method are described elsewhere [1] and in other chapters of this book.
3. *Transepidermal water loss:* TEWL was measured by evaporimetry, initially using an EP 1 (Servomed, Stockholm) and later on with a Tewameter (Courage and Khazaka, Cologne), according to the recently published guidelines [17].

Measurements for TEWL and BFV are taken on normal skin before exposure to the irritant, providing a baseline value of nonirritated skin. On irritated skin a minimum of two measurements are taken, one from each side of the back. If there is a marked deviation, the measurements are repeated on another area and the mean is taken as the final value of that recording.

Skin Protective Creams

Three protective creams were chosen:

1. Stokoderm Salbe (Stockhausen, Krefeld, FRG). Oil in water emulsion containing stearate, lanolin, and eucoriol as active ingredients. Eucoriol is a tanning agent and consists chemically of sodium–bis–chlorophenyl sulfamine. Recommended use: Universal protection against various irritants at work, particularly against organic solvents.
2. Contra alkali Creme (Basotherm, Biberach/Riss, FRG). Oil in water emulsion with an agent that is supposed to bind alkali ions and liberate hydrogen ions, thus restoring the normal pH of the skin. Recommended use: "Special cream for the prevention of the skin damage induced by alkalis and solvents."
3. Marly Skin (Quinta, Merzhausen, FRG). Biphasic formulation (lipophilic and hydrophilic) containing stearic acid and dimethylpolysiloxane (lipophilic groups) as well as propylene glycol, glycerol and sorbitol (hydrophilic groups) and a propellant gas producing a creamy foam. According to the manufacturer it is supposed to be effective against various chemically aggressive substances, particularly acids, alkalis, detergents, irritating body secretions such as blood and urine, and even against allergens. A twice daily application is considered to be sufficient due to 4 h lasting protection.

Results

The results are shown in Figs. 1–3. The product Stokoderm was effective in reducing the SLS-induced erythema, BFV, and TEWL. The differences in the Stokoderm group in comparison to the control group were significant regarding all test parameters. In contrast, Contra Alkali failed to suppress the irritation completely.

Sodium hydroxide cause only very little visible irritation in the control group due to the low concentration used. The product Contra Alkali caused a remarkable aggravation of the skin damage. There was marked erythema in all animals accompanied by large scales and fissure. BFV and TEWL were also markedly elevated. The differences were significant in week 2 and week 1 (data not shown). The product Stokoderm did not enhance the skin damage caused by NaOH. The very slight trend to do so was not

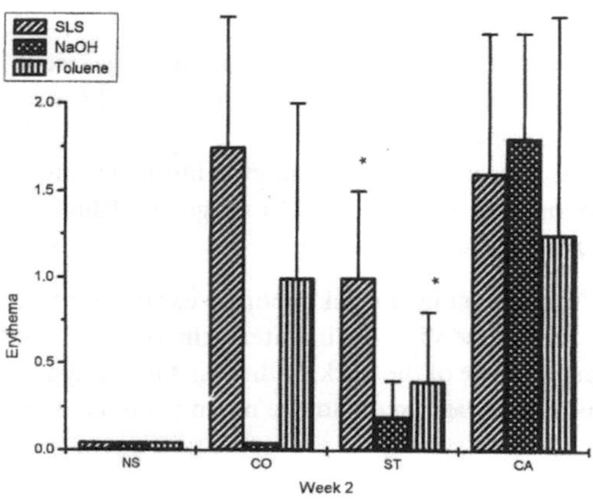

Fig. 1. The effect of two barrier creams: Stokoderm Salbe (*ST*) and Contra Alkali Creme (*CA*) in the guinea pig model after 2 weeks of treatment with three irritants (sodium lauryl sulfate, *SLS*; sodium hydroxide, *NaOH*; toluene). *CO*, control animals; *NS*, normal skin (untreated). Shown are the data of the clinical parameter erythema (score: 0 to 3+). Significant differences from control animals and barrier cream treated animals are indicated by * ($p < 0.05$)

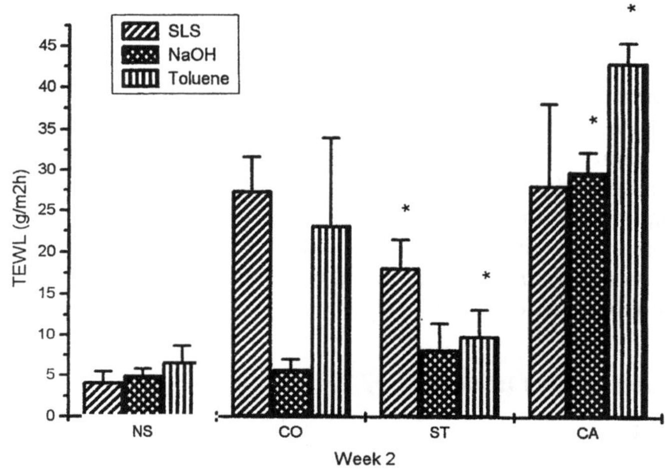

Fig. 2. Test results obtained from measurements of transepidermal water loss (TEWL). For further details, see Fig. 1 legend

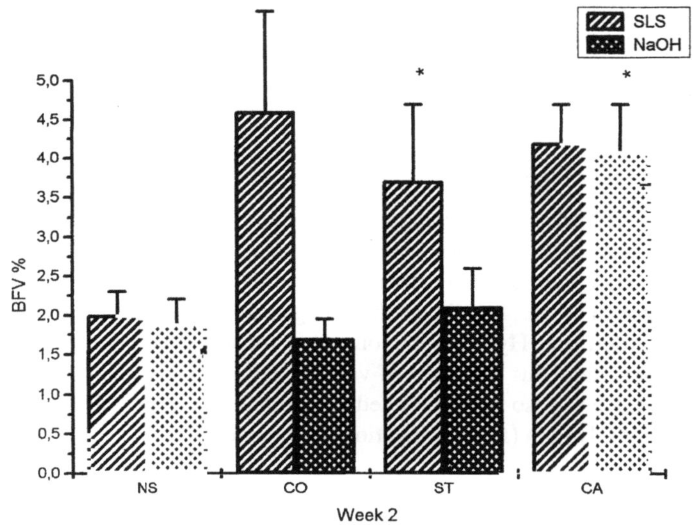

Fig. 3. Test results obtained from measurements of blood flow volume (*BFV*). For further details, see Fig. 1 legend (BFV not measured for toluene)

significant. The data shown in Fig. 2 are pooled from two experimental groups, five animals each. The experiment was repeated in order to rule out an experimental error. The organic solvent Tol produced an erythema of slight to moderate degree in all animals. TEWL in the control group was markedly elevated. Stokoderm was capable of suppressing the irritant response regarding all three test parameters in a significant way. Contra Alkali failed to do so – the TEWL was nearly twofold over the control and the difference obtained significance.

In another experiment the product Marly Skin was evaluated [9]. Marly Skin was unable to reduce the irritation due to SLS and Tol. Erythema, BFV, and TEWL were significantly higher than in the not pretreated control group (differences significant for all parameters in week 2).

The Repetitive Irritation Test in Humans

Materials and Methods

The method has been described in detail elsewhere [8]. Briefly, the test is performed on healthy volunteers. A test panel for the evaluation of one product consists of a minimum of ten subjects. The irritant is applied to the volar aspect of the forearm using glass cylinders of 2.5 cm diameter. Aqueous solutions of SLS (1%, 5%, and 10%) are pipetted into the cylinders and left in place for 30 min. The SPC is applied to one forearm 30 min before contact with SLS. The other forearm receives SLS only and serves as control. The exposures are repeated in the first week five times and in the second week four times.

Assessment of Irritation

Cutaneous irritation is evaluated as described above. In this experiment colorimetry was also performed using a Minolta Chroma Meter CR-100 (Minolta, Osaka). The *La** value (red-green axis) was considered to be the most reliable one for erythema quantification [23]. Scoring and measurement with biophysical techniques were performed on the 1st, 5th, and 12th day of the experiment after the subject had adapted to room conditions for 20 min.

Evaluated Products

The following two protective skin creams were evaluated:
1. Taktosan Salbe (Stockhausen, Krefeld, FRG). Water in oil emulsion with eucoriol as active ingredient. Further constituents: water, petrolatum, mineral oil, ozokerite, glycerol oleate, lanolin alcohol, magnesium sulfate, fragrance and bronopol. Recommended use: Hydrophobic ointment for work with water miscible oils and cooling fluids, aqueous solutions of various nature, acids, alkalis, salts, cement, chalk and fertilizers. Also recommended as an emollient against dry and fissured skin.
2. Marly Skin (for specifications see above).

Results

There was a clear dose-response relationship regarding the score for erythema and the concentration of SLS. Differences between day 5 and day 12 were significant for 5% and 10% SLS (Fig. 4a). The results of TEWL measurements are shown in Fig. 4b. Compared to the baseline values on day 0 the increase of TEWL was already significant on day 5 for 5% and 10% SLS. BFV also showed a good dose-response relationship – the differences were significant for the 12th day in comparison to the baseline values (Fig. 4c). The chromameter *La** values showed the highest variation on day 0 before the application of the irritants. They increased slightly in the first week and markedly in the second week at the two highest concentrations of SLS. Only for 5% and 10% SLS the differences in La* values were significant (Fig. 4d).

Taktosan reduced the irritation caused by SLS; this effect was clearly visible in markedly reduced erythema scores on day 5 and 12 (Fig. 5a). Significance was obtained

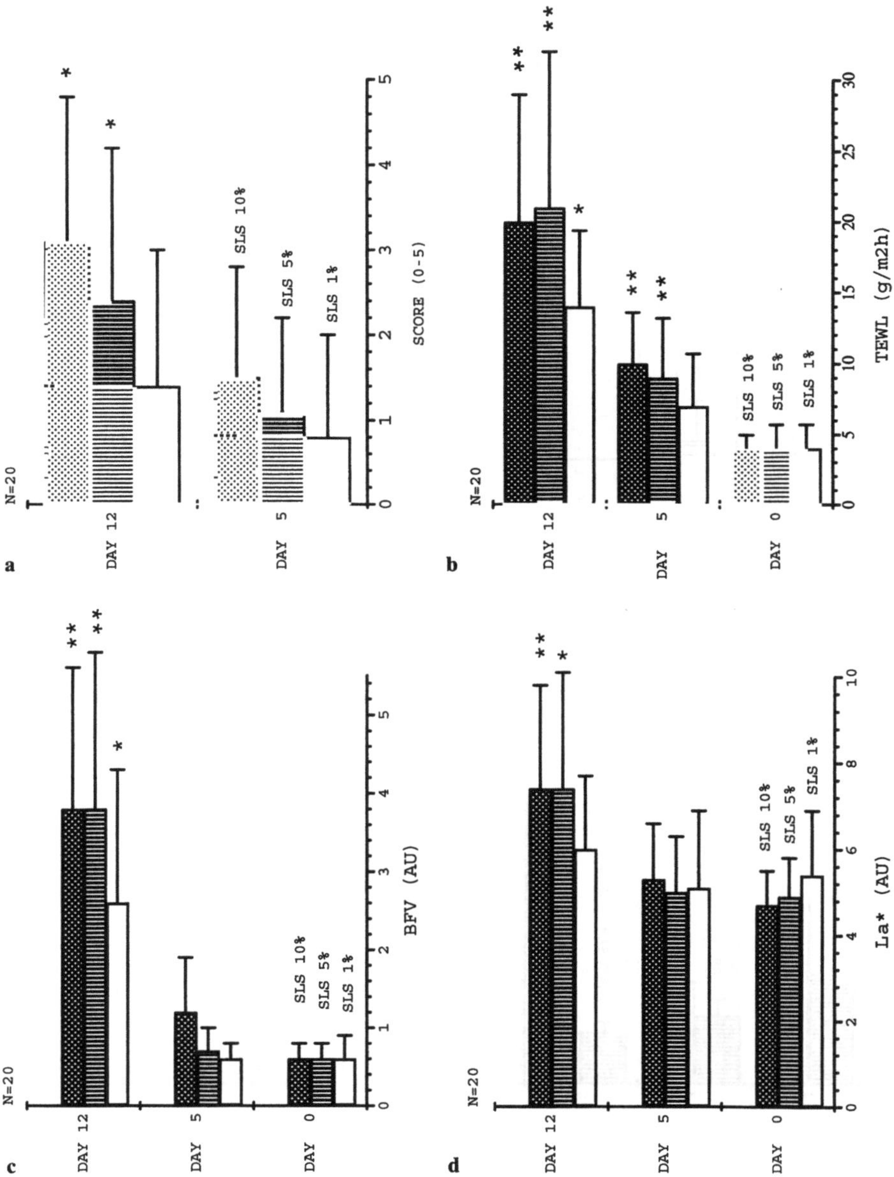

Figs. 4a–d. Dose-response relationship with sodium lauryl sulfate (SLS) and various test parameters. Mean values of 20 subjects. **a** Score for erythema; **b** TEWL (transepidermal water loss); **c** BFV (blood flow volume, arbitrary units, AU); **d** *La**skin color reflectance values

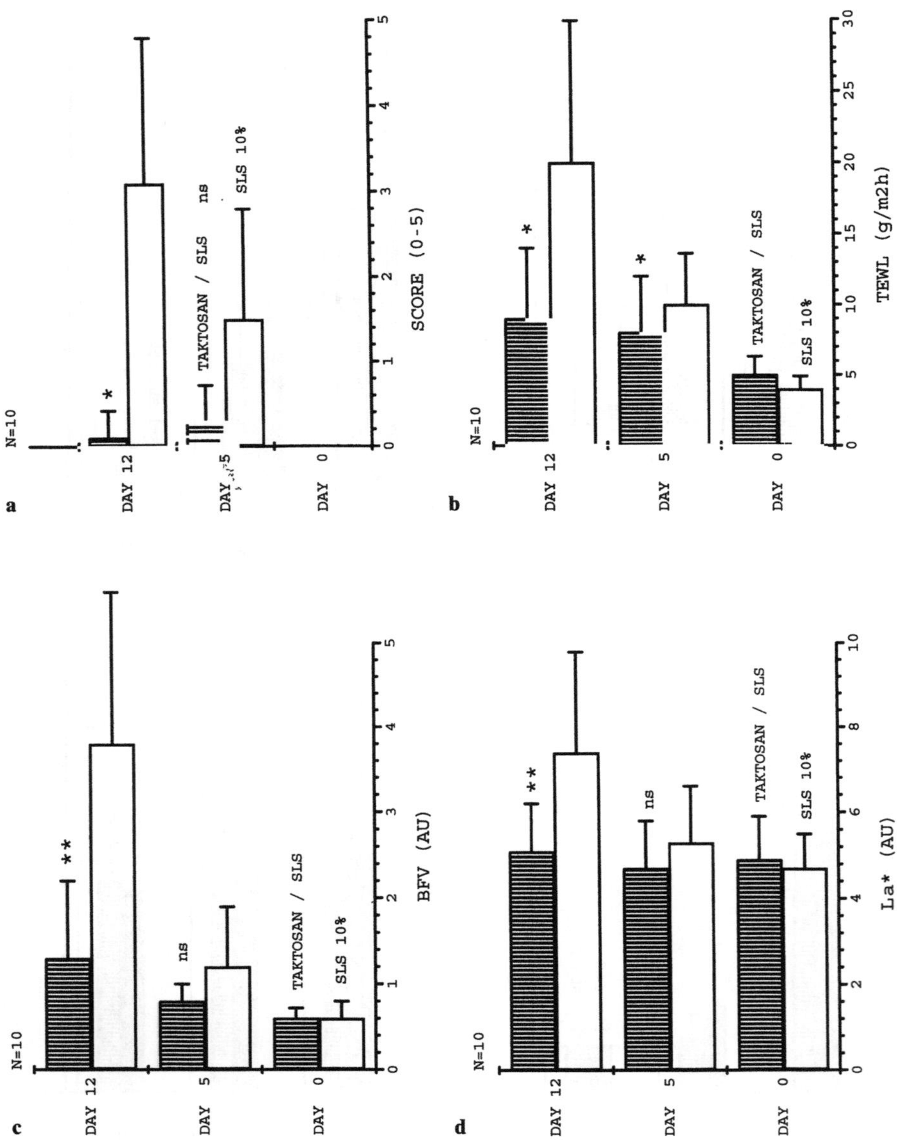

Figs. 5a–d. The effect of pretreatment with Taktosan Salbe on the irritation due to 10% sodium lauryl sulfate (*SLS*). Test parameters **a–d** as in Fig. 4. Statistical differences in comparison to the control indicated by * ($p < 0{,}05$) to *** ($p < 0.001$); *ns*, not significant

only for the 12th day. TEWL was significantly lower on the Taktosan pretreated side, both on day 5 and day 12 regarding the highest concentration of SLS (Fig. 5b). Measurements of BFV and skin color revealed significant differences on day 12 (Fig. 5c, d).

The results were similar for the lower concentration of SLS (data not shown). For Taktosan the erythema scores, TEWL, and BFV values were significantly lower on day 12 (no significance on day 5) in comparison to the SLS control. The *La** values for 1% and 5% SLS plus Taktosan were lower on days 5 and 12 but failed to reach statistical significance at both time periods in comparison to the control.

In contrast, Marly skin was unable to inhibit the irritation due to SLS. Scores for erythema and measured values for TEWL, BFV, and *La** were slightly lower but altogether failed statistical significance. This was also true for the lower concentrations of SLS.

Discussion

In these models we have provided evidence that some SPCs, such as Stokoderm Salbe and Taktosan Salbe, are effective in reducing the inflammation due to various irritants. In contrast, other products such as Contra Alkali and Marly Skin were not effective against the used irritants. To our surprise these products even aggravated the response to sodium hydroxide. Thus, under certain circumstances some so-called barrier creams may even be harmful.

There is little information on the mechanisms of action of SPCs. The frequently quoted general rule is that water in oil emulsions are effective against aqueous solutions of irritants and oil in water emulsions are effective against lipophilic materials. We have shown that there are exceptions to this rule. In the guinea pig model the oil in water emulsion Stokoderm Salbe was extremely effective against an aqueous solution of the detergent SLS. We attribute this action not only to the vehicle, but also to the tanning agent Eucoriol. Komp [11] could demonstrate a dose-dependent effect of this agent on human skin in a repetitive occlusive chamber test.

The paradoxical aggravating effect observed with two commercial SPCs may be explained by an interaction of the irritant with the ingredients of the SPC. Marly Skin contains a relatively high concentration of stearic acid. The subsequent exposure to sodium hydroxide will form sodium stearate, which is a soap and an irritant by itself.

The experiments show that clinically visible irritation can be quantified by biophysical techniques. Measurements of TEWL seem to be of great value in particular. With SLS this parameter showed the greatest differentiating power, revealing statistical significance at lower concentrations of the irritant and at an earlier time period of the experiment than the other parameters. Subclinical irritation is well recognized by measurement of TEWL. This holds true at least for surface active irritants which damage the stratum corneum barrier [20].

The measurement of BFV correlated well with the clinical scores of erythema. The *La** values obtained by colorimetry seem to have less differentiating potential then TEWL when assessing irritants such as SLS. This may be different when irritants are evaluated which produce intense fiery erythema already at low concentrations (e.g., tretinoin, anthralin).

In summary, noninvasive biophysical techniques are extremely valuable in quantifying the inflammatory response to various irritants when SPCs are to be evaluated. The described models might be very useful in developing new active ingredients.

Furthermore, various aspects for the optimal use of SPCs can be studied: application time before exposure to irritant, concentration and best vehicle for the active ingredient, specificity of the protective agent against a series of chemically different irritants, and optimal treatment regimens for the irritant–free exposure interval necessary to repair the stratum corneum barrier.

References

1. Berardesca E, Maibach HI (1988) Bioengineering and the patch test. Contact Dermatitis 18: 3–9
2. Boman A, Wahlberg JE, Johansson G (1982) A method for the study of the effect of barrier creams and protective gloves on the percutaneous absorption of solvents. Dermatologica 164: 157–160
3. Burckhardt W (1947) Neuere Untersuchungen über die Alkalieempfindlichkeit der Haut. Dermatologica 94: 73–85
4. Carrié C (1955) Zur Wirksamkeit von Hautschutzsalben. Hautarzt 6: 363–365
5. Dicke W, Mehlem P (1987) Alles über Hautschutz, Hautreinigung, Hautpflege. Wirtschaftsverlag, Bremerhaven
6. Estlander T, Jolanki R (1988) How to protect the hands. Dermatol Clin 6: 105–114
7. Frosch PJ (1922) Cutaneous irritation. In: Textbook of contact dermatitis. Rycroft RJG, Menné T, Frosch PJ, Benezra C (eds), Springer, Berlin, Heidelberg, New York p. 28–61
8. Frosch PJ, Kurte A, Pilz B (1993) Evaluation of skin barrier creams: III. The repetitive irritation test (RIT) in humans. Contact Dermatitis (in press)
9. Frosch PJ, Schulze-Dirks A, Hoffmann M, Axthelm I (1993) Evaluation of skin barrier creams: II. Ineffectiveness of a popular "skin protector" against various irritants in the repetitive irritation test of the guinea pig. Contact Dermatitis (in press)
10. Frosch PJ, Schulze-Dirks A, Hoffmann M, Axthelm I, Kurte A (1922) Efficacy of skin barrier creams: I. The repetitive irritation test (RIT) in the guinea pig. Contact Dermatitis 28:94–100
11. Komp B (1985) Hautschutzsalben. Dermatosen 33: 20–26
12. Mahmoud G, Lachapelle JM (1985) Evaluation of the protective value of an antisolvent gel by laser Doppler flowmetry and histology. Contact Dermatitis 13: 14–19
13. Mahmoud G, Lachapelle JM, Van Nesté D (1984) Histological assessment of the skin damage by irritants: its possible use in the evaluation of a "barrier Cream". Contact Dermatitis 11: 179–185
14. Maibach HI, Lowe NJ (eds) (1987) Models in dermatology, vol 3. Karger, Basel
15. Malten KE, den Arend JACJ (1985) Irritant contact dermatitis. Traumiterative and cumulative impairment by cosmetics, climate and other daily loads. Dermatosen 33: 125
16. Mellström GA, Boman A (1992) Comparative evaluation of Permeation testing of protective gloves to solvents. Contact Dermatitis 26: 120–127
17. Pinnagoda J, Tupker RA, Agner T, Serup J (1990) Guidelines for transepidermal water loss measurement (TEWL). Contact Dermatitis 22: 164–178
18. Savalides A, Schultz T, Salce L (1990) The evaluation of gloves for protection against cosmetic ingredients. J Soc Cosmet Chem 41: 267–273
19. Tronnier H, Kresken J, Jablonski K, Komp B (1989) Haut und Beruf. Grosse, Berlin
20. Tupker RA, Pinnagoda J, Nater JP (1990) The transient and cumulative effect of sodium lauryl sulphate on the epidermal barrier assessed by transepidermal water loss: interindividual variation. Acta Derm Venereol (Stockh) 70: 1–5
21. Ummenhofer B (1982) Beruflicher Hautschutz , Dermatologische Probleme und Möglichkeiten. Zentrabl Haut Geschlechtskr 147: 287–297
22. Wahlberg JE (1971) Absorption-inhibiting effect of barrier creams. Berufsdermatosen 19: 37
23. Wilhelm KP, Maibach HI (1989) Skin color reflectance measurement for objective quantification of erythema in man. J Am Acad Dermatol 21: 574–576

Assessing Treatment of Psoriasis and Eczema by Noninvasive Methods

L. DUTEIL, C. QUEILLE-ROUSSEL, and J. CZERNIELEWSKI*

Introduction

The efficacy of treatments for inflammatory skin diseases such as psoriasis and eczema is currently assessed using clinical scoring systems based on a gradation of erythema, scaling, and infiltration. These clinical assessments, although easy and rapid to use, are never objective and seldom reproducible. Skin biopsies and other biological samples are very useful, but, since they are generally obtained by invasive methods, their use must remain exceptional.

Currently, several noninvasive biophysical techniques are available which allow an objective and quantitative assessment of the various components of lesioned skin. Information which is directly related to the physiological cutaneous parameters such as skin blood flow (SBF) or transepidermal water loss (TEWL) can be obtained with these techniques. Other less specific techniques provide quantitative data on the severity of a lesion, such as the surface extension of a psoriasis plaque or the thickness of edematous skin.

Psoriasis

Psoriasis is a common chronic skin disease which affects approximately 2% of the population. It is characterized by a hyperplastic epidermis with a thickened parakeratotic stratum corneum that gives rise to exfoliated silvery colored scales. The erythematous aspect of psoriatic plaques is caused dilated, elongated, coiled, and tortuous papillary capillary loops which come very close to the skin surface [1]. These drastic abnormalities lead to the modification of various parameters which can be assessed noninvasively and objectively with readily available biophysical methods. Some of these parameters can be used as markers, either to study the physiopathology of psoriasis, or to monitor treatment efficacy and safety and to compare the activity of different treatments. Typical values of such parameters recorded [2] at two untreated skin locations (forearm and legs and their respective uninvolved controls) are shown in Table 1.

* Centre International de Recherches Dermatologiques Galderma (cird Galderma), 635 Route des lucioles, Sophia Antipolis, 06565 Valbonne Cedex, France

Table 1: Psoriasis vulgaris biophysical pretreatment values (means ± S.D.)

	Forearm ($n = 10$)		Leg ($n = 8$)	
	Uninvolved	Involved	Uninvolved	Involved
SBF (V)	0.17 ± 0.1	1.39 ± 0.8	0.1 ± 0.05	0.95 ± 0.8
TEWL (g/m²/h)	5.2 ± 1.3	18.7 ± 11	7.6 ± 3.5	10.9 ± 5
$tcpO_2$ 37°C (mm Hg)	7.4 ± 4	38.8 ± 20	14.6 ± 9	49.7 ± 30
$tcpO_2$ 44°C (mm Hg)	67.5 ± 10	46.3 ± 5.5	61.9 ± 20	46.9 ± 24
tcp CO_2 44°C (mm Hg)	53 ± 7.8	57 ± 7	48.3 ± 5	53.2 ± 6

SBF, skin blood flow; TEWL, transepidermal water loss; $tcpO_2$, transcutaneous pressure of oxygen.

Microvascular changes play an essential role in the pathogenesis of psoriasis [3, 4]; the modification of the psoriatic capillaries seems to precede the other known histological and biochemical abnormalities in the psoriatic lesions. Nonetheless, psoriatic capillaries respond very early after the initiation of an antipsoriatic therapy. Therefore SBF and related parameters are choice markers to monitor antipsoriatic treatments.

Skin Blood Flow

Due to extensive modifications to the microcirculatory network SBF is greatly increased in psoriasis. Many methods have been utilized to measure cutaneous blood flow in psoriasis (see [5] for review). Quantitative data have been obtained [6–8] using the radioactive ^{133}Xe washout technique. The main disadvantage of this method is that it involves repetitive applications of radiotracer to the patient's skin. Using the ^{133}Xe washout method, Klemp and Staberg [6] found a mean cutaneous blood flow of 63.5 ± 9.0 ml $(100\text{g min})^{-1}$ in untreated psoriatic plaques on the forearm ($n = 20$ patients), which was significantly higher than the corresponding value on the contralateral nonaffected forearm, 11 ± 1.3 ml $(100\text{ g min})^{-1}$.

Laser Doppler velocimetry (LDV) [9] is presently the most widely used technique for measuring SBF. This noninvasive and objective method is easy to handle and can be used routinely to monitor antipsoriatic therapies. It is based on the principle of the optical Doppler shift: a laser light beam (red or infrared domain) is directed onto the skin by an optical fiber. The beam is scattered by both the mobile red blood cells and the fixed structures of the skin, down to a depth of 1–1.5 mm. A second fiber collects the backscattered light, of which a small fraction undergoes a shift in frequency (Doppler shift) caused by the flowing red blood cells (RBC). The size of the frequency shift is proportional to the velocity of the RBC. The shifted and unshifted beams are mixed onto the surface of a photodetector which produces a voltage. After electronic treatment of this voltage, the output signal is proportional to the number of RBC multiplied by their velocity, i.e., to the SBF. This method does not call for a complicated procedure such as tedious calibrations or curve fitting to extrapolate the

SBF value, but simply involves a single averaging of the real time SBF signal that has been recorded on a chart recorder or by means of a computer.

Table 2 summarizes some of the studies in which LDV has been used to investigate the antipsoriatic activity of different therapies. As can be seen in this table, the untreated psoriatic SBF is found to be 5 to 12.8 times higher than the SBF level measured in the uninvolved control skin. Figure 1 illustrates the evolution of the ratio involved/uninvolved SBF that we observed during PUVA bath therapy [10]. This ratio decreases progressively during the course of treatment. Depending on the therapy and on the severity of the investigated psoriasis, this ratio can be reduced to one third of its initial untreated value within either a few days or a few weeks of treatment. In general, and irrespective of the therapy, the response of SBF to treatment follows two phases: a rapid reduction to almost 50% of its initial value in the first few days (or the first week) of treatment and, thereafter, a somewhat slower decrease, falling to the uninvolved SBF level in a quasi linear manner. This difference in kinetics may be related to differences in response between superficial and deeper vessels. Indeed, psoriatic superficial capillaries are known to respond very early to treatment [11], 3–7 days prior to the normalization of the basal cell layer labeling index, and preceding clinical improvement.

Table 2. Laser Doppler velocimetry investigations in antipsoriatic therapies

Antipsoriatic therapy	Number of patients	Before treatment SBF involved/non-involved ratio	Time to decrease to 2/3 untreated value	Correlation with clinical score	Reference
Goekerman	6	5	5–8 days	Poor linearity	[15]
Goekerman	4	9	3–4 weeks	Good	[14]
or beech tar	4	9	3–4 weeks	Good	[14]
Ingram regimen with or without coal tar	11	7	1–2 weeks	Good	[12]
Costicosteroid					
with occlusion	10	N.D.	2 > days	Good	[13]
without occlusion			>7 days		
PUVA bath	10	9.7	4 weeks	Good	[10]
Beech tar	8	12.8	3 weeks	N.D.	[7]

SBF, skin blood flow; N.D., not determined.

LDV monitoring combined with other biophysical methods allows an objective comparison between treatments to be made in intraindividual clinical trials. For example, Frödin et al. [12], using two psoriatic lesions, one on each arm of the same patient and of comparable size, site, and clinical aspect, was able to conclude that the traditional addition of a coal tar bath in the Ingram regimen had no advantage over a single oil emulsion. Using a very similar method, Broby-Johansen and Kristensen [13] treated chronic plaques of psoriasis with a potent corticosteroid applied topically for 7 days, both with and without occlusion. The corticosteroid (clobetasol propionate) + occlusion (hydrocolloid dressing) had a very pronounced effect on all the measured

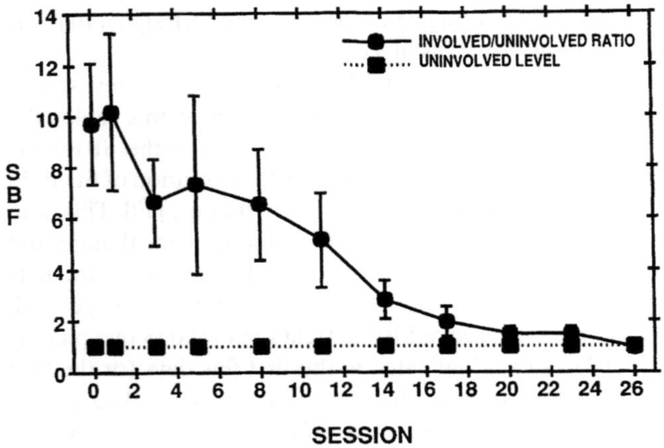

Fig. 1. Evolution of the ratio involved/uninvolved skin blood flow (SBF) during PUVA bath therapy (lesions are located on forearm; $n = 10$; mean ± SEM)

parameters which was apparent after 24 h, whereas the steroid alone was only marginally effective after 7 days. The authors concluded that this type of short course corticosteroid therapy appears harmless and relevant for clinical dermatology. Staberg and Klemp [14], comparing beech tar and Goekerman therapy in an interindividual study, detected no difference between the two treatments with respect to their effect on SBF.

Correlation between LDV readings and clinical scores of psoriasis is generally satisfactory (see Table 2). However, Kahn et al. [15], using a fine analysis performed on each subject separately, found no significant linear relationship between LDV values and clinical assessments under Goekerman therapy. In this study, throughout most of the treatment period, these two indices were in good agreement. The only striking difference was that SBF values diminished significantly faster than visual scores from days 4 to 8 inclusive ($p < 0.05$). These results, if confirmed, suggest that LDV measurements can provide advance knowledge of clinical improvement, an asset that may prove valuable in the design of topical chemotherapy and drug dosage.

Klemp and Staberg [7] reported SBF in involved psoriatic skin, as measured by ^{133}Xe washout, to be twice as high as at measured on similarly located skin of normal individuals ($n = 10$, $p < 0.0002$), whereas no statistical difference could be detected between LDV measurements in the same study. Moreover, other authors [15, 16] reporting on comparisons of SBF between healthy skin and uninvolved psoriatic skin using LDV have observed no significant differences. These discrepancies between LDV and^{133}Xe could be attributed either to a different level of investigation or to a methodological problem (probe positioning, duration of signal averaging, etc.). In addition, the ratio between uninvolved psoriatic and normal SBF depends on the state of activity of psoriasis: from a value of close to 2 in active psoriasis, it decreases to 1.4 in chronic stable psoriasis, and no statistical difference exists in patients with minimal psoriatic skin manifestations [17].

Variability of SBF inside a given psoriatic plaque is an important factor to be taken into consideration when monitoring this parameter during antipsoriatic therapy. Hull et al. [18] have described a single graphic technique for detecting the most active (advancing) edge of psoriatic plaques. Using LDV, they found a 2.5– to 4.5– fold increase in SBF at the active edge compared with the inactive edge of each plaque (Fig. 2).

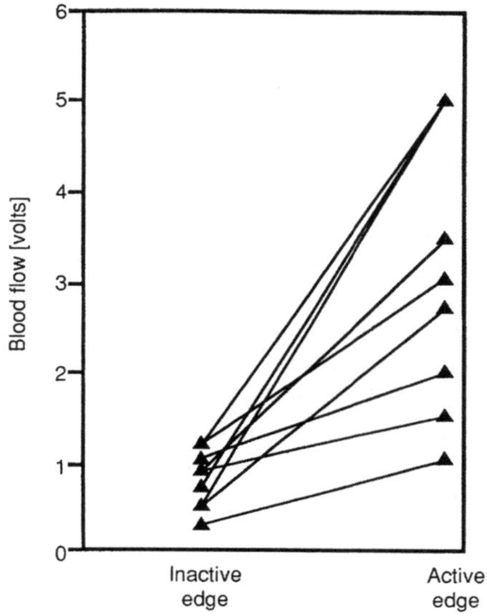

Fig. 2. Blood flow at the active and inactive edges of psoriatic plaques. (From [18])

The Transcutaneous Pressure of Oxygen

Oxygenation of tissues is perhaps the most important physiological process. The commercial available devices designed for transcutaneous pressure of oxygen ($tcpO_2$) measurements are based on a Clark-type oxygen electrode [19]. The probe is attached to the skin via a fixation ring filled up with a liquid contact. Oxygen diffusing from the skin passes through the membrane of the probe and is reduced at the cathode. After an equilibration phase (about 15 min), the current generated in the anode-cathode system is proportional to the number of oxygen molecules coming from the skin and is converted into a pressure value (mm Hg). The probe is also equipped with a temperature controlled heating element.

In normal skin, the standard procedure for measuring $tcpO_2$ is to produce hyperemia by heating the electrode to 44° C in order to achieve maximal vasodilation. In this state of maximal hyperemia, the capillary blood of the skin becomes arterialized, and a close correlation is obtained between $tcpO_2$ and arterial PO_2. The maximal vasodilation induces a state of flow independency, and only severe vascular disturbance or local skin alterations (edema, hyperkeratosis) will alter the outcome of the measurement. Several factors can affect $tcpO_2$, such as local SBF, epidermal thickness [20], density and morphologic characteristics of superficial capillaries [21], O_2 skin conductivity, and local O_2 consumption [22]. Most of these factors are modified in psoriasis. However, it has been shown [23] that $tcpO_2$ measured at 37°C (skin temperature about 35°C) is closely correlated to capillary blood flow.

In 1979, Tronier et al. [24] reported a decreased $tcpO_2$ value in the psoriatic lesion compared to uninvolved skin, which returned to the nonaffected level after UV therapy. Ott and Stüttgen [25] also found a reduction in $tcpO_2$ (44° C) in psoriatic plaques. They showed that measurement of the decrease in $tcpO_2$ per minute ($\Delta\ PO_2/\Delta t$) following inhalation of pure oxygen and after arterial occlusion with a cuff could be used as a gauge for skin O_2 consumption. They found a $\Delta PO_2/\Delta t$ that was 70% higher in involved than in uninvolved skin, indicating a higher O_2 consumption in psoriatic plaques. Using the same method, Broby-Johansen and Kristensen [13] found a significant reduction in O_2 consumption in involved skin as early as 24 h after occluded corticosteroid application, whereas the steroid treatment alone produced the same effect but to a lesser degree and only after 7 days of application.

Figure 3 illustrates the results which we obtained with $tcpO_2$ at 37°C during PUVA bath therapy of ten patients (forearm). At 37°C, the $tcpO_2$ is higher in involved than in uninvolved skin (see Table 1). The ratio involved/uninvolved $tcpO_2$ at 37°C showed a decrease of 75% in the first 3 weeks of treatment and returned more slowly thereafter to the control level. As can be seen in Fig. 1, the SBF measurement made on the same skin location (just before $tcpO_2$ measurements) evolves in a manner similar to that of $tcpO_2$ at 37°C. A very good correlation exists between the two parameters ($r = 0.93$). Thus, it is likely that, at least in psoriasis, the main factor affecting $tcpO_2$ at 37°C is SBF.

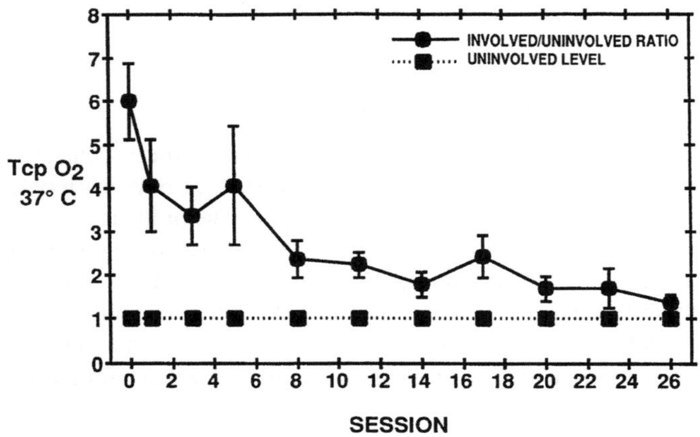

Fig. 3. Evolution of the ratio involved/uninvolved ($tcpO_2$) at 37°C during PUVA bath therapy (lesions are located on forearm; $n = 10$; mean ± SEM)

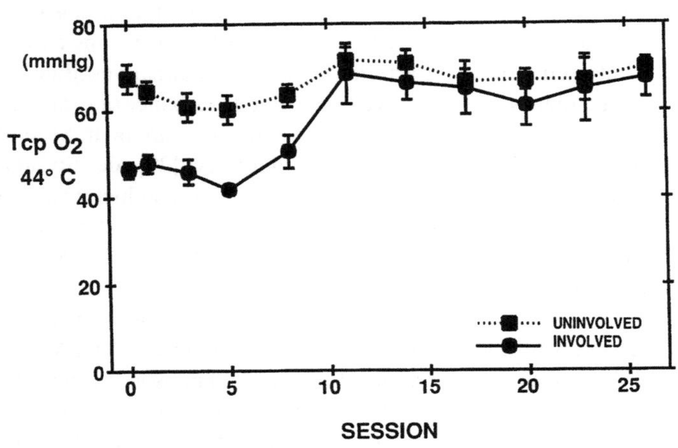

Fig. 4. Evolution of the transcutaneous pressure of oxygen $tcpO_2$ at 44°C in involved and uninvolved psoriatic skin during PUVA bath therapy (lesions are located on forearm; $n = 10$; mean ± SEM)

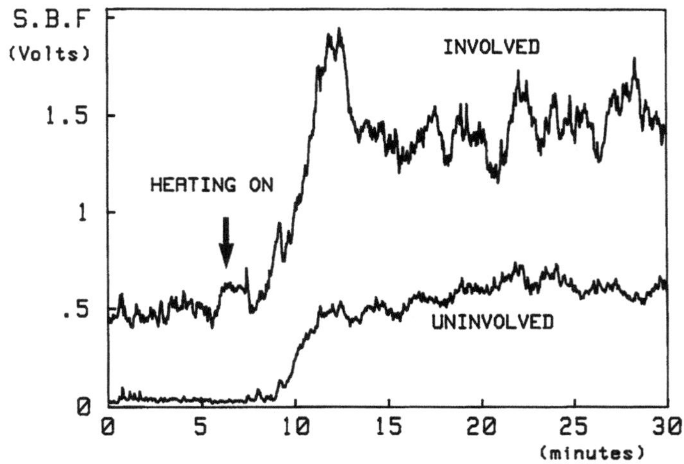

Fig. 5. Typical heating effect on blood flow of involved and uninvolved psoriatic skin (forearm)

The tcpO_2 measured at 44°C (Fig. 4), just after 37°C measurements, evolved in a very different manner. Starting from a decreased value on involved skin, and after a lag time, there was a rapid increase in tcpO_2 between treatment sessions 5 and 10 (2 weeks) such as that a value close to the uninvolved level was attained (normal value).

As shown in Table 1, heating the untreated psoriatic skin from 37°C to 44°C induced a small and nonsignificant increase ($p > 0.05$) in tcpO_2. This could suggest either a maximally dilated vascular bed in psoriasis or a malfunctioning vascular reactivity to a heat stimulus in involved skin. Therefore, the low tcpO_2 values at 44°C in psoriatic plaques could be explained by a lower SBF than in uninvolved skin. In order to check this assumption, LDV measurements of SBF were performed at 37°C and 44°C on the forearm of 15 untreated psoriatic patients.

The behavior typical of SBF in heated involved and uninvolved skin is shown in Fig. 5, and the results are shown in Table 3. Heating from 37°C to 44°C increased the uninvolved SBF by a factor of six and more than doubled the involved SBF. Thus, whatever the temperature, the SBF is always higher in plaques. The results are in agreement with those of Klemp and Bojsen [26], who showed that the psoriatic skin vasculature is not maximally dilated but capable of further dilation. Using a vasodilator (tetrahydrofurfuryl nicotinate, Trafuryl) a 1.5− fold increase in psoriatic SBF was found. Concerning epidermal thickness, Faltsie-Jensen et al. [20] have shown that the gradient of tcpO_2 across the viable epidermis is −0.26 mm Hg/μ m. Due to the hyperproliferation, the psoriatic epidermis is thickened. Thus, under these conditions, the high O_2 consumption in psoriasis is due to the increased number of epidermal cells,

Table 3. Skin blood flow at 37°C and 44°C in psoriasis (LDV values, mean ± S.D. in volts)

	37°C	44°C
Uninvolved skin	0.12 ± 0.02	0.79 ± 0.1
Involved skin	0.65 ± 0.1	1.74 ± 0.2

to the increase in mitotic activity of each single cell, and probably also to the presence of extravasated inflammatory cells in the epidermis. It should be noted as well that we have observed a significant increase in transcutaneous carbon dioxide pressure ($tcpCO_2$ 44°C, see Table 1) in untreated psoriatic skin.

Therefore, $tcpO_2$ at 44°C could be considered as a metabolic activity index in psoriasis. Under PUVA bath therapy, this index seems to return to normal earlier than do other parameters.

Skin Transepidermal Water Loss and Hydration

When sweating is avoided, the transepidermal water loss (TEWL) corresponds to the continuous passive diffusion of water vapor through the epidermis and stratum corneum. It depends on the skin temperature and ambient air humidity [27]. Among the existing techniques to measure TEWL (see [28] for review), the open chamber water evaporation gradient method is the most convenient. The evaporimeter probe is a cylindrical chamber (12 mm diameter) open at each end. It contains two pairs of sensors (hygrosensor and thermistor) for the determination of relative humidity and temperature at two levels above the skin surface, i.e., at 3 and 9 mm. From this differential measurement, the water evaporation rate from the skin is derived and expressed in $g/m^2/h$ by the control unit. Excepted for the palm, sole, and forehead, the normal values are less than 10 $g/m^2/h$. The TEWL measurement is used for characterization of the skin barrier function which depends mainly on the stratum corneum integrity.

For the skin hydration determination, the most widely used techniques are those involving cutaneous electrical properties, in particular the skin impedance Z. The impedance, which is the total electrical opposition to the flow of an alternating current, depends on two components: resistance (R) and capacitance (C). Most of the existing methods (see [29] for review) are based on the measurements of Z, R, or C and concern either the whole of the stratum corneum or its superficial layers, depending on the current frequency used. The hydration state of the stratum corneum influences its electrical properties by acting on the electrical mobility of all its charged entities such as ions, keratin chains, and matrix proteins, which have a dipolar moment, and water molecules themselves (proton exchange).

Psoriatic lesions, which are generally thick and scaly, are known to produce high TEWL values compared to nonaffected skin. Thus, the altered stratum corneum in psoriasis has a defective water-barrier function. Paradoxically, this kind of skin appears dry and scaly, although higher values of TEWL would indicate the presence of water in the stratum corneum. In fact, combined measurements [30, 31] of TEWL and stratum corneum hydration in psoriasis and eczema have shown an inverse relationship between water-barrier and reservoir function, i.e., the higher the TEWL the lower the skin hydration. Tagami et al. [48], using the sorption-desorption test (water-droptest), evaluated the waterholding capacity in several pathologic scaly skin conditions. They argued that scaly stratum corneum is always dry because it is less hygroscopic and markedly less capable of binding water than normal skin. They found that, even in the inconspicuous eczematous lesions, normalization of the decreased water holding capacity under treatment took place at the end of successful therapy, whereas the hygroscopicity of stratum corneum returned gradually to normal.

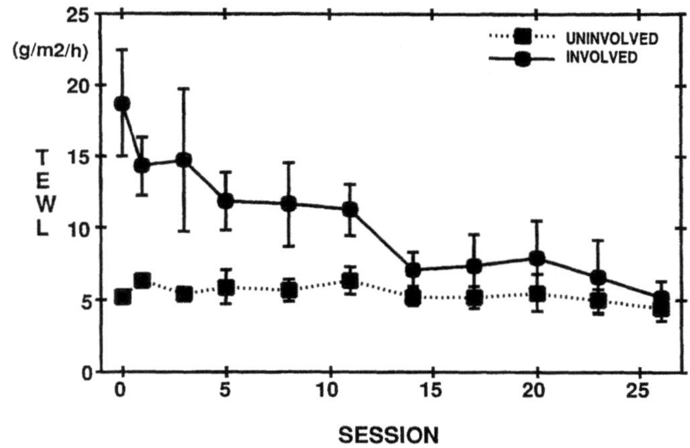

Fig. 6. Evolution of transepidermal water loss (TEWL) in involved and uninvolved psoriatic skin during PUVA bath therapy (lesions are located on forearm; $n = 10$; mean $\pm$ SEM)

No clear-cut differences were observed between uninvolved psoriatic skin and normal skin, either with TEWL or with hydration measurements [12, 32].
TEWL measurements have been used [10] to follow normalization of psoriatic stratum corneum on the forearm during PUVA bath therapy (Fig. 6).

In the same study the leg lesions (mainly around the knees) of another group of psoriatic patients were investigated. In this group of patients ($n = 7$), due to a great inter- and intrasubject variability in TEWL measurements, no difference between involved and uninvolved skin could be detected. Correlation between TEWL and clinical assessment of scaling was found to be satisfactory on the forearm ($r = 0.96$), whereas on the legs the relationship was less straightforward ($r = 0.85$). Serup and Blichmann [31] reported that neither TEWL nor stratum corneum hydration (conductance measurements) was correlated to scaling. They concluded that low conductance of psoriatic skin is probably a manifestation of abnormal keratinization.

Comparing two antipsoriatic therapies, anthralin and PUVA, Marks et al. [33] found that TEWL lags behind clinical clearance in anthralin-treated patients; in those treated with PUVA, clinical and TEWL progressions were parallel. Hartop et al. [34] found no significant reduction of TEWL on psoriatic involved skin after 1–4 weeks of linoleic acid treatment whereas subsequent treatment with clobetasol propionate reduces the TEWL value to the uninvolved level within 2 weeks.

Some authors have proposed a biological interpretation of the electrophysiological measurements in psoriasis. Clar et al. [35] suggested that skin impedance is essentially linked to the physicochemical state of the stratum corneum and that transcutaneous potential is related to the metabolic activity of the germinative cells of the epidermis. Borroni et al. [36] derived from the impedance locus (Z as a function of current frequency) the skin external resistance Ro, and internal resistance $R\ \alpha$ and the capacity-loss angle α. They considered that the angle α mainly reflects the metabolic and proliferative activity of epidermis: the higher the renewal of epidermal cells, the lower the value of α. Ro is referred to as the resistance of external layers of the epidermis, namely, the stratum corneum and granulosum, and as the epidermal barrier function. $R\ \alpha$, the resistance of deeper layers in epidermis, is not modified in psoriatic plaques when compared to uninvolved and normal skin. Angle α measured in psoriatic uninvolved skin was also significantly decreased ($p < 0.02$) in comparison to healthy control skin. This technique was successfully used to discriminate between the effect to two different corticosteroids [37].

Besides measurements of Z and phase angle to monitor three antipsoriatic therapies, Cambrai et al. [38] also used the phoreographic index, which is obtained from the change in skin resistance observed when an electrical current of increasing intensity is applied to the skin. This index behaved differently from other electrical parameters during therapies and was considered to reflect the membrane properties of living epidermal cells.

Ultrasound Skin Thickness Measurements

The high-frequency ultrasound technique for skin thickness measurement was introduced by Alexander and Miller [39] in 1979. In this technique (see [40] for review), high-frequency (15–25 MHz) ultrasound pulses are emitted from a transducer and directed towards the skin surface. These waves are partially reflected at every boundary that limits two media with different acoustic impedances, namely, the air-skin surface, dermis-hypodermis, and hypodermis-muscle fascia interfaces. The echoes are reflected toward the transducer and visualized as a series of peaks on an oscilloscope. Knowing the sound velocity in the tissue (about 1580 m/s), the skin thickness can be calculated from the temporal distance on the scope between the peaks representing the skin surface and the dermis-hypodermis interface. This one-dimensional skin thickness measurement is called an A-scan.

In normal skin, the differentiation between epidermis and dermis is difficult (except on palm), but in pathologic skin where epidermis thickened, such as in psoriasis, an estimation of epidermal thickness can be obtained.

Serup [41] reported a mean increase in psoriatic plaque skin thickness of 55% when compared to uninvolved skin. The absolute increase in thickness of psoriatic lesions was larger in skin locations having a comparatively low habitual thickness. Thus, plaques located on the extremities were proportionally more thickened (mean increase 77%) than plaques situated on the trunk (mean increase 33%). After successful tar treatment, the thickness of the lesions returned to values found in clinically normal looking skin, even if slight sequels of psoriatic plaques could be still recognized.

Broby-Johansen et al. [42] have used A-scan skin thickness, LDV blood flow, and skin color measurements to evaluate the antipsoriatic effect of various topical corticosteroids applied for 7 days under a hydrocolloid dressing. The ranking of drug effects, calculated from the differences between pre- and posttreatment values of the parameters, was identical to the rank order generally accepted for topical steroids. In this study, colorimetric measurements showed more variability than the two other techniques, and A-scan appeared to be the most accurate method, although its dynamic range was smaller.

Today, commercially available B-scan and C-scan devices allow two- and three-dimensional ultrasound imaging of the skin, respectively. In B-scan, the acquisition of successive A-scans on a line and the conversion of the echo amplitudes into gray levels enable one to visualize an ultrasonic image representing the echostructure of the skin.

With a lateral scanning system, it is possible to combine multiple B-scans to obtain a 3-D image of the skin, which is the so-called C-scan mode.

Recently, Vaillant et al. [43], using a B-scan system to evaluate skin modifications in psoriasis, found a 51% increase in whole skin thickness (when compared to uninvolved skin) which could be accounted for by a 120% increase in epidermal thickness and a 47% increase in thickness of the dermis. At the end of successful therapy, the thicknesses of epidermis, dermis, and whole skin were decreased by 34%, 70%, and 67%, respectively.

Boroni et al. [44] have monitored by B-scan the psoriatic plaques on the forearm and lumbosacral area of 20 patients during PUVA therapy. On the forearm, psoriatic skin showed a significant reduction ($p < 0.02$) in the epidermal thickness after clearing of the lesion, while no significant changes were detectable in the thickness of the dermis. Psoriatic skin in the lumbosacral area underwent a significant reduction with respect to the thickness of both the epidermis ($p < 0.001$) and the dermis ($p < 0.005$).

These data suggest that ultrasound skin imaging techniques are very promising and reliable methods for monitoring the resolution of psoriatic lesions under therapy.

Eczema

Eczema is an inflammatory skin disease which is expressed in a wide variety of forms and has multiple origins. The common clinical characteristics are the early appearance of erythema, sometimes edematous, which precedes vesiculation. These signs are followed later by scaling and occasional lichenification. Although eczema has a greater incidence than psoriasis, noninvasive methods have been much less often used to characterize this disease. The reason is probably because of the nonhomogeneous aspect of eczema lesions, which are generally sparse and scattered and therefore can lead to a great variability in the measurements. Most noninvasive assessments of eczema have concerned either the barrier function properties of the skin in atopic eczema or the characterization of experimentally induced contact dermatitis.

Noninvasive methods have demonstrated that various forms of eczema show increased TEWL [45–47] with decreased stratum corneum hydration [48, 49].

Numerous studies including noninvasive techniques have been undertaken to investigate the pathophysiology of uninvolved skin in patients with atopic dermatitis. Baseline TEWL has been reported to be increased in both dry noneczematous skin and clinically normal skin [50] as compared to normal controls. These results have been confirmed by others [32, 51]; an inverse relationship between TEWL and skin hydration in apparently normal atopic skin has been found. The data suggest that clinically normal skin of atopic patients may be functionally abnormal, resulting in a defective barrier which could lead to a higher risk of irritant or contact dermatitis.

Table 4 illustrates the results obtained by Watanabe et al. [52] in atopic xerosis, the dry skin of patients with atopic dermatitis. Besides the increase in TEWL and the decrease in skin hydration, this table lists the various stratum corneum functional impairments in atopic xerosis. These account for the greatly increased susceptibility of atopic patients to develop dry skin and to react to both chemical and physical irritation, as observed elsewhere [53, 54].

Objective noninvasive methods have been used in allergic patch-test reactions (con-

Table 4. Characteristics of the stratum corneum in atopic xerosis (from [52])

Investigation	n	Atopic xerosis (mean ± SE)	n	Controls (mean ± SE)	(paired t test)
TEWL (g/m2/h)	28	6.4 ± 0.4	18	4.8 ± 0.2	< 0.01
Skin surface hydration (μ mho)	28	21 ± 2	18	35 ± 2	< 0.01
Soluble amino acids (nmol/mg of protein)	20	186 ± 24	19	290 ± 27	< 0.01
Parakeratotic cells (%)	10	0.4	10	0.4	N.S.
Corneocyte surface area (μm^2)	13	875 ± 29	10	1032 ± 32	< 0.01
Turnover time (days)	7	7 ± 2	5	14 ± 2	<0.01
Number of cell layers in stratum corneum	7	21 ± 4	6	15 ± 1	< 0.05

tact eczema) either to provide objective and quantitative assessments of lesion intensity or to evaluate the anti-inflammatory activity of drugs.

Most of the objective methods used to quantify allergic patch-test reactions do not discriminate between the whole range of reaction intensity. For example, Staberg et al. [55] found that LDV was able to separate doubtful and positive patch-test reactions, but was unable to differentiate between the different positive test intensities. The $tcpO_2$ measurement can be regarded as complementary to the LDV in this domain, since it lacks sensitivity over the range of negative to weak positive reactions, but it does discriminate between medium and stronger reactions [56]. A-scan echographic skin thickness measurements are also unsuitable for distinguishing between strong and very severe reactions [57].

A method [58] combining ultrasound B-scanning and image analysis seems to provide a sensitive and reproducible system for evaluation of patch-test reactions. This method is based on the quantification of the edema and infiltration in the B-scan image.

Due to its structure, the dermis appears highly echogenic on the B-scan image. The presence of edema and inflammatory infiltration is expressed by a decrease in the dermal echogenicity and the appearance of a hyporeflective band. B-scan image processing allows the selection of an amplitude band of the ultrasound reflection peaks. For evaluation of edema and infiltration, a low amplitude band is chosen. The degree of inflammation is quantified by the average amplitude of peaks within the hypoechogenic area, by the size of this area, and by the number of peaks whose amplitude is in the selected band. In allergic patch-test, the variations of these parameters run parallel to the intensity of the induced reactions. The Spearman rank correlation coefficient r was -0.739 ($p<0.001$) for amplitude values (Fig. 7) and 0.903 ($p<0.001$) for surface area values, indicating that there was good correlation between visual scoring and echographic assessment.

This method has been successfully applied to assess the activity of three corticosteroids in experimentally induced contact eczema [59]. Experimental lesions were

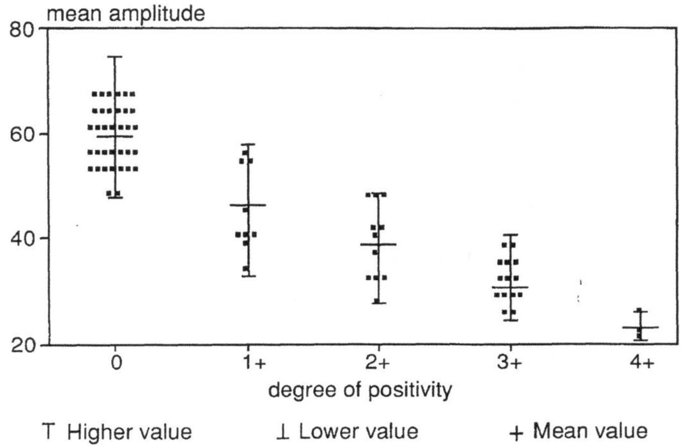

Fig. 7. Correlation between visual scoring and mean amplitude value of ultrasound peaks in the inflammatory region of the B-scan skin image. Rank Spearman test for mean amplitude values. (From [58])

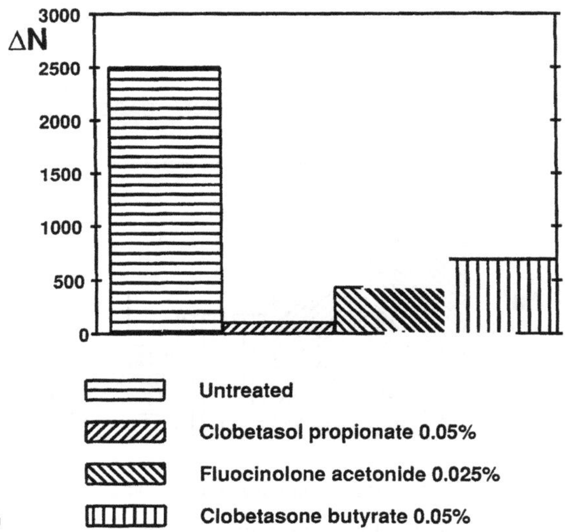

Fig. 8. Rank order of nickel patch-test reaction: Increase (between baseline and 64 h after eczema induction) in the mean number of low reflecting ultrasound peaks in B-scan image. (The greater this number is, the greater the skin edema and infiltration). (From [59])

induced by patch-tests with nickel sulfate (5%) in petrolatum in ten sensitized subjects. The drugs were applied at 16 and 40 h after nickel patch-test application. Therapeutic response was assessed as the difference between values obtained before and 64 h after induction. Figure 8 shows the results expressed as the mean number of peaks reflecting in the low amplitude range. This number increased less on the treated sites and is a sign of inhibition of the inflammation. The rank order of the efficacy of the test substances as determined echographically was identical to the rank order generally accepted for these steroids.

In a similar test, we have investigated the activity of four topical anti-inflammatory drugs [60]. Nickel dermatitis was induced by a 48h patch-test application, and then the lesions were treated twice daily with the tested drugs. To quantify drug activities

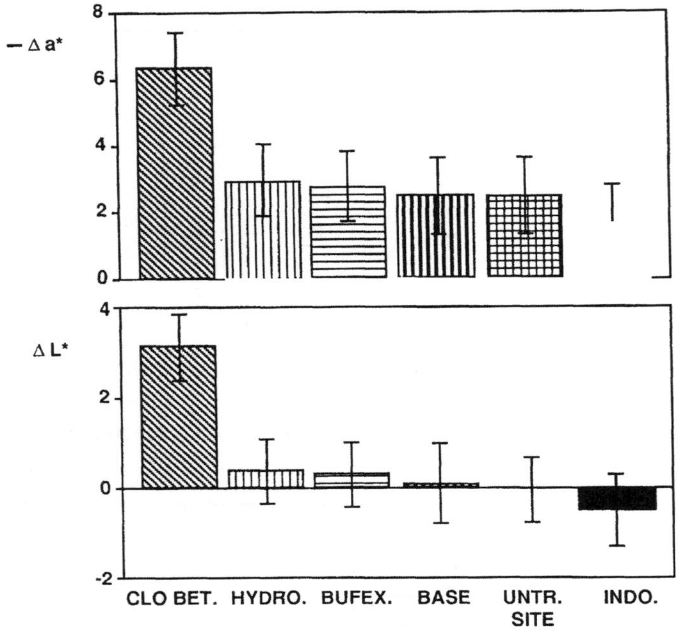

Fig. 9. Nickel patchtest reactions: Rank order obtained from the delta values (between before and after 4 days of b.i.d. treatment) of the colorimetric parameters a^* and L^* (± S.D.). Tested drugs were clobetasol propionate (*CLOBET*) 0.05%; hydrocortisone, (*HYDRO*) 1%; bufexamac (*BUFEX*) 5%; indomethacin (*INDO*) 2.5%

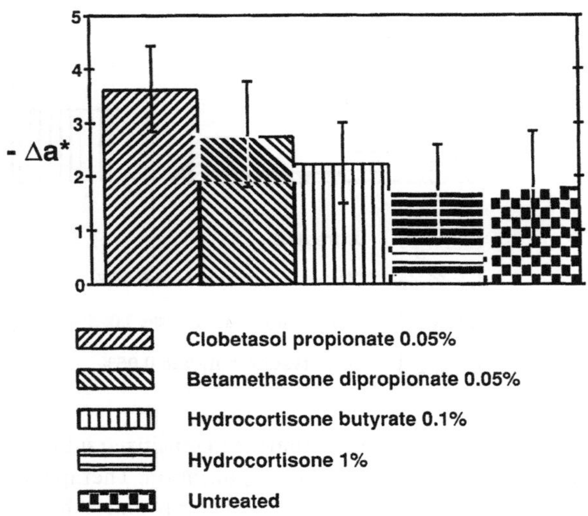

Fig. 10. Nickel patch-test reactions: rank order of topical corticosteroids determined by the variation in the colorimetric component a^* (between before and after 4 days of b.i.d. treatment)

objectively, skin color (colorimetry), SBF (LDV), and TEWL were measured before drug application (day 3), and then 6 h after the last application (day 7). The colorimetric measurements were made using the $L^*a^*b^*$ CIE system (Commission Internationale de l'Eclairage, 1976). In this system, a color is expressed by three components: L^* (luminance) represents the brightness, a^* represents the color range from green (−) to red (+) and b^* the color range from blue (−) to yellow (+). The presence of erythema is manifested by an increase of a^* and a decrease in L^*. As expected, only clobetasol propionate cream significantly improved the spontaneous clinical evolution in comparison to other creams, indomethacin cream even being aggravating (already reported). The rank order obtained from the delta colorimetric values (Δa^*, ΔL^*) is shown in Fig. 9. Statistical analysis (analysis of variance followed by multiple comparison Student-Newman-Keuls test) showed that Δa^* and ΔL^* were the most discriminating parameters in this study and gave the best correlation with visual scoring.

We confirmed these last results in a study (unpublished) using the same design and dealing with the assessment of four corticosteroids belonging to different classes of therapeutic activity. The best rank order corresponding to the known rank order of corticosteroids was obtained with colorimetric parameters, as shown in Fig. 10 for Δa^*.

Conclusion

Noninvasive objective investigations of psoriasis and eczema are increasing in number. Most of the reported results are in good agreement; however, some are contradictory. Therefore, there is still a need to standardize the use of these techniques with respect to the different sources of variability which can affect the validity of the results. The causes of variability include the methodology itself and the heterogeneity of patient populations. Nevertheless, in clinical pharmacology, the investigator has a set of noninvasive techniques at his disposal to objectively measure lesion severity and to quantify the efficacy of treatments. For the dermatologist, technology cannot replace clinical inspection of the patient's lesions. However, it is likely that objective methods will very soon enable him to reinforce his diagnosis, to modify the treatment regimen during therapy, or to predict a possible relapse.

References

1. Braverman IM, Yen A (1977) Ultrastructure of the capillary loops in the dermal papillae of psoriasis. J Invest Dermatol 68:53–60
2. Duteil L, Schalla W (1987) Evolution of cutaneous parameters during antipsoriatic therapy (PUVA): comparison according to the measuring site. Fundam Clin Pharmacol 1: 395
3. Klemp P (1987) Cutaneous and subcutaneous blood flow measurements in psoriasis. Dan Med Bull 34: 147–159
4. Ryan T (1980) Micorcirculation in psoriasis: blood vessels, lymphatics and tissue fluid. Pharmacol Ther 10: 27–64
5. De Lacharrière O, Kalis B (1989) Measurement of skin microcirculation. In: Lévèque JL (ed) Cutaneous investigation in health and disease. Dekker, New York, pp 385–420
6. Klemp P, Staberg B (1983) Cutaneous blood flow in psoriasis. J. Invest. Dermatol 81: 503–506
7. Klemp P, Staberg B (1985) The effects of antipsoriatic treatment on cutaneous blood flow in psoriasis measured by 133Xe washout method and laser Doppler velocimetry. J Invest Dermatol 85: 259–263
8. Klemp P. (1985) Regulation of local subcutaneous blood flow in patients with psoriasis and effects of antipsoriatic treatment on subcutaneous blood flow. J Invest Dermatol 85: 175–178
9. Nilson GE, Tenland T, Öberg A (1980) A new instrument for continuous measurement of tissue blood flow by light beating spectroscopy. IEEE Trans Biomed Engin 271: 12–19

10. Schalla W, Duteil L (1987) Sequence of change during resolution of psoriatic lesions. J Invest Dermatol 89: 441
11. Bravermann IM, Sibley J (1982) Role of the microcirculation in the treatment and pathogenesis of psoriasis. J Invest Dermatol 78: 12–17
12. Frödin T, Skogh M, Molin L (1988) The importance of the coal tar bath in the Ingram treatment of psoriasis. Evaluation by evaporimetry and laser Doppler flowmetry. Br J Dermatol 118: 429–434
13. Broby-Johansen U, Kristensen JK (1989) Antipsoriatic effect of local corticosteroids – 02 cosumption and blood flow measurements compared to clinical parameters. Clin Exp Dermatol 14: 137–140
14. Staberg B, Klemp P (1984) Skin blood flow in psoriasis during Goeckerman or beech tar therapy. Acta Derm Venereol (Stockh) 64: 331–334
15. Khan A, Schall LM, Tur E, Maibach HI, Guy RH (1987) Blood flow in psoriatic skin lesions: the effect of treatment. Br J Dermatol 117: 193–201
16. Trevisan G, Dal Canton M (1991) Laser-Doppler evaluation of cutaneous blood flow in psoriasis. G Ital Dermatol Venereol 126: 71–74
17. Klemp P, Staberg B (1986) Cutaneous and subcutaneous blood flow in nonlesional skin of patients with minimal psoriatic skin manifestations. J Invest Dermatol 86: 582–584
18. Macdonald Hull S, Goodfield M, Wood EG, Cunliffe WG (1989) Active and inactive edges of psoriatic plaques: identification by tracing and investigation by laser Doppler flowmetry and immunocytochemical techniques. J Invest Dermatol 92: 782–785
19. Huch R, Huch A, Lübbers DW (1981) Transcutaneous PO^2. Thieme-Stratton, New York
20. Falstie-Jensen N, Spaun E, Brochner-Mortensen, Falstie-Jensen (1988) The influence of epidermal thickness on transcutaneous oxygen pressure measurements in normal persons. Scand. J Clin Lab Invest 48: 519–523
21. Franzeck UK, Bollinger A, Huch R, Huch A (1984) Transcutaneous oxygen tension and capillary morphologic characteristics and density in patients with chronic venous incompetence. Circulation 70: 806–811
22. Severinghaus JW, Stafford M, Thunstrom AM (1978) Estimation of skin metabolism and blood flow with $tcpO^2$ and $tcpCO^2$ electrodes by cuff occlusion of the circulation. Acta Anaesthesiol Scand Suppl 68: 9–15
23. Rooth G, Ewald U, Caligara F (1987) Transcutaneous PO^2 and PCO^2 monitoring at 37°C; cutaneous PO^2 and PCO^2. Adv Exp Med Biol 220: 23–32
24. Tronnier H, Böttger EM, Hoffmann E (1979) Transcutane PO^2-Messung unter UV-Therapie von Psoriasis und Akne (Vorläufige Mitteilung). Z Hautkr 54: 546–550
25. Ott A, Stüttgen G (1984) Microcirculation in psoriasis. Acta Derm. Venereol Suppl Stockh 113: 99–102
26. Klemp P, Bojsen J (1986) Local variation in cutaneous and subcutaneous blood flow measured by CdTe(Cl) minidetectors in normal and psoriatic skin. J Invest Dermatol 86: 109–114
27. Pinnagoda J, Tupker RA, Agner T, Serup J (1990) Guidelines for transepidermal water loss (TEWL) measurement. Contact Dermatitis 22: 164–178
28. Wilson DR, Maibach H (1989) Transepidermal water loss: a review. In: Lévèque JL (ed) Dekker, New York, pp 113–134
29. Tagami H (1989) Impedance measurement for evaluation of the hydration state of the skin surface. In: Lévèque JL (ed) Dekker, New York, pp 79–112
30. Tagami H, Yoshikuni K (1985) Interrelationship between water-barrier and reservoir functions of parhologic stratum corneum. Arch Dermatol 121: 642–645
31. Serup J, Blichmann C (1987) Epidermal hydration of psoriasis plaques and the relation to scaling. Acta Derm. Venereol (Stockh) 67: 357–366
32. Berardesca E, Fideli D, Borroni G, Rabbiosi G, Maibach H (1990) In vivo hydration and water retention capacity of stratum corneum in clinically uninvolved skin in atopic and psoriatic patients. Acta Derm Venereol (Stockh) 70: 400–404
33. Marks J, Rogers S, Chadkirk B, Shuster S (1981) Clearance of chronic plaque psoriasis by anthralin- subjective and objective assessment and comparison with photochemotherapy. Br J. Dermatol 105 S 20: 96–99

34. Hartop PJ, Allenby CF, Prottey C (1978) Comparison of barrier function and lipids in psoriasis and essential fatty acid-deficiency rats. Clin Exp Dermatol 3: 259–267
35. Clar EJ, Cambrai M, Heid E, Grosshand E (1976) Electrophysiology of the epidermis in psoriasis (preliminary study). Ann. Dermatol Syph 103/3: 291–295
36. Borroni G, Berardesca E, Gabba P, Rabbiosi G (1988) Skin impedance in psoraitic epidermis. Bioeng. Skin 4: 15–22
37. Borroni G, Berardesca E, Gabba P, Vignoli GP, Rabbiosi G (1987) Can the use of powerful topical corticosteroids at high concentrations be justified in psoriasis? An in vivo electrophysiological study. Pharmacol Skin 1: 261–264
38. Cambrai M, Clar EJ, Grosshans E, Altermatt C (1979) Skin impedance ans phoreographic index in psoriasis. Arch Dermatol Res 264: 197–211
39. Alexander H, Miller D (1979) Dertermining skin thickness with pulsed ultrasound. J Invest Dermatol 72: 17–19
40. Payne P (1989) Skin thickness measurement and cross sectional imaging. In: Lévèque JL (ed) Dekker, New York, pp 183–214
41. Serup J (1984) Non-invasive quantification of psoriasis plaques-measurements of skin thickness with 15 MHz pulsed ultrasounds. Clin. Exp. Dermatol 9: 502–508
42. Broby-Johansen U, Karlsmark T, Petersen LJ, Serup J (1990) Ranking of the antipsoriatic effect of various topical corticosteroids applied under a hydrocolloid dressing-skin-thickness, blood flow and colour measurements compared to clinical assessments. Clin Exp Dermatol 15: 343–348
43. Vaillant L, Berson M, Machet L, Bertram A, Pourcelot L, Lorette G (1991) Ultrasound imaging of psoriatic skin: a non invasive technique to evaluate treatments of psoriasis. Proceedings of the 2nd International congress on ultrasound and the skin, Modena (Italy), Sept 1991, p 14
44. Boroni G, Vignati G, Zaccone C, Vignoli GP, Zanetta R, Beradesca E, Brazzelli V, Perinti A, Rabbiosi G (1991) Monitoring of psoriatic plaque during photochemotherapy by 20 MHz-Sonography. Proceeding of the 2nd international congress on ultrasound and the skin, Modena (Italy), Sept 1991 p 15
45. Grice K, Sattar H, Baker H, Sharrat M (1975) The relationship of transepidermal water loss to skin temperature in psoriasis and eczema. J Invest Dermatol 64: 313–315
46. Abe T, Ohkido M, Yamamoto K (1987) Studies on the skin barrier function: skin surface lipids and transepidermal water loss in atopic skin during childhood. J Dermatol 5: 223–229
47. Rajka G (1974) Trnsepidermal water loss on the hands in atopic dermatitis. Arch Dermatol Frosch 251: 111–115
48. Tagami H, Kanamaru Y, Inoue K, Suehisa S, Inoue F, Iwatsuki K, Yoshikuni K, Yamada M (1982) Water Sorption-desorption test of the skin in vivo for functional assessment of the stratum corneum. J Invest Dermatol 78: 425–428
49. Thune P (1989) Evaluation of the hydration and the water-holding capacity in atopic skin and so-called dry skin. Acta Derm Venereol (Stockh) S 144: 133–135
50. Werner Y, Lindberg M (1985) Transepidermal water loss in dry and clinically normal skin in patients with atopic dermatitis. Acta Derm Venereol (Stockh) 65: 102–105
51. Lodén M, Olsson H, Axéll T, Werner Linde Y (1992) Friction, capacitance and transepidermal water loss (TEWL) in dry atopic and normal skin. Br J Dermatol 126: 137–141
52. Watanabe M, Tagami H, Horii I, Takahashi M, Kligman A (1991) Functional analyses of the superficial stratum corneum in atopic xerosis. Arch Dermatol 127: 1689–1692
53. Tupker RA, Pinnagoda J, Coenraads PJ, Nater JP (1990) Susceptibility to irritants: role of barrier function, skin dryness and history of atopic dermatitis. Br J Dermatol 123: 199–205
54. GöllHausen R, Göttersberg K, Winter H, Przybilla B, Ruzicka T, Ring J (1988) Skin sensitivity in patients with atopic eczema and normals. Evaluation by visual assessment, evaporimeter and laser Doppler flowmeter. J Invest Dermatol 90: 241
55. Staberg B, Klemp P, Serup J (1984) Patch test response evaluated by cutaneous blood flow measurements. Arch Dermatol 120: 741–743
56. Prens EP, Van Joost, Steketee J (1987) Quantification of patch test reactions by ranscutaneous PO^2 measurement. Contact Dermatitis 16: 142–146
57. Serup J, Staberg B, Klemp P (1984) Quantification of cutaneous oedema in patch test reac-

tions by measurements of skin thickness with high frequency pulsed ultrasound. Contact Dermatitis 10: 88–93
58. Seidenari S, Di Nardo A, Pepe P, Giannetti A (1991) Ultrasound B scanning with image analysis for assessment of allergic patch test reactions. Contact Dermatitis 24: 216–222
59. Seidenari S, Di Nardo A (1991) Echographic evaluation of the acitvity of topical corticosteroids Proceedings of the 2nd international congress on ultrasound and the skin, Modena (Italy) Sep 1991, p 50
60. Queille Roussel C, Duteil L, Padilla JM, Poncet M, Czernielewski J (1990) Objective assessment of topical anti-inflammatory drug acitivity on experimentally induced nickel contact dermatitis: comparison between visual scoring, colorimetry, laser Doppler velocimetry and transepidermal water loss. Skin Pharmacol 3: 248–255

Use of Noninvasive Methods in Evaluating Different Treatments of Psoriasis and the Effects of UV Exposure on Normal Skin

T. Frödin*

Introduction

In this article I will review and comment on two studies which exemplify the use of different noninvasive methods in clinical dermatology research. In one of the studies we followed the healing of psoriasis and evaluated two slightly different treatments. In the other we followed the effect of a single exposure of ultraviolet light on normal skin. The methods used were evaporimetry, laser-Doppler flowmetry, and optothermal infrared spectrometry (OTIS).

Evaporimetry was used to measure the transepidermal water loss (TEWL). The barrier for TEWL is localized to the deeper layer of the stratum corneum and is highly effective [5, 12]. TEWL is a passive diffusion process. Damage to the barrier leads to an increase in TEWL. Measurements of TEWL can therefore be used for assessment of the skin barrier function and for elucidating how it is affected by damage or skin disease [10, 12]. Laser-Doppler flowmetry was used to measure the skin blood flow. Changes in blood flow and its distribution are major components of inflammation. Inflammation and/or changes in microvascular morphology are prominent features of many skin diseases and of skin damage [25].

OTIS was used to measure the skin water content. The water content of the stratum corneum is of consequence for the appearance and function of the skin. Reduced water content of the stratum corneum is a feature of dry skin in atopic states and senile xerosis, in eczema, in psoriasis, and in other scaly dermatoses, and has also been reported after exposure to solvents and surfactants [5, 8, 29, 31, 33]. In this study OTIS has been used to indicate changes in the stratum corneum.

The principles of evaporimetry and laser-Doppler flowmetry have already been described and discussed in previous chapters. OTIS was introduced fairly recently and is a special form of optothermal spectrometry [13], a technique derived from photoacoustic spectroscopy [24]. Both techniques are based on the detection of heat generated in a sample as a result of absorption of periodic radiation. The principle originates from the discovery by Alexander Graham Bell, in 1880, that an acoustic signal is produced when a sample is illuminated with intensity-modulated light [1]. In photoacoustic spectroscopy, variations in temperature are detected as pressure variations in a closed cell. In OTIS the heat generated in the sample is transferred by conduction to a thin solid sapphire plate, and the subsequent thermal expansion of the plate is transformed to an electric signal by a piezoelectric crystal cemented to the plate.

* Department of Dermatology, University Hospital, Linköping, Sweden

Assessment of skin hydration with photoacoustic spectroscopy mainly involves analyzing the thermal inertia, a characteristic influenced by the degree of hydration. In OTIS the water content of the skin is instead assessed on the basis of its optical properties [5, 7].

The psoriasis study [11] was initiated in order to evaluate the importance of the coal tar bath component in the Ingram treatment of psoriasis. Ingram's combination of coal tar bath, ultraviolet radiation (UVB), and dithranol in a stiff paste is highly efficient in clearing psoriasis [14]. The three components of this regimen were not evaluated separately until 1966, when Bowers et al. [2] cast doubt on the value of coal tar. Nevertheless, the Ingram regimen gives such satisfactory results that it has usually been strictly adhered to. However, there are good reasons for simplifying methods used in treating psoriasis, not least with regard to time and cost. We used evaporimetry and laser-Doppler flowmetry as complements to the clinical assessment in following the effect of treating plaque psoriasis with full Ingram treatment and modified treatment (tar bath replaced by oil emulsion bath).

Sunlight and artificial ultraviolet (UV) radiation produce a variety of biological effects in the skin and are widely used in the treatment of conditions such as psoriasis and eczema. In appropriate doses UV radiation causes inflammation with increased blood flow and vasodilatation in the dermis, giving rise to visible erythema. It induces visible pigmentation by oxidation of melanin precursors, redistribution of preformed melanosomes, and initiation of synthesis of new melanin. It causes histological and histochemical changes related to damage to epidermal cells and secondary epidermal hyperplasia with hyperkeratosis and scaling. All wavelengths of UV light are capable of inducing these reactions, but with differing efficacy and depth profiles, penetration being deeper with longer wavelengths. Thus, the effect of UV light on the skin varies with its spectral distribution [15].

The short-term effects of single exposures to UV light and the long-term effects of multiple exposure have been studied extensively [15], but the long-term effects of single exposures have been afforded less attention. The aim of the present study [9] was to monitor noninvasively for 1 month the effects of a single exposure to UVA, UVB, and UVC, using evaporimetry, laser-Doppler flowmetry, and OTIS as complements to the clinical assessment.

Methods

Evaporimetry. A prototype of the EP 1 evaporimeter (Servomed, Stockholm, Sweden) [20] was used. The method is discussed R. Tupker et al. (this volume, pp 56–70)

Laser-Doppler Flowmetry. A prototype of the Periflux laser-Doppler flowmeter (Perimed, Stockholm, Sweden) [32] was used. However, the standard probe was substituted with a multichannel probe, which integrates the skin blood within an area of approximately 1 cm in diameter [6, 26], in the UV challenge study.

Optothermal Infrared Spectrometry. The OTIS unit is shown in Fig. 1. The chopping frequency of the radiation can be chosen by adjusting the speed of the chopper. The periodic radiation passes through the transparent sapphire plate resting on the skin. It

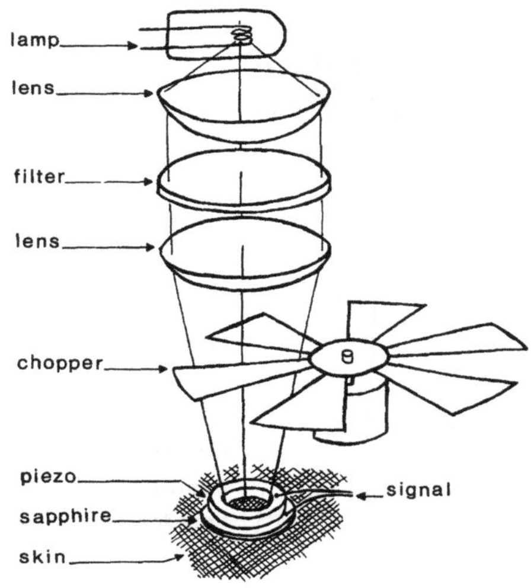

Fig. 1. The optothermal infrared spectrometry (OTIS) unit. Light from the lamp is collimated, filtered, chopped, and directed onto the sample through the piezo electric ring and sapphire. The thermal expansion of the sapphire changes the tension in the piezo electric ring, resulting in an electric signal

is absorbed in the tissue, giving rise to a temperature change of the same periodicity as that of the incident radiation. The heat is conducted to the sapphire plate. The signal produced is processed in a lock-in amplifier, and the phase angle and amplitude are registered by a pen recorder. Only thermal expansions of the same periodicity as the incident radiation are registered; no other temperature fluctuations in the sample will influence the signal.

The amplitude of the OTIS signal is approximately proportional to the product of the optical absorption coefficient and the thermal diffusion length [5, 7]. In the present application the optical absorption coefficient is directly proportional to the concentration of water, because infrared radiation of wavelength 1940 nm was chosen. In this region water has a specific absorption band, caused by the stretching-bending vibration of the water molecule, in which no other constituents of the skin would be likely to interfere [7]. The chopping frequency used here is 30 Hz, which gives a theoretical measuring depth in skin down to 24 μm. However, since water in the layer closest to the probe is responsible for the greater part of the integrated OTIS signal, this will mainly respond to changes in the most superficial layer, i.e., stratum corneum.

Study Design

In the psoriasis study [11] we included 11 inpatients with stable plaque psoriasis. They had symmetrical lesions on their forearms. In the morning six of the patients were given a coal tar bath with the right arm in a separate container with oil emulsion, and the other five patients were given an oil emulsion bath with their right arm in the container with a corresponding concentration of coal tar. After towel drying they received UVB irradiation and after this dithranol in Lassar's paste was applied to the lesions. Thus, each patient had two contralateral lesions treated identically in all aspects but one, that is coal tar bath on one side and oil emulsion bath on the other prior to the UVB irradiation.

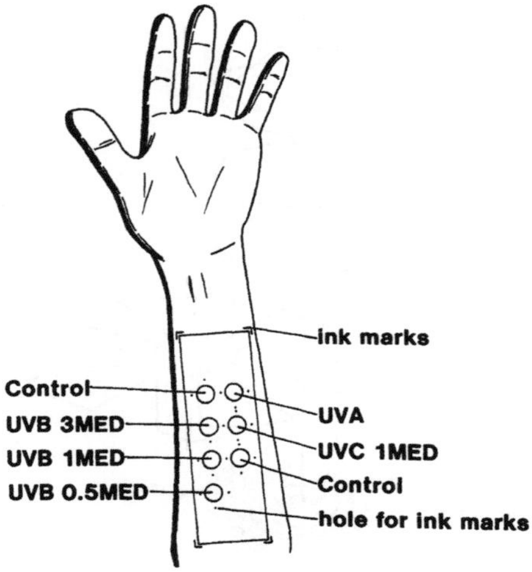

Fig. 2. Test areas with template, marking system, and doses

The lesions and control areas from adjacent normal appearing skin were evaluated before start of treatment and then once a week for 4 weeks.

Clinically the lesions were assessed with regard to erythema, palpable infiltration, and desquamation to a three degree scale. Evaporimetry was used for measurement of TEWL and laser-Doppler flowmetry for skin blood flow.

In the UV challenge study [9], six healthy men of skin type III took part. Test areas, transparent template for identifying the test areas, and irradiation doses are shown in Fig. 2. The minimal erythema doses (MEDs) were determined by pretesting on the contralateral arm. UVA was given at a fixed high dose, 150 J/cm^2. Test areas were followed clinically and by measurements before irradiation and afterwards repeatedly for a month. Clinically they were assessed for erythema, pigmentation, and scaling. TEWL, skin blood flow, and skin water content were measured with evaporimetry, laser-Doppler flowmetry, and OTIS, respectively.

Results

Psoriasis Study

Figure 3e shows the results of the clinical assessment; successive healing can be seen. After the first 3 weeks, only slight erythema remained in most lesions. There was no difference between the two treatment areas. Figure 3 a shows the Δ TEWL values ($TEWL_{test\ area} - TEWL_{control\ area}$) which decrease with clinical healing. There was no significant difference between the two treatment areas. The large discrepancy between the two areas at week 0 (before start of treatment) is explained by an unusually high TEWL value in one patient for the lesion selected for oil emulsion. The TEWL values for the control areas varied very little during the study period (Fig. 3b).

Figure 3c, shows the Δ blood flow values ($\text{blood flow}_{test\ area} - \text{blood flow}_{control\ area}$). The rate of fall in blood flow was comparable to the rate of fall in TEWL. After 3 weeks

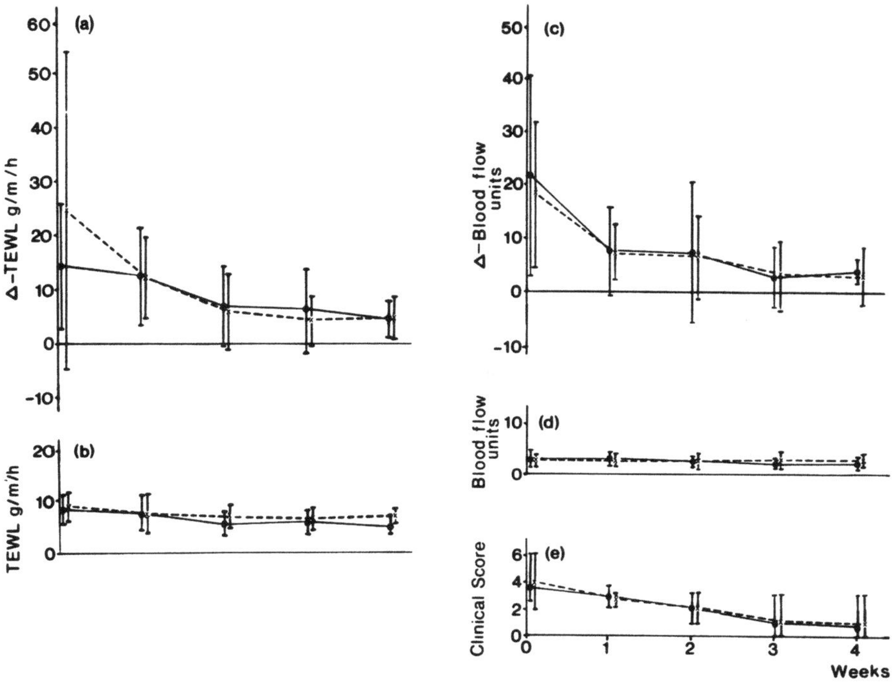

Figs. 3a–e. Transepidermal water loss (TEWL) laser-Doppler flowmetry, and clinical scores in psoriatic lesions treated with the full Ingram regimen (——) and the modified Ingram regimen, i.e., tar substituted with oil emulsion (- - - - -). **a** Mean difference between psoriasis lesion and control area (Δ TEWL) ± SD; **b** mean TEWL for control areas ± SD; **c** mean difference in blood flow (Δ blood flow) between psoriasis lesion and control area ± SD; **d** mean blood flow for control areas ± SD; **e** clinical score, mean, and range. Week 0, before start of treatment; weeks 0 and 1, $n = 11$; weeks 2 and 3, $n = 10$; week 4, $n = 8$

Fig. 4. Laser-Doppler flowmetry, results in arbitrary units. Mean values for the Δ SBF (skin blood flow) for the six test subjects. Δ SBF, $SBF_{\text{test area}} - \text{mean } SBF_{\text{control areas}}$; Δ SBF value on Day 0 is adjusted to zero for each test area. I, range of the mean for the two control areas; the value on day 0 is set at zero. Irradiation indicated by *arrow*. Figures before interruption (//) indicate hours

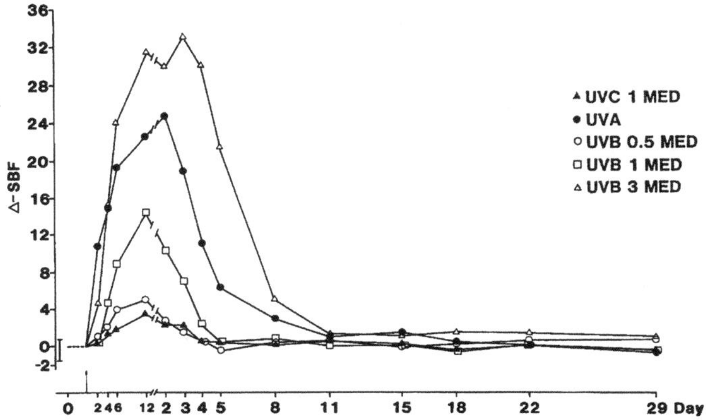

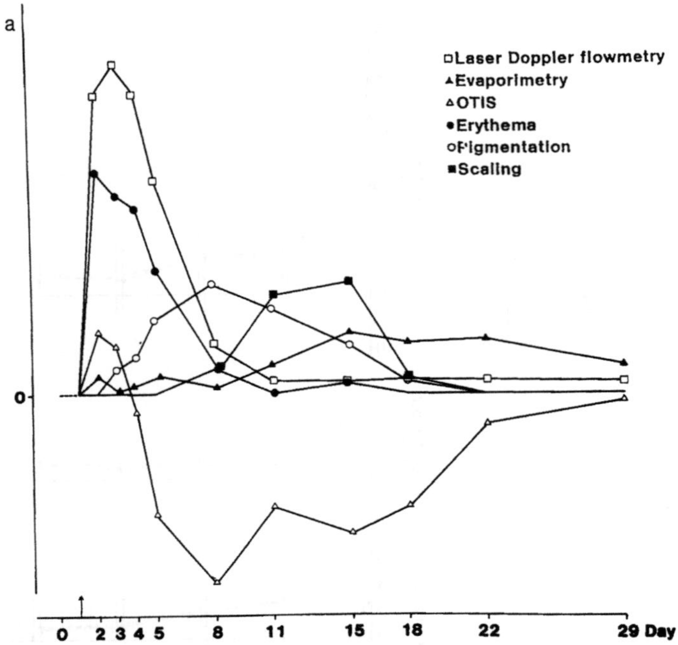

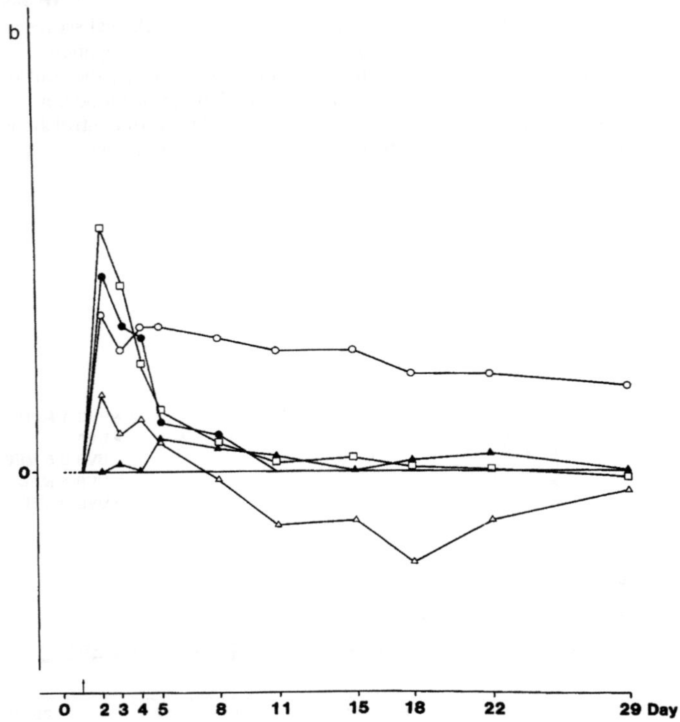

Fig. 5 a, b. Overview of all findings for **a** UVB 3 MED and **b** UVA. Note only one ordinate is shown; no units are given. Irradiation indicated by *arrow*

of treatment the blood flow values for the psoriasis lesions were only slightly greater than those for the control areas. The values for the two treatment areas did not differ significantly. Figure 3d shows that values for the control areas remain stable. The greater scatter around the means of the Δ TEWL and Δ blood flow values in the early part of the study period reflects the interindividual variations in the initial state of the lesions.

UV Challenge Study

Based on this study, single doses of UV light appeared to produce increased mean blood flow values for all test areas (Fig. 4). These were most pronounced for 3 MED of UVB, and for UVA 150 J/cm^2 and only moderate for 1 MED UVC. The increase in skin blood flow was most pronounced 12–24 h after irradiation and coincided with the clinical erythema score. The mean Δ TEWL values were hardly affected, except for a moderate increase in the areas irradiated with 3 MED UVB but not until a week after irradiation, which roughly corresponds to the onset of scaling. The mean values of skin water content measured with OTIS were slightly elevated 2 days after irradiation, followed by a marked decrease which was most pronounced 8 days after irradiation with 3 MED UVB. The other areas showed less remarkable changes, but a minimum was recorded 18 days after irradiation. For comparison, Fig. 5a and b shows all the mean values for the areas irradiated with 3 MED UVB and UVA, respectively.

Discussion

In psoriasis lesions the epidermal water barrier is damaged and TEWL is found to increase, sometimes 10- to 20-fold [12].

In the present study the mean TEWL values in psoriasis lesions before treatment were three to four times higher, and in some cases up to ten times higher, than in the uninvolved skin of the control areas. These values tally with those found in psoriasis plaques by Marks et al. [19], who used the same evaporimetric method. The initially high Δ TEWL values successively decreased with clinical healing and also paralleled the restitution of skin blood flow. This fall in TEWL with clinical improvement confirms the findings of others [12, 19, 22].

In a few plaques, higher TEWL values were noted after the first week of treatment despite clinical improvement, possibly the result of the removal of a thick layer of scales causing occlusion. The same finding was reported by Rajka and Thune [22], but Serup and Blichmann [27] found no correlation between TEWL and degree of scaling.

In psoriatic skin the capillaries are morphologically abnormal, and skin blood flow is considerably higher than in normal skin [17]. Klemp and Staberg, who used the epicutaneous ^{133}Xe wash-out technique, found a 10- to 14-fold increase in skin blood flow in untreated psoriatic lesions compared to skin of normal individuals [17, 18]. Laser-Doppler flowmetry has shown the skin blood flow in untreated psoriasis lesions to be approximately 10 times greater than in skin of normal individuals [18, 28]. The skin blood flow measured by laser-Doppler flowmetry is apparently similar in uninvolved skin of psoriatics and skin of normal individuals [16, 18]. In this study the mean skin blood flow before treatment was eight to nine times higher (for individual lesions up to

20 times higher) than in the control areas. This accords with other studies [18, 28], in which the decrease in skin blood flow with healing during Goeckerman or beech tar treatments measured with laser-Doppler flowmetry was also similar to that found by us. Khan et al. [16] found decreasing laser-Doppler values during Goeckerman treatment, but recorded values comparable to the control areas at a much earlier stage than we did, and before clinical resolution had taken place. Several factors not directly related to skin blood flow changes due to the healing process might influence the laser-Doppler values. Laser-Doppler flowmetry is assumed to record skin blood flow down to about 1 mm, but the response could be influenced by changes taking place in the skin during treatment, including the degree of acanthosis and the amount of scales accumulated on the surface, which in turn influence the distance between the probe and the various strata of the vascular network. An increase in skin blood flow occurred in a few psoriasis lesions after the first week of treatment, possibly owing to thinning of the scaly layer and resulting augmentation of the contribution of deeper and larger vessels to the signal. The same phenomenon was observed by Klemp and Staberg 18]. Further, both UV light [9] and dithranol can induce inflammation with increased skin blood flow. In the present study a small increase in the laser-Doppler signal was occasionally recorded in the control area; this could be explained by the UVB exposure or by a toxic reaction following accidental contamination with dithranol. Khan et al. [16] found no change in basal skin blood flow in normal skin after multiple UV exposure as part of the Goeckerman therapy.

Despite these considerations the conclusion to be drawn from the present results is that both laser-Doppler flowmetry and evaporimetry are well suited for following the healing process of the psoriatic lesion; further, they are excellent aids to monitor and compare different methods of treatment.

The coal tar bath component in the Ingram treatment proved to be of no advantage over an oil emulsion bath; there was no difference between the treatments as assessed clinically or by evaporimetry or laser-Doppler flowmetry.

If UV-light is given at a high enough dose, the epidermal barrier may be damaged, leading to increased TEWL. In the present study the mean Δ TEWL values after single doses of UV light were hardly affected, except by the highest UVB dose (3 MED), which was followed by a small increase from the end of the second week after exposure. The results indicate that UVB and UVC in doses of approximately 1 MED cause no functional damage to the epidermal barrier. After a UVB dose of about 3 MED a moderate increase in TEWL is usual, indicating epidermal barrier damage. In a separate experiment provocation with UVB at the high dose of 5 MED resulted in a four fold increase in TEWL, indicating marked barrier damage. A UVA dose of 150 J/cm^2 was high enough to cause initial edema but no barrier function damage as judged by the TEWL. Although TEWL was raised in the UVB 3 MED area, the skin water content measured by OTIS was diminished (Fig. 5a). This conforms with the findings of Tagami and Yoshikuni [30] and Serup and Blichmann [27]: in the presence of scaly pathological stratum corneum the water content of that layer is lower than in normal skin and the TEWL is increased. Note, however, that the barrier function remains intact even during the first few days following irradiation, when the inflammatory reaction (Fig. 5) is maximal.

Evaporimetry can clearly be useful in assessing acute UV damage to the skin, especially as it distinguishes the different potentials of UVA, UVB, and UVC for causing damage to the epidermal barrier, and it is also useful for monitoring the recovery period.

If UV light is given at a high enough dose it will cause inflammation, a prominent feature of which is increased skin blood flow. The latter is conveniently measured by laser-Doppler flowmetry [3, 4]. The clinical sign related to vasodilatation and increased skin blood flow is erythema, which by definition occurs after a UV dose of at least 1 MED. In the present investigation the mean skin blood flow values for all test areas increased; the increase was pronounced for UVB 3 MED and UVA and moderate for UVC and UVB 0.5 MED, reaching a maximum after 12–24 h (Fig. 4). The greater the intensity of the reaction the earlier the increase appears and the longer it persists. From day 11 after irradiation the skin blood flow values are almost normal. The conformity of these results with the clinical assessment of erythema (Fig. 5) is striking.

The present findings confirm the correlation between degree of UV erythema and the laser-Doppler signal reported by others [3, 4, 34]. An approximately linear response has been demonstrated 24 h after irradiation between laser-Doppler value and the logarithm of the dose of UVB [4, 34], UVC [4], and UVA [3], at least for erythema doses and for UVB up to 5 MED [34]. Diffey and Farr concluded that there was no qualitative difference in the vascular response after irradiation with UVA, UVB, or UVC and that the same dermal blood vessels were involved [3, 4].

We believe that laser-Doppler flowmetry is highly useful for studying the inflammatory component of UV reactions. The increase in skin blood flow values corresponds closely with the intensity of erythema, but it must be kept in mind that the method is not generally applicable for the assessment of erythema of any cause.

UV-induced changes in the stratum corneum might also affect its water content. For example in the scaly skin seen in certain dermatoses [29] and the clinically dry skin of atopic eczema [33] the water content of the stratum corneum is lower than normal. In the present investigation OTIS was used to detect changes in skin water content as an indicator of disorder in the stratum corneum after single exposure to UV light.

The OTIS values (Fig. 5) tended to increase during the first days after irradiation in all areas, after which a statistically significant fall, greatest in the area exposed to UVB 3 MED, occurred. In this area the OTIS value reached a minimum earlier (day 8) than in the others (day 18). Having reached the minimum, values gradually approached the pretreatment levels.

The slightly raised skin water content values during the first days may have been due to the acute sunburn reaction with spongiosis and intracellular edema. The subsequent fall in skin water content could possible be explained by one or both of the following theoretical considerations:

1. UV irradiation induces cellular damage, leading to a defect in the stratum corneum with impaired ability to retain water. Scaling occurred on the area exposed to UVB 3 MED, the very area showing the most pronounced decrease in skin water content. Scaly skin has a water content lower than normal [29, 30].
2. Hyperkeratosis is a sequel of UV irradiation, and it has been shown to occur from the third day after single doses of UVB and UVC [23]. For UVA it has so far only been demonstrated after repeated doses [21]. The measuring depth of OTIS with the chosen chopping frequency is about 24 μm. The keratin layer in induced hyperkeratosis might

be thick enough to totally prevent the stratum spinosum, with its higher water content, from influencing the signal; if so, a lower water content value would be registered. The decrease in skin water content could at least partly depend on increased thickness of the stratum corneum.

OTIS, as a specific detector of water in vivo, is a valuable method for studying changes in skin water content, mainly in the stratum corneum, induced by, e.g., UV irradiation.

To conclude, the psoriasis study illustrates that objective noninvasive methods, such as the ones used here, i.e., evaporimetry and laser-Doppler flowmetry, are valuable complements to the clinical assessment when studying the effect of treatment and in comparing the efficacy of different topical preparations. The study of the effect of single doses of UV light also demonstrates that the use of different, noninvasive, in vivo methods in combination is useful in elucidating different components of the response such as changes in skin blood flow, influence on the barrier function, changes in the stratum corneum, and in particular the dynamics of the different components. The elucidation of these different components will bring new information and hopefully a better understanding of the studied phenomena.

References

1. Bell AG (1880) On the production and reproduction of sound by light. Am J Sci 20: 305–324
2. Bowers RE, Dalton D, Fursdon D, Knowelden J (1966) The treatment of psoriasis with UVR, dithranol paste and tar baths. Br J Dermatol 78: 273–281
3. Diffey BL, Farr PM, Oakley AM (1987) Quantitative studies on UVA-induced erythema in human skin. Br J Dermatol 117: 57–66
4. Farr PM, Diffey BL (1986) The vascular response of human skin to ultraviolet radiation. Photochem Photobiol 44: 501–507
5. Frödin T (1988) Evaluation of the state of the skin by assessing cutaneous barrier function, blood flow, and water content. Studies in vivo using evaporimetry, laser-Doppler flowmetry, and optothermal infra-red spectrometry. Medical dissertation no 265, Linköping University
6. Frödin T, Andersson C (1987) Multiple parameter assessment of skin irritancy. Contact Dermatitis 17: 92–99
7. Frödin T, Helander P, Molin L, Skogh M (1988) Optothermal infrared spectrometry (OTIS) – a specific method for assessing the hydration of stratum corneum in vivo. Bioeng Skin 4: 115–130
8. Frödin T, Helander P, Molin L, Skogh M (1988) Hydration of human stratum corneum studied in vivo by optothermal infrared spectrometry, electrical capacitance measurement, and evaporimetry. Acta Derm Venereol (Stockh) 68: 461–467
9. Frödin T, Molin L, Skogh M (1988) Effects of single doses of UVA, UVB and UVC on skin blood flow, water content, and barrier function measured by laser-Doppler flowmetry, optothermal infrared spectrometry, and evaporimetry. Photodermatology 5: 187–195
10. Frödin T, Skogh M (1984) Measurement of transepidermal water loss using an Evaporimeter to follow the restitution of the barrier layer of human epidermis after stripping the stratum corneum. Acta Derm Venereol (Stockh) 64: 537–540
11. Frödin T, Skogh M, Molin L (1988) The importance of the coal tar bath in the Ingram treatment of psoriasis. Evaluation by evaporimetry and laser Doppler flowmetry. Br J Dermatol 118: 429–434
12. Grice KA (1980) Transepidermal water loss. In: Jarret A (ed.) The physiology and pathophysiology of the skin, vol 6. Academic, London, pp 2115–2155

13. Helander P (1983) Optical spectroscopy using an open photoacoustic cell. Dissertation in science and technology no 90, Linköping University
14. Ingram JT (1953) The approach to psoriasis BMJ 2: 591–594
15. Johnson BE (1984) Reactions of normal skin to solar radiation. In: Jarret A (ed.) The physiology and pathophysiology of the skin, vol 8. Academic London, pp 2413–2492
16. Khan A, Schall LM, Tur E, Maibach HI, Guy RH (1987) Blood flow in psoriatic skin lesions: the effect of treatment. Br J Dermatol 117: 193–201
17. Klemp P, Staberg B (1983) Cutaneous blood flow in psoriasis. J Invest Dermatol 81: 503–506
18. Klemp P, Staberg B (1985) The effects of antipsoriatic treatment on cutaneous blood flow in psoriasis measured by ^{133}Xe washout method and laser Doppler velocimetry. J Invest Dermatol 85: 259–263
19. Marks J, Rogers S, Chadkirk B, Shuster S (1981) Clearance of chronic plaque psoriasis by anthralin subjective and objective assessment and comparison with photochemotherapy. Br J Dermatol 105 [Suppl 20]: 96–99
20. Nilsson GE (1977) Measurement of water exchange through skin. Med Biol Engl Comput 15: 209–218
21. Pearse AD, Gaskell SA, Marks R (1987) Epidermal changes in human skin following irradiation with either UVB or UVA. J Invest Dermatol 88: 83–87
22. Rajka G, Thune P (1976) The relationship between the course of psoriasis and transepidermal water loss, photoelectric plethysmography and reflex photometry. Br J Dermatol 94: 253–261
23. Rosario R, Mark GJ, Parrish JA, Mihm MC (1979) Histological changes produced in skin by equally erythemogenic doses of UV–A, UV–B, UV–C and UV–A with psoralens. Br J Dermatol 101: 299–308
24. Rosencwaig A (1973) Photoacoustic spectroscopy of biological materials. Science 181: 657–658
25. Ryan TJ (1983) Cutaneous circulation. In: Goldsmith LA (ed) Biochemistry and physiology of the skin, vol II. Oxford University Press, Oxford, pp 817–877
26. Salerud EG, Nilsson GE (1986) Integrating probe for tissue laser Doppler flowmeters. Med Biol Eng Comput 24: 415–419
27. Serup J, Blichmann C (1987) Epidermal hydration of psoriasis plaques and the relation to scaling; measurement of electrical conductance and transepidermal water loss. Acta Derm Venereol (Stockh) 67: 357–359
28. Staberg B, Klemp P (1984) Skin blood flow in psoriasis during Goeckerman or beech tar therapy. Acta Derm Venereol (Stockh) 64: 331–334
29. Tagami H, Kanamaru Y, Inoue K, Suehisa S, Inoue F, Iwatsuki K, Yoshikuni K, Yamada M (1982) Water sorption-desorption test of the skin in vivo for functional assessment of the stratum corneum. J Invest Dermatol 78: 425–428
30. Tagami H, Yoshikuni K (1985) Interrelationship between water-barrier and reservoir functions of pathologic stratum corneum. Arch Dermatol 121: 642–645
31. Takenouchi M, Suzuki H, Tagami H (1986) Hydration characteristics of pathologic stratum corneum – evaluation of bound water. J Invest Dermatol 87: 574–576
32. Tenland T (1982) On laser Doppler flowmetry; methods and microvascular applications. Linköping studies in science and technology. Medical dissertation no 136, Linköping University
33. Werner Y (1986) The water content of the stratum corneum in patients with atopic dematitis; measurement with the corneometer CM 420. Acta Derm Venereol (Stockh) 66: 281–284
34. Young AR, Guy RH, Maibach HI (1985) Laser Doppler velocimetry to quantify UV-B induced increase in human skin blood flow. Photochem Photobiol 42: 385–390

A Novel Fluorimetric Method to Investigate Sebaceous Glands in Humans

G. SAUERMANN, A. HERPENS, U. HOPPE[1], and A. KLIGMAN[2]

[1] Beiersdorf AG, Forschungszentrum, Unnastraße 48, 2000 Hamburg 20
[2] Department of Dermatology, University of Pennsylvania, Philadelphia, USA

Comedogenicity of Raw Materials and Consumer Products

Propionibacteria are gram-positive anaerobic bacteria which inhabit the deeper parts of sebaceous follicles, normally low in oxygen. They produce porphyrins which are probably partially dispersed into the surrounding medium composed of sebaceous lipids and desquamating cells from the follicular wall [1]. Porphyrins are strongly fluorescent; their excitation maximum is located around 400 nm, emission bands are mainly in the range between 600 and 700 nm [2]. Illumination of the skin with light of the appropriate wavelength allows visualization of fluorescent glands within facial areas and the upper back [3] (Fig. 1). Assuming that fluorescence intensity and porphyrin content are related, which has been proven in the case of uptake of porphyrins by propionibacteria in culture [4], and knowing that fluorescence intensity is strongly related to the population density of at *P. acnes* the skin surface [5] and that comedones are densely populated with propionibacteria [6], fluorescence intensity of individual glands could be a marker for comedonal content and for the comedogenic potential of

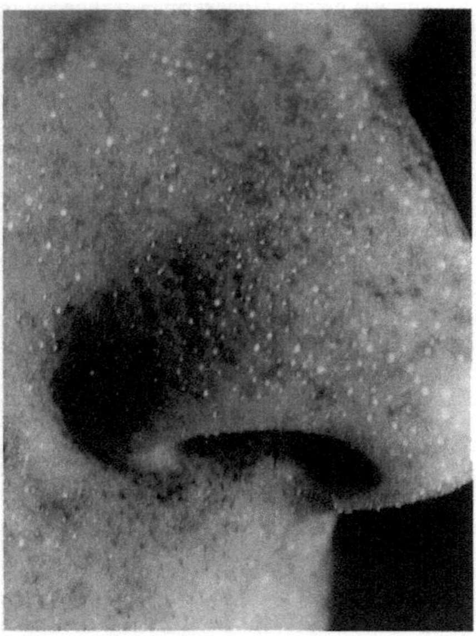

Fig. 1. Fluorescent sebaceous follicles of the nose (illuminated by UVA 1)

various products (Figs. 2, 3). Previous work has indicated such a link [7, 8]. One of the goals of the present investigations was to establish a relationship between comedogenicity according to the rabbit ear model [9–12] and human porphyrin fluorescence data quantified by image analysis, i.e., the suitability of this noninvasive in vivo method to classify the comedogenic potential of substances in humans while avoiding animal testing.

Investigations by Kjelstad et al. [13] indicated a maximal porphyrin synthesis rate by propionibacteria around pH 6.1, whereas the maximum of bacterial growth peaks at pH 6.7. More acidic or basic pH values restrict growth of propionibacteria and syn-

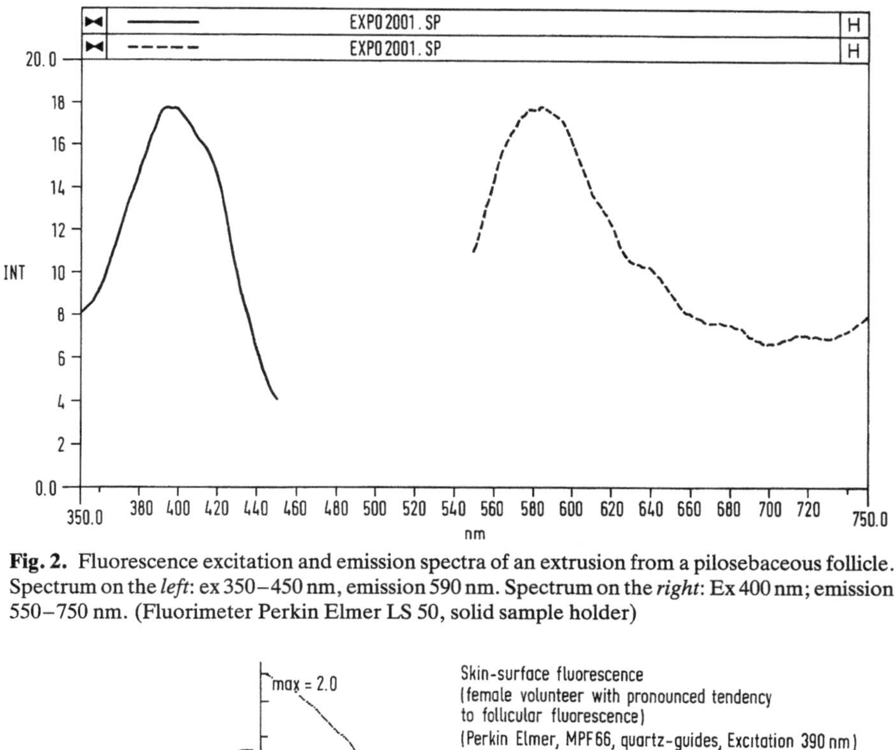

Fig. 2. Fluorescence excitation and emission spectra of an extrusion from a pilosebaceous follicle. Spectrum on the *left*: ex 350–450 nm, emission 590 nm. Spectrum on the *right*: Ex 400 nm; emission 550–750 nm. (Fluorimeter Perkin Elmer LS 50, solid sample holder)

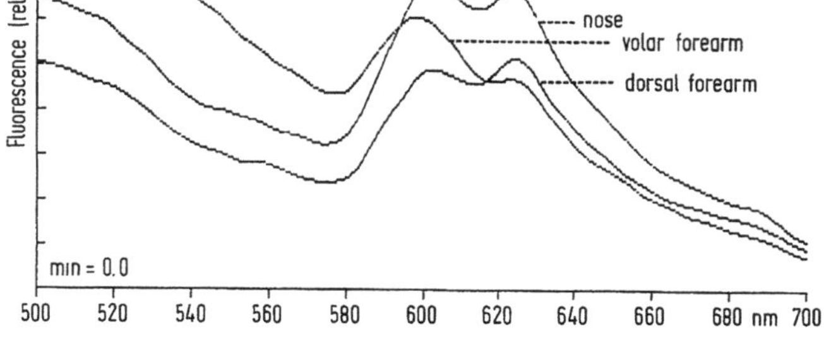

Fig. 3. Integral measurement of the in situ fluorescence emission from sebaceous follicles in different locations on human skin

thesis of porphyrins. Thus, it seems of interest to investigate the influence of products with different pH values and sufficient buffer capacity on the development of comedones. Product preservatives, which have a broad range of antibacterial activity, are also likely to influence comedo formation.

Follicles are penetration paths not only for substances which are molecularly dispersed by diffusion, but also for microcrystalline particles pumped into the follicle by mechanical agitation [14]. Pigmentary titanium dioxide, a physical sunscreen, could function as a sensitizer of type II – like porphyrins if it was transfered to deeper living parts of the skin and if oxygen was available [15].

α-Hydroxypalmitic acid is a metabolite of epidermal ceramides and an active antimicrobial substance of the skin surface [16].

α-Hydroxy fatty acids of short chain length, e.g., lactic acid enforce desquamation [17]. Increasing chain length often enhances antimicrobial activity. Therefore the influence of this class of compounds seem worth investigating for their comedogenic potential.

6-cis-Hexadecanoic acid (HD) is a natural ingredient of sebaceous lipids. Its content rises with the increasingly pathogenic state of the gland and supposedly substitutes for deficient linoleic acid. Oleic acid or 6-*cis*-octadecanoic acid acts, as penetration enhancer by liquifying epidermal lipid membranes [18, 19] for decreasing the stratum corneum barrier. HD probably shows a similar potential, it i.e., might increase transepidermal water loss of the follicular wall, supplying an essential ingredient for bacterial growth.

Materials and Methods

To compare the effect of different products on comedogenicity, product application and instrumental investigations were performed on the upper back. Up to 12 of the products listed in Table 1 were applied once daily (Monday Friday) for 6 weeks. Measurements were performed before the first product application, 3 (not always reported here) and 6 weeks after starting, and always 24 h after preceding product application the last.

All volunteers were between 20 and 40 years of age. Their backs normally showed a moderate density of fluorescent follicies.

Equipment

1. Monochromatic illumination (398 ± 5 nm, flux rate < 0.01 mW/cm^2; 1 kW Xe arc; Müller-Electronic, Moosinning, FRG)
2. Highly sensitive camera C 2400/09 Hamamatsu Corp., Japan) held vertically above investigated skin site (17 x 17 mm^2) (Fig. 4)
3. Cut-off filter (T_{50} = 610 nm)
4. Sensitivity control (regularly checked look-up-tables)
5. Macro optic (UV-Micro Nikor 4.5/105 mm; Nikon) (theoretical resolution 33 μm^2/pixel)
6. Image analysis (Zeiss-Kontron VIDAS AT 386) (Fig. 5)
7. Reflection standard (Teflon) (Spectralon/LOT; Darmstadt, FRG)

Table 1. Products used to assess comedogenicity

products	concentration/vehicle	number of volunteers/study		
		Study I	Study II	Study III
Isopropylmyristate	100%	10	4	12
Isopropylmyristate	50% in vaseline	10		
Isopropylmyristate	25% in vaseline	10		
Sodiumdocylsulfate	7,5% in H_20	10		
Lanolin		10		12
Benzalkoniumchloride	5% in H_20	10		
Cocoabutter	100%	10	4	
Oleic acid	100%	10		
Oleic acid	50% in vaseline	10		
Acetylated lanolin (Acetulan)	100%		4	12
Olive oil	100%		4	12
Evening primrose oil	100%		4	
Isopropylpalmitate	100%			12
Avocado oil	100%			12
Decyloleate	100%			12
2-Octyldodecanol	50% in mineral oil		10[a]	
Myristylmyristate	50% in mineral oil		10[a]	
Octylmethoxycinnamate	50% in mineral oil		10[a]	
Vehicle-lotion A containing citricacid/citrate buffer adjusted to ph 4			12[a]	
Vehicle lotion A containing citric acid/citrate buffer adjusted to pH 5.5			12[a]	
Vehicle lotion B containing preservatives phenoxyethanol + parabenes s			10[a]	
Vehicle lotion free of preservatives (according to European Community positive list)			10[a]	
Mineral oil containing 10% TiO_2 powder (coated) applied on one half of the forehead			7[a]	
Mineral oil containing 10% TiO_2 powder (uncoated) applied on one half of the forehead)			7[a]	
6-*cis*-Hexadecanoic acid (10% in ethanol)			10[a]	
α-Hydroxy palmitic acid (10% in ethanol)			7[a]	
Ethanol 100%			7[a]	

TiO_2, titanium dioxide.
[a] Data taken from several different studies.

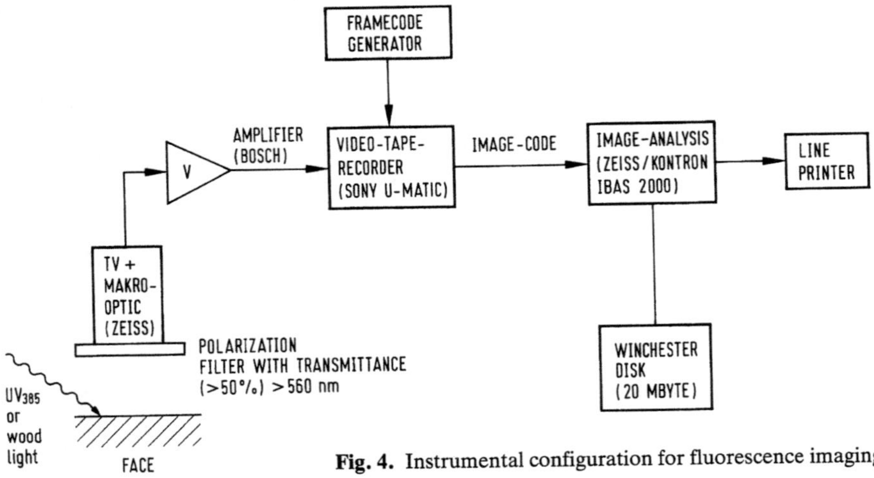

Fig. 4. Instrumental configuration for fluorescence imaging

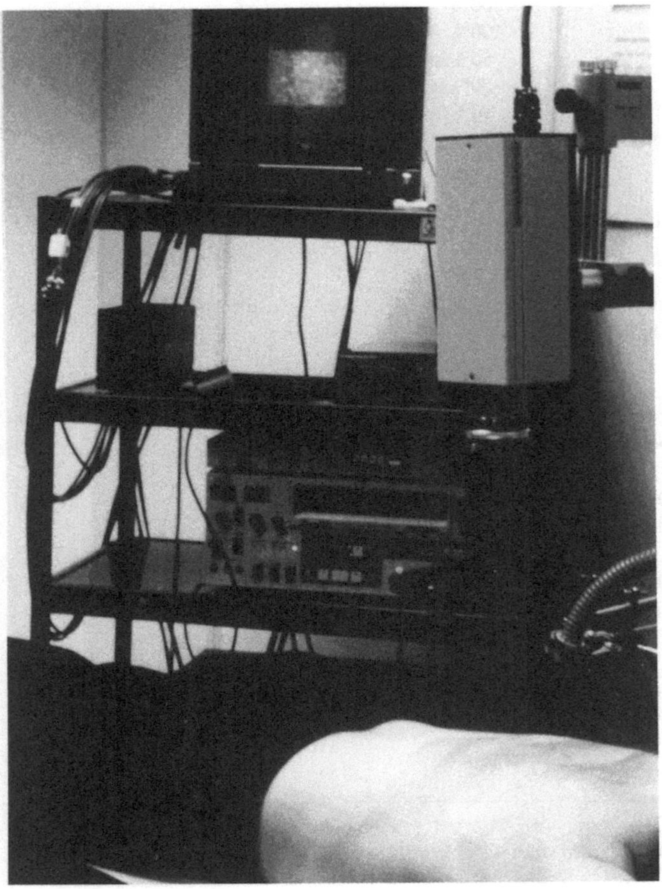

Fig. 5. Instumental set-up for image analysis of fluorescent follicles

Image Analysis

The following software packages were used for analysis:

1. Camera sensitivity maximized by LUT "Porphyr"
2. AVERAGING (suppression of noise by several digitalization procedures) (Figs. 6, 7)
3. Storage of picture (1 GByte erasable optical disc)
4. MEDIAN filtration (elimination of noise)
5. SHADING correction (elimination of uneven illumination)
6. LINEAR GREY SCALING (adjustment of grey value scale)
7. DYNAMIC THRESHOLD segmentation (elimination of gradients of brightness) (Fig. 8)
8. OPEN-function (erosion of small nonspecific objects)
9. CONTOUR (visual quality control parameters) (Fig. 7)

Parameters

1. number of fluorescent spots/area. Criteria: minimal size, minimal fluorescence intensity above background level, emission wavelength > 610 nm, delta count ($= d_6 - d_o$, where d_6 is the density of fluorescent glands after 6 weeks of treatment (and d_o is the density of fluorescent glands at test start) (Fig. 8).
2. Size (μm^2) of individual glands (Fig. 9).
3. fluorescence intensity (relative units) of individual glands (Fig. 10).

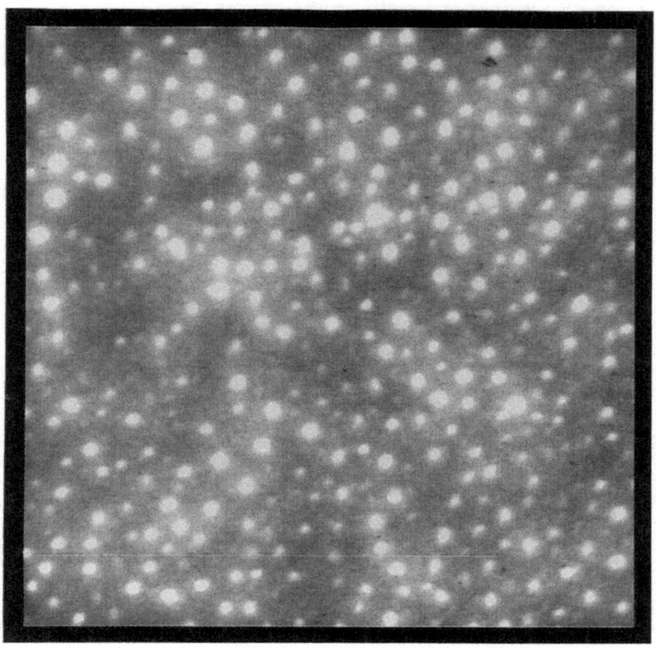

Fig. 6. Original image of a skin site rich in fluorescent follicles before further image processing has taken place

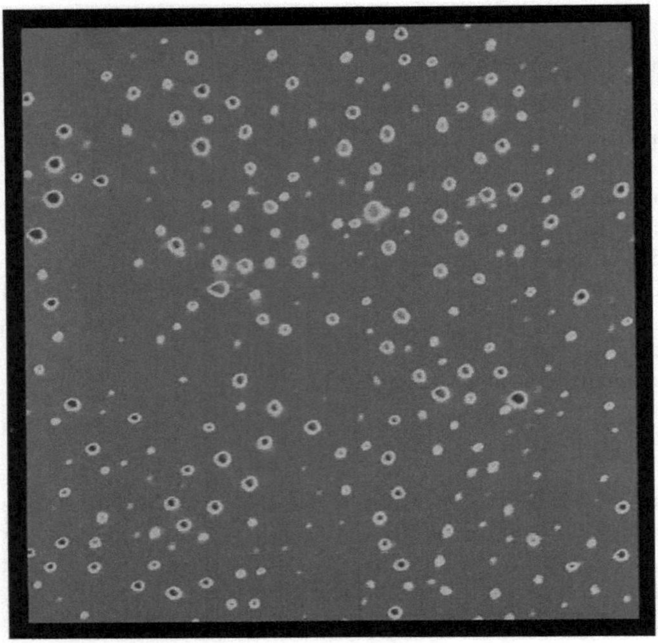

Fig. 7. Image of Fig. 6 after AVERAGING (see text for details)

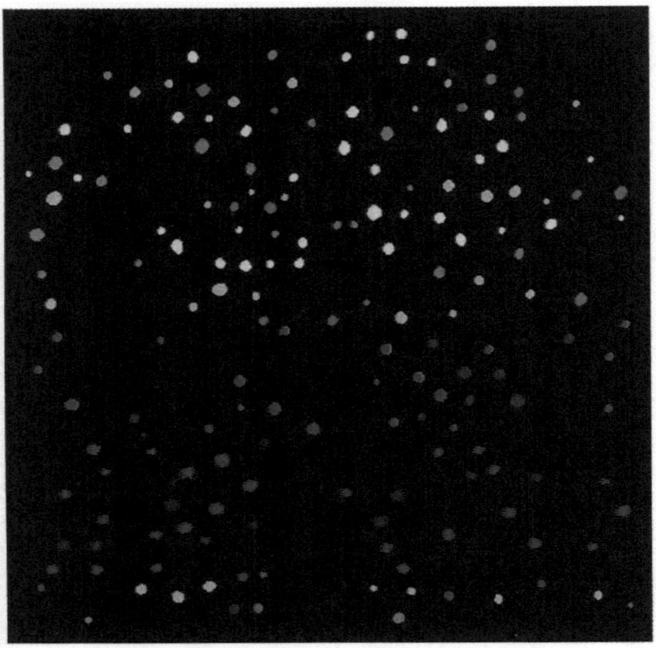

Fig. 8. Image of Fig. 7 after further processing

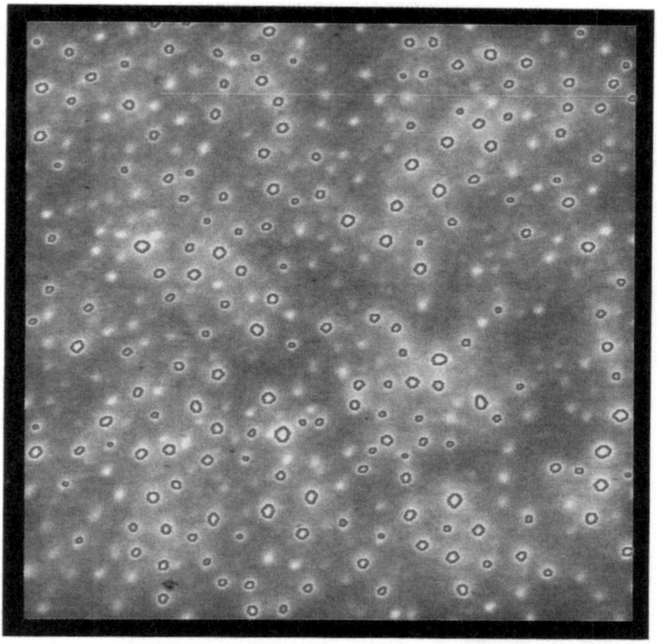

Fig. 9. Data of Fig. 6 with contour lines of minimal intensity determining size

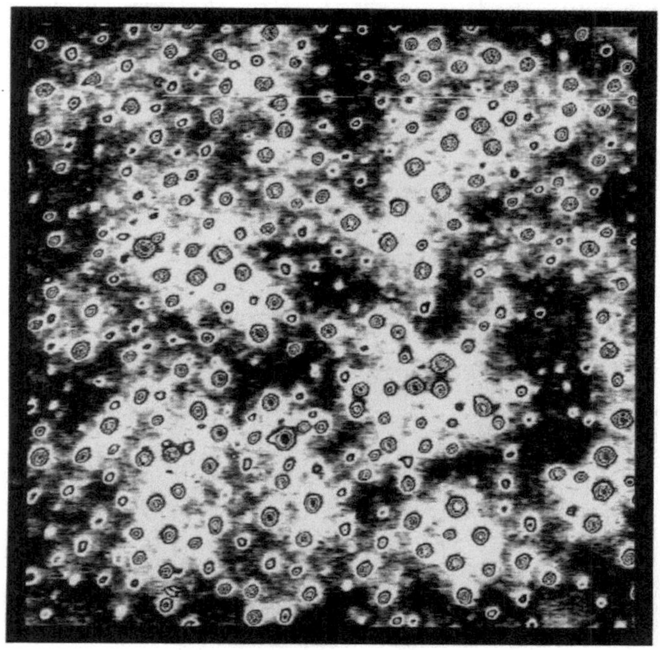

Fig. 10. Image of Fig. 6 with equidistant contour lines illustrating fluorescence intensity

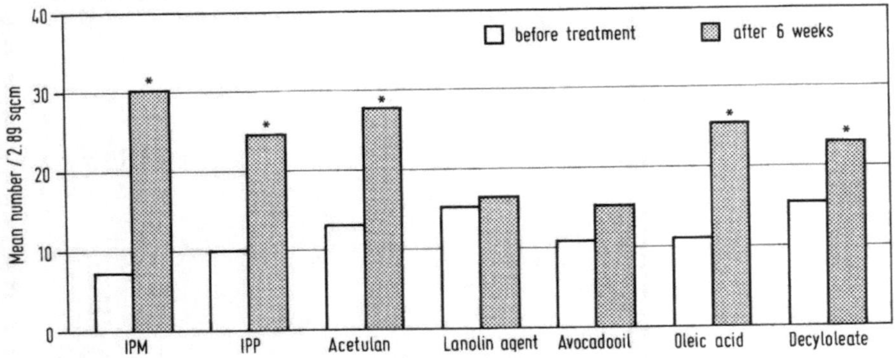

Fig. 11. Change of density of fluorescent follicles after daily treatment for 6 weeks; *x* statistically significant compared with starting conditions; *IPM*, isopropyl myristate; *IPP*, isopropyl palmitate

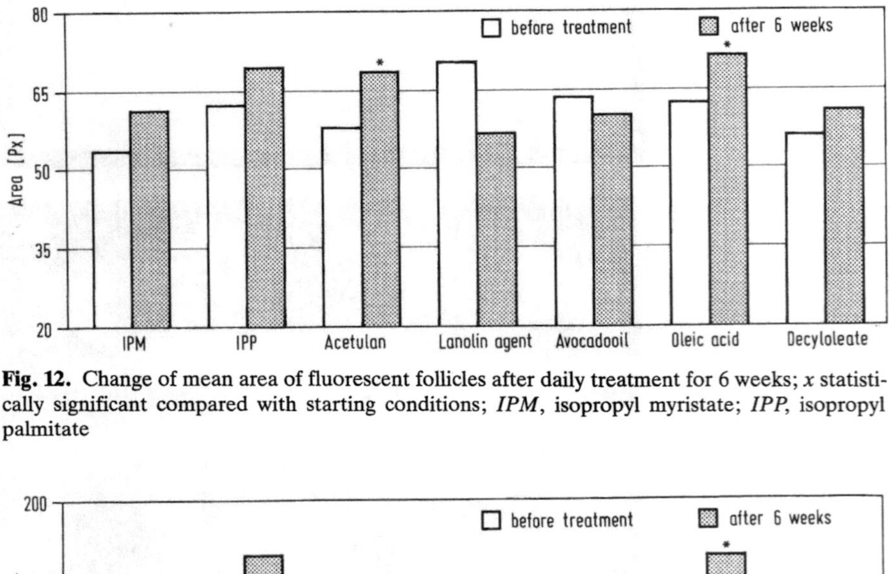

Fig. 12. Change of mean area of fluorescent follicles after daily treatment for 6 weeks; *x* statistically significant compared with starting conditions; *IPM*, isopropyl myristate; *IPP*, isopropyl palmitate

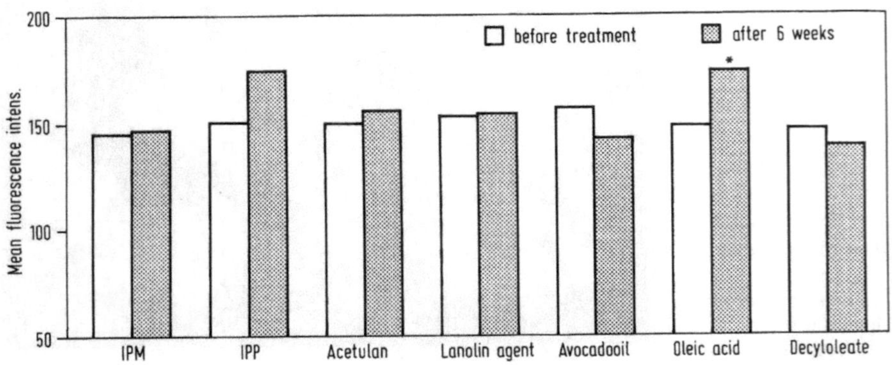

Fig. 13. Change of mean intensity of fluoresscent follicles after daily treatment for 6 weeks; *x* statistically significant compared with starting conditions; *IPM*, isopropyl myristate; *IPP*, isopropyl palmitate

Results

Analytical Importance of Delta Count, Comedonal Size (Area), and Fluorescence Intensity

The most sensitive parameter turned out to be the change in the density of fluorescent glands (delta count) during the test period (Fig. 11). Size and especially intensity of the spots were of less analytical value (Figs. 12, 13). The relation between area and inten-

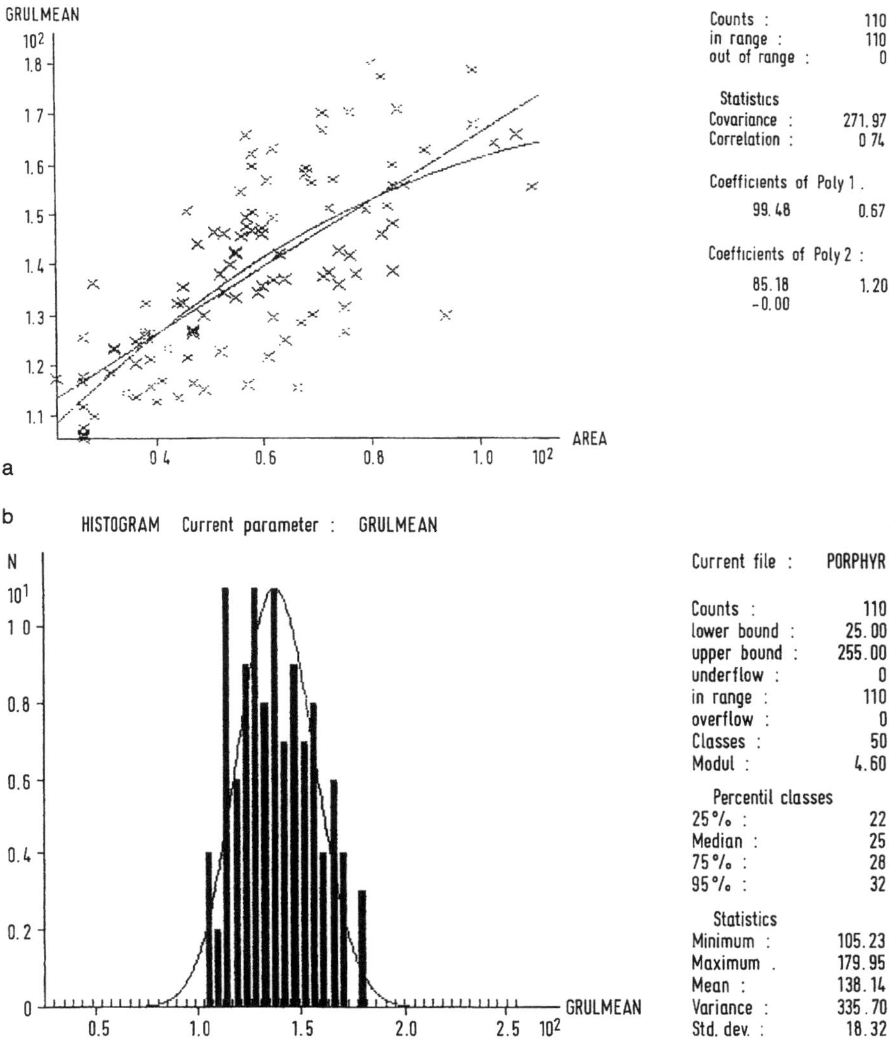

Fig. 14. Relation between area and intensity of fluorescent follicles of an arbitrarily chosen image **b** Histogram of individual grey values (intensities) (minimum threshold for fluorescent follicles to be identified = 100). **c** Histogram of individual areas (pixel) (1 pixel = 1000 μm^2)

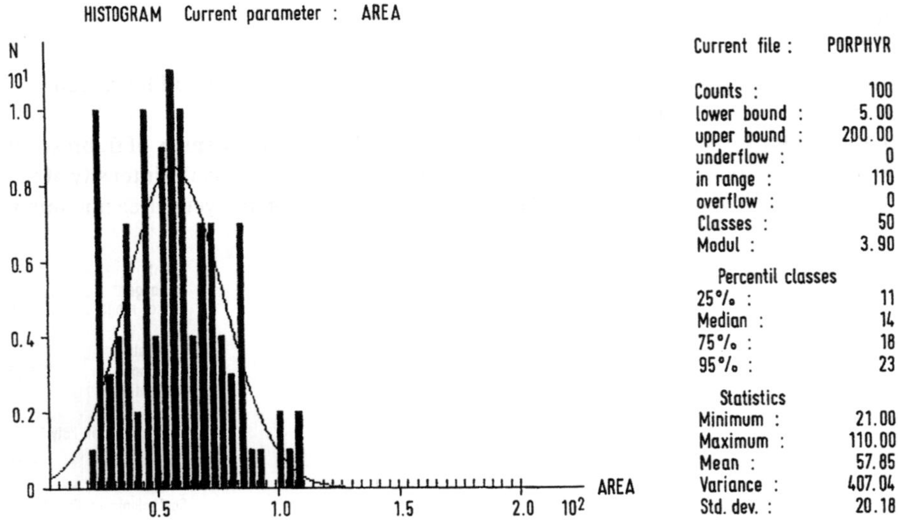

Fig. 14c

sity of fluorescent follicles (Fig. 14) indicates a lack of correlation between these two parameters.

Comedogenicity of Raw Materials

Figure 15 shows the increased delta count during the test period in relation to scores characterizing comedogenicity derived from the rabbit ear model [10, 11].

Looking at the different concentrations of isopropyl myristate, a maximum at 75% and a steadily decreasing count parallel to decreasing concentrations were found. Oleic acid did not show decreasing comedogenicity with decreasing concentration in the range 50%–100%. Lanolin was ineffective, and acetylated lanolin showed relatively high comedogenicity. Sodium dodecy sulfate (SDS) weakly induced comedones contrary to some [10] and in accordance with other [12] studies. Benzalkonium chloride strongly decreased the delta count below the starting level, probably a consequence of its antimicrobial action causing a decrease in either porphyrin-producing propionibacteria or in its porphyrin-producing activity.

2-Octyl dodecanol, myristyl myristate, and octyl methoxycinnamate are probably weakly comedogenic when painted on the skin as a 50% solution in mineral oil based upon a moderate increase of the mean fluorescent follicle area; the density of comedones and mean intensity of fluorescence did not change.

Influence of Preservative-Containing Products

Some so-called preservative-free cosmetic lotions were observed to be comedogenic, in contrast to their preservative-containing (phenoxyethanol/parabenes) variants.

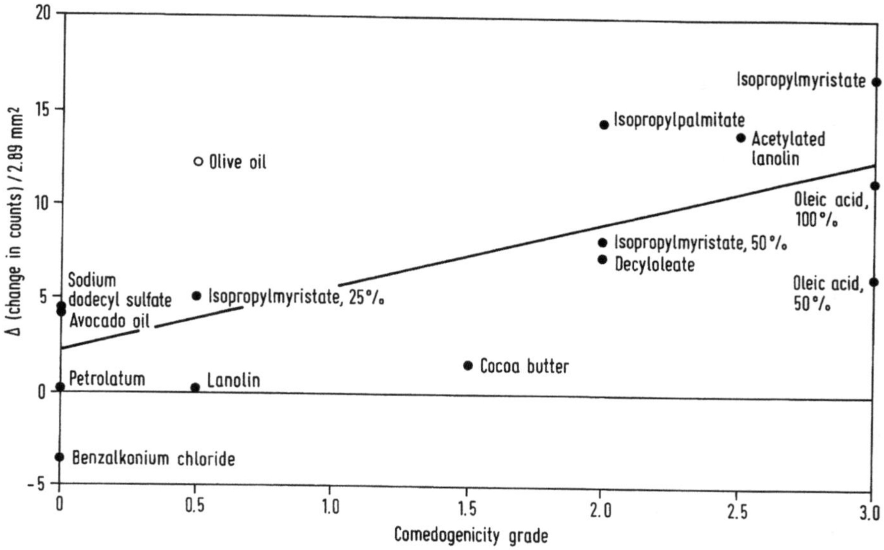

Fig. 15. Correlation of the number of fluorescent follicles per unit area with rabbit ear model of comedogenicity

Influence of ph Value of Products

The influence of the pH value of the topically, applied product on the generation or dissolution of comedones was studied by topical application of a vehicle adjusted to a pH value of 5.5 (A) and to pH 4 (B). While product A moderately reduced the number and area of fluorescent spots, product B was significantly more effective.

Influence of Titanium Dioxide-Containing Products

The influence of titanium dioxide powder, an effective sunscreen, on comedogenicity was studied on the forehead (sun exposed, February) and on the back (well protected against sun, February). The uncoated material caused slight shifts to lower numbers of comedones and smaller areas on the back (not significant). On the forehead (light exposed) there was a slight increase. The coated version did not cause any changes on the back, while on the forehead a minor increase was detected after 7 days of regular use.

Influence of Skin Surface Lipids

An effect of HD was not observable up to a concentration of 10% (in ethanol). The influence of α-hydroxypalmitic acid was found to be strongly dependent on concentration, reaching a maximum regarding comedogenicity at around 1%.

Relation Between Fluorescence-Detected Comedones and Cyanoacrylate Biopsies

Figure 16 shows the relation between numbers of comedones found by the cyanoacrylate technique [20] and fluerescence techniques before biopsying the skin. Even after cyanoacrylate stripping, almost the same number of fluorescent spots are detectable, indicating the location of propioniobacteria's habitat and demonstrating the methods extensive scope of the method (Fig. 17).

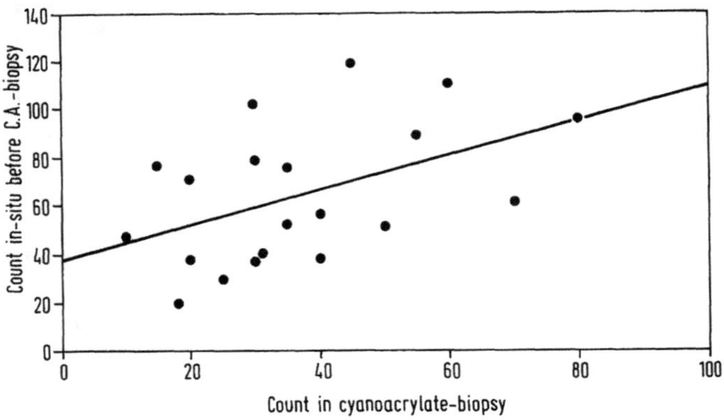

Fig. 16. Correlation between numbers of fluorescent follicles determined in situ versus counts determined on cyanoacrylate biopsies (20 samples)

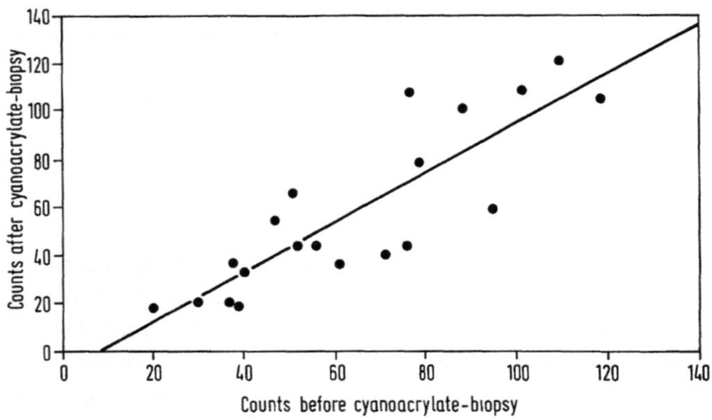

Fig. 17. Correlation between numbers of fluorescent follicles determined in situ before cyanoacrylate stripping versus fluorescent follicles determined in situ after cyanoacrylate stripping

Discussion

The finding that mainly the difference of identified glands – necessary criteria are fulfilled when the constant threshold value of intensity is surpassed by that of individual spots – show a development analogue to comedogenicity data derived from rabbit ear results may be the consequence of a still imperfect method. Based on the dose-effect results of oleic acid and isoproyl myristate, it is to be assumed that this parameter is sensitive enough to discriminate between relatively large changes of concentration. Size and intensity do not sufficiently change to be discriminative. The results of benzalkonium chloride or the effect of the ph value of topically applied products may be influenced by an additional phenomenon, the change of fluorescence yield [21]; this has not been investigated yet.

The parallel behavior of animal and human data support the assumption that the comedogenicity of topically applied products may be classified in humans by porphyrin fluorescence.

Comedolytic and Antibacterial Substances

Formation of comedones may be considered as a retention hyperkeratosis caused by incomplete desquamation. Assuming that propionibacteria causally influence the formation of comedones and the appearance of acne [22], application of proper antibacterials should decrease bacterial count and subsequently porphyrin fluorescence.

Materials and Methods

Antibacterial and Desquamating Agents

The influence of vitamin A acid or antibiotics presently used in acne therapy and of some antimicrobial preservatives used in topical products was investigated in a similar way as described above. The density of fluorescent follicles was determined after 10 and 20 days of product application. A total of 12 volunteers (6 femates, 6 males), age 20–40, participated. A series of products were applied once daily (10 µl/cm^2; Monday-Friday) for 3 weeks (Table 2, study A). In another study the influence of several other (miscellaneous) comedolytic substances were investigated in an analogous manner (Table 2), study B.

Table 2. Comedolytic and antibacterial substances

Study A	
Vitamin A acid	(0.65%)
Clindamycin	(1.28%)
Tetracycline	(3%)
Erythromycin	(2%)
Benzoyl peroxide	(5%)
Salicylic acid	(5% in ethanol)
Bronidox	(0.1% in xanthan gum gel)
Octhilione	(Kathon; 0.1% in xanthan gum gel)
Untreated	(six female volunteers)
Study B	
Human lysozyme	(0.1% from milk; Sigma)
Linolenic acid	(0.1% in gel base)
Nisin	(Nisaplin, 0.1%)
Short chain fatty acids	(10% in mineral oil; from wool wax acid)
Lipid-absorbing silica	(TaKallophane; pure)
C8 triglyceride	(Tricaproine; 10% in cream base)
Ethanol	(50% in water)

Results

Antibacterial Compunds

Vitamin A acid, clindamycin, benzoyl peroxide, and salicyclic acid decreased porphyrin fluorescence within the observation period of 3 weeks (Fig. 18). The results after us of erythromycin were not conclusive. The effect of tetracycline could not be evaluated due to strong autofluorescence of the product. Bronidox and Kathon had no effect. The size of the fluorescent spots also decreased (Fig. 19).

The effect of regular applications of Clindamycin is clearly demonstrated in Fig. 20. Within the treated area fluorescent spots are almost absent, while the neighboring untreated sites show normal porphyrin-containing glands.

During the treatment period large follicles shrunk considerably, with a concomitant decrease in fluorescence intensity.

Miscellaneous

Lysozyme linolenic acid, and especially nisin preparations reduced the density of comedones. Tricaproine did not change the density but reduced the mean area previously high of the comedones (Fig. 21).

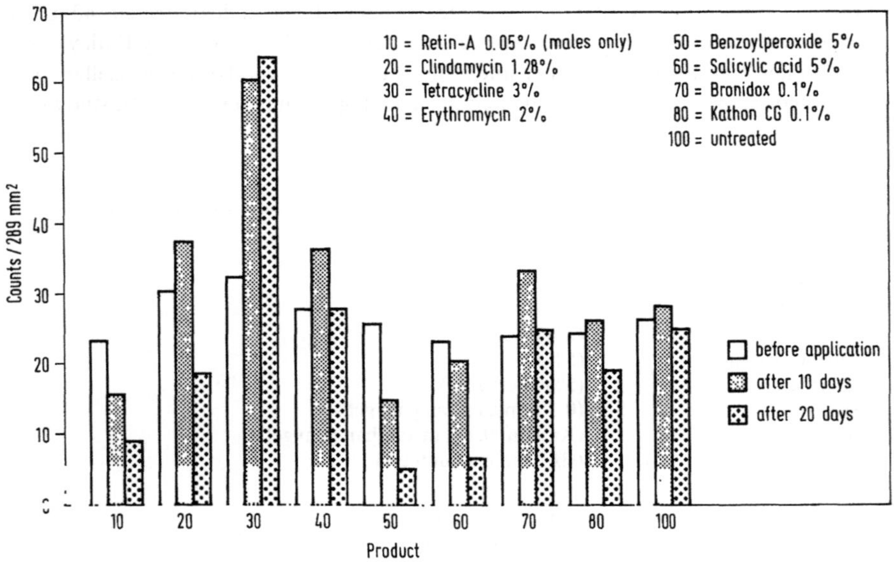

Fig. 18. Influence of topically applied antibacterials and desquamating agents on the density of fluorescent follicles. *10*, Retin A (0.05%, males only); *20*, clindamycin (1.28%); *30*, tetracycline (3%); *40*, erythromycin (2%); *50*, benzoyl peroxide (5%); *60*, salicylic acid (5%); *70*, (Bronidox, 0.1 %); *80*, octhilinone (Kathon CG, 0.1%); *100*, untreated

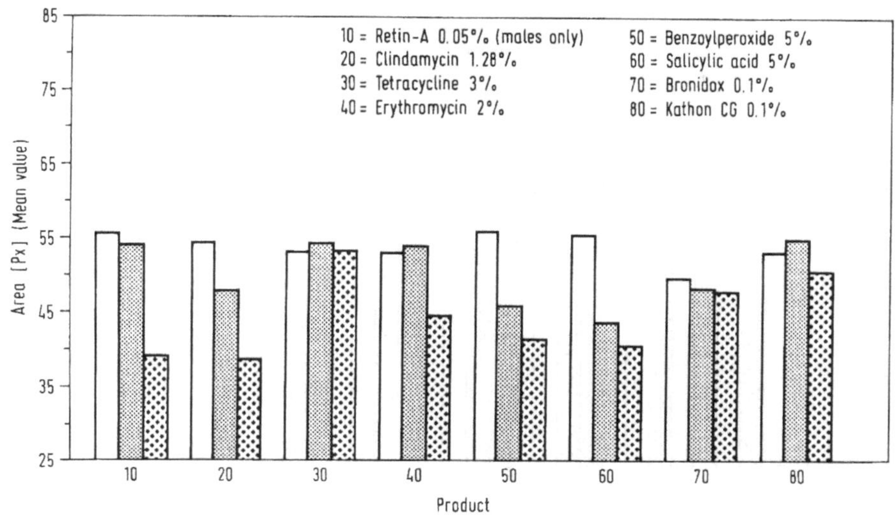

Fig. 19. Influence of topically applied antibacterials and desquamating agents on the mean area of fluorescent follicles. *10*, Retin A (0.05%, males only); *20*, clindamycin (1.28%); *30*, tetracycline (3%); *40*, erythromycin (2%); *50*, benzoyl peroxide (5%); *60*, salicylic acid (5%); *70*, (Bronidox, 0.1%); *80*, octhilinone (Kathon CG, 0.1 %)

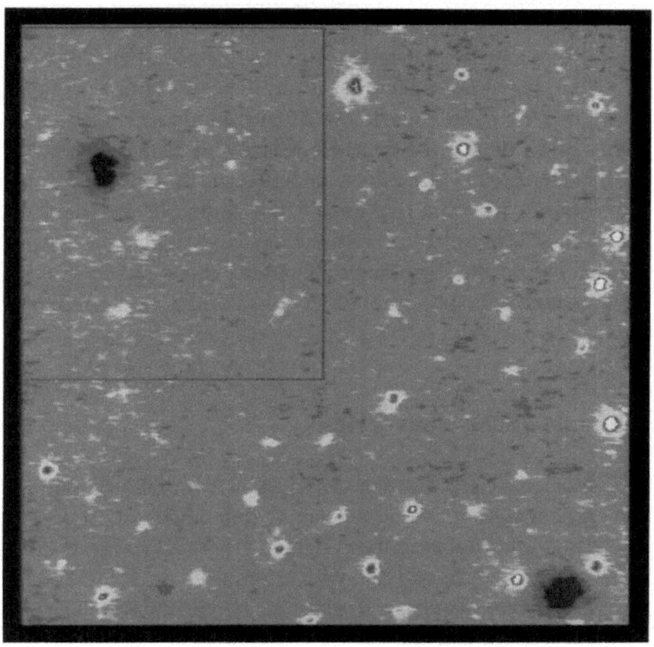

Fig. 20. Skin site after a treatment period of 3 weeks with clindamycin (*upper left* side, indicated by frame) vs untreated control area (*lower right*)

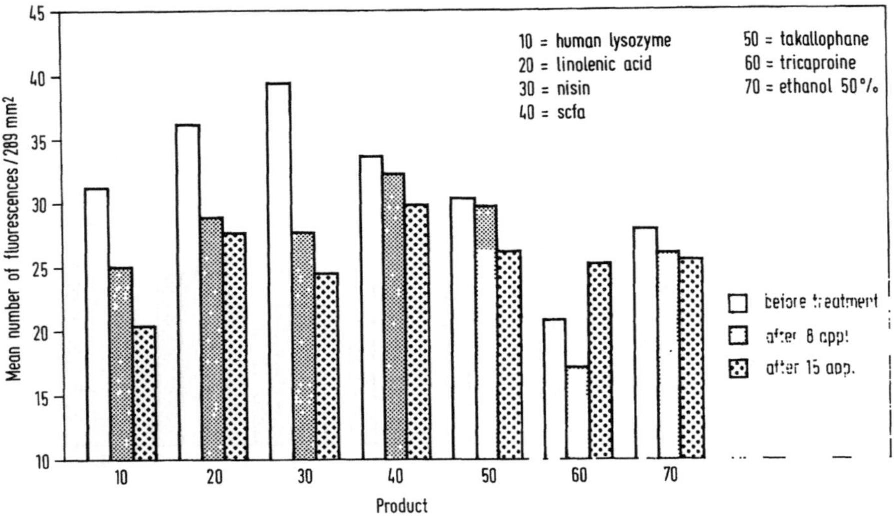

Fig. 21. Influence of miscellaneous topically applied products on the density of fluorescent follicles. *10*, Human lysozyme; *20*, linolenic acid; *30*, nisin; *40*, short chain fatty acids; *50* lipid-absorbing silica (Takallophane, 5%); *60*, C 8 triglyceride (Tricaproine, 5%); *70* ethanol (50%)

Discussion

The growth rate of propionibacteria and synthesis of porphyrins correlate fairly well [13]. Therefore it is to be expected that antibacterial substances will diminish porphyrin synthesis. Porphyrins already present in the gland, probably leak into surrounding tissue and are transported to the skin surface by flowing sebum, which is oxidized by singlet oxygen produced by porphyrin sensitization. If neosynthesis of porphyrins is diminished by antibacterials or if the amount of sebum increases due to desquamation-promoting agents, the comedonal size and count will shrink.

The density of comedones quickly decreases during treatment with linolenic acid, in accordance with the hypothesis that comedo formation and follicular hyperkeratinization are linked to essential fatty acid deficiency [23]. The irregularly changing densities and the shrinking mean area caused by short chain triglycerides may reflect the melanogenic potential of 1,2-diglycerides generated in situ by bacterial hydrolysis [24, 25].

Inflamed Sebaceous Glands

Sunburned skin is strongly fluorescent; when illuminated with radiation of 280 nm, strong emission of > 350 nm can be detected (Fig. 22).

Visibly inflamed sebaceous glands show a fluorescence pattern in the UVA range (340 nm) when illuminated with UV-B (290 nm) (Fig. 23).

The efficacy of anti-acne treatment should also be clearly visible using this part of the fluorescence spectrum.

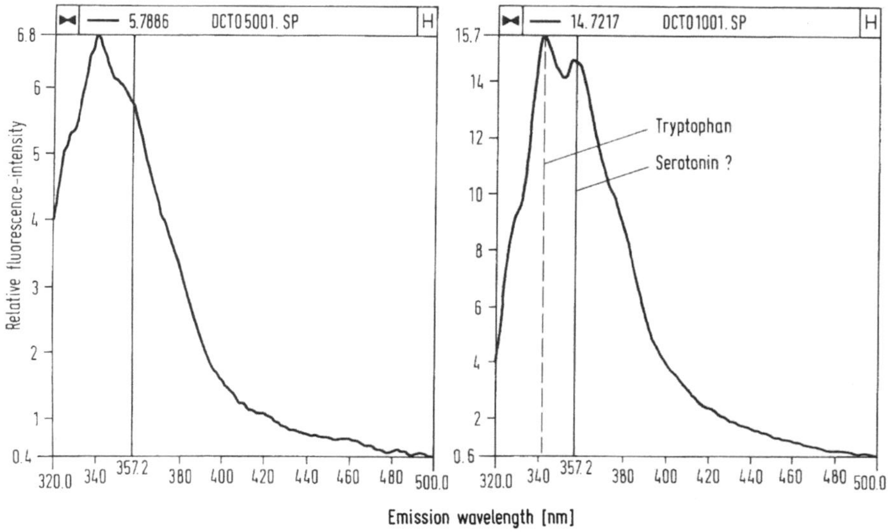

Fig. 22. Fluorescence spectra of non irradiated (*left*) and sunburned (*right*) lower forearm (excitation 290 nm, emission 320–500 nm)

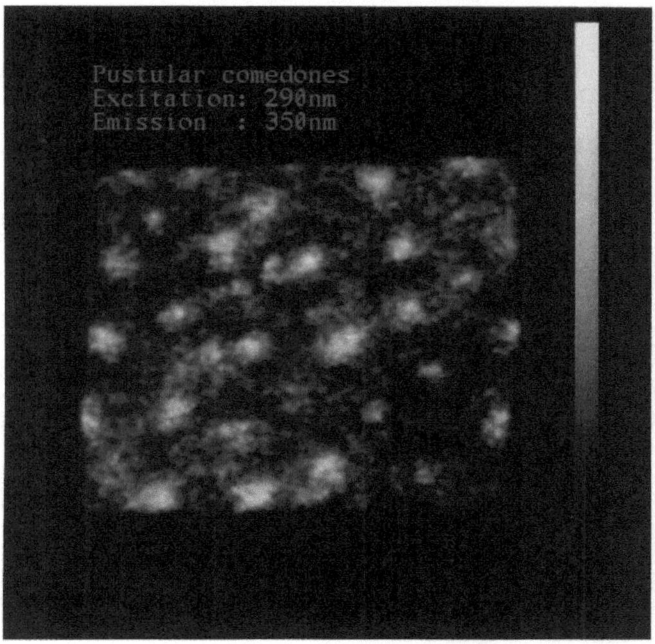

Fig. 23. Fluorescence emission (excitation 290 nm, emission 350 nm) of inflamed sebaceous glands (upper back)

Conclusions

The increase in number and area of fluorescent follicles was found to parallel the comedogenic ratings of the test substances in the rabbit ear model. Mean area and mean fluorescence intensity were not correlated with comedogenicity.

This method may provide a noninvasive human model for determining the comedogenicity of topically applied cosmetics and drugs.

The efficacy of antibiotics against *P. acnes* can be readily monitored by frequent measurement of porphyrin fluorescence.

The comedolytic activity of vitamin A acid and salicylic acid is clearly visible.

References

1. Fanta D et al. (1981) Porphyrin synthesis by propionibacteria in dependence on external factor. Arch Dermatol Res 271: 127–133
2. Meloe TB et al. (1982) In vivo porphyrin fluorescence from Propionibacteria acnes. A characterization of the fluorescing pigments. Dermatologica 164: 167–174
3. Bommer S (1927) Hautuntersuchungen in gefiltertem Quarzlicht. Klin. Wochenschrift 6: 1142–1144
4. Kjelstad B, et al. (1986) Uptake of hematoporphyrin derivative in bacteria and photosensitization of Propionibacterium acnes bacteria. Photobiochem Photobiophys 10: 163–173
5. McGinley KJ et al. (1988) Facial follicular porphyrin fluorescence: correlation with age and density of Propionibacterium acnes. Br J Dermatol 102: 437–441
6. Kligman AM et al. (1970) Bacteriology of acne comedones. Arch Dermatol 102: 397–399
7. Sauermann G et al. (1989) Analysis of facial comedos by porphyrin fluorescence and image analysis. J. Toxicol. Cut Ocul Toxicol 8 4: 369–385
8. Sauermann G et al. (1990) A novel fluorimetric method for assaying comedogenic substances in humans. 49th annual meeting of the American Academy of Dermatol, Dec 1990
9. Kligman AM et al. (1982) A human model for assessing human comedogenic substances. Arch Dermatol 118: 903–905
10. Lanzet M Comedogenic effects of cosmetic raw materials Cosmet Toil 101: 63–72
11. Morris WE et al. (1983) Use of the rabbit ear model in evaluating the comedogenic potential of cosmetic ingredients. J Soc Cosmet Chem 34: 215–225
12. Fulton JE et al. (1986) J Am Acad Dermatol 10: 96–105
13. Kjelstadt B et al. (1984) Influence of pH on porphyrin production in Propionibacterium acnes. Arch Dermatol Res 276: 396–400
14. Schäfer H (1992) In: (ed) Empfindliche Haut. Diesbach, Berlin, p 159
15. Degussa AG (1989) Schriftenr Pigmente 56;
16. Millers et al. (1988) In vitro and in vivo antistaphylococcal activity of human stratum corneum lipids. Arch Dermatol 124: 209–215
17. Van Scott EJ et al. (1984) Hyperkeratinization, corneocyte cohesion and alpha hydroxy acids. J Am Acad Dermatol 11 5: 867–879
18. Stewart ME et al. (1989) The effect of changes in sebaceous gland activity on the fatty acid composition of sebum. In: Marks, Plewig G (eds) Acne und related disorders. Dunitz, London, pp 63–66
19. Francoeur ML et al. (1990) Oleic acid: its effects of stratum corneum in relation to transdermal drug delivery. Pharm Res 7 6: 621–627
20. Marks R et al. (1971) Skin surface biopsy: an improved technique for the examination of the horny layer. Br J Dermatol 84: 117–123
21. Polo CF et al. (1988) Factors influencing fluorescence spectra of free porphyrins. Clin Chem 34 4: 7757–760

22. Pochi PE (1988) Acne: androgens and microbiology. Drug Dev Res 13: 157–168
23. Wertz PW et al. (1985) The composition of the ceramides from humanan stratum corneum and from comedones. J Invest Dermatol 84: 410–412
24. Kligman AM et al. (1974) Pigmentation in comedones. Arch Dermatol 109: 60–62
25. Gordon PR et al. (1989) Human melanogenesis is stimulated by diacylglycerol. J Invest Dermatol 935: 700–702

Assessing Impaired Blood Supply of the Skin in Peripheral Arterial Occlusion Using Heat Flow Calorimetry

V. WIENERT and N. OYOUN-NIEPEL*

Introduction

Heat flow calorimetry is a quantitative, noninvasive, and simple method of assessing the skin's thermal conductivity, either when the vessels of the capillary system are stationary or when the vessels are dilatated after being stimulated by heat. The tissue blood supply is recorded by measuring locally applied heat as it diffuses.

This chapter describes how the blood supply of the skin in the lower leg was examined by means of this method. The patients chosen for the examination included some healthy persons, some patients from risk groups, and some patients with manifest peripheral occlusion, both before and after surgical recanalization. We were particularly interested in analyzing the feedback mechanism of the skin's microcirculation under both normal and chronic restricted circulation conditions.

Methods

The principle of heat flow calorimetry is based on the fact that tissue absorbs more heat from a heated sensor when it is well supplied with blood [3]. Model experiments have shown that thermal conductivity of tissue has a certain value when circulation is interrupted and increases as perfusion increases: at first as marked increase, then not so pronounced [4].

The computer-controlled heat flow calorimeter which we used can measure the heat flow (Q') between a source of heat fixed on the skin's surface (sensor) and the skin. The sensor has a constant temperature (T) and a contact area of 1 cm^2. Figure 1 shows the sensor attached to the skin and Figure 2 the bridging circuit of the heat flow calorimeter. The sensor temperature, which is freely adjustable is held constant electrically and the electrical power needed to warm the surface of the sensor is recorded. In steady-state thermal conditions this electrical power corresponds to the heat flow from the sensor into the skin. The thermal conductivity coefficient, determined from the differential of the heat flow Q' according to the sensor temperature T, indicates the conductive part of the thermal conduction in skin with no blood supply and increases because of convection with increasing circulation. Thus, the coefficient is proportional to perfusion [5] and will be referred to here as the perfusion index.

---

* Department of Dermatology, University of Aachen, Division of Dermatological Phlebology, Pauwelsstraße 30, 5100 Aachen, FRG

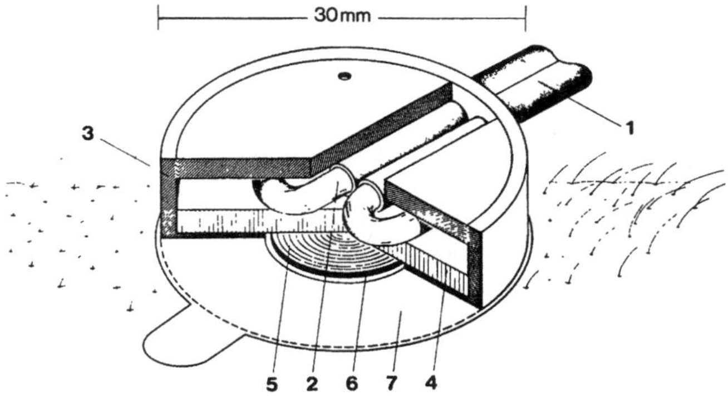

Fig. 1. Section through the probe attached to the skin. *1*, two-stranded cable with silicon insulation; *2*, extremely flexible fine-stranded cable core; PVC casing; *4*, mounting plate (quartz), gold plated on both sides; *5*, gilded copper plate; *6*, surface contacting the skin; *7*, double-sided adhesive ECG electrode ring

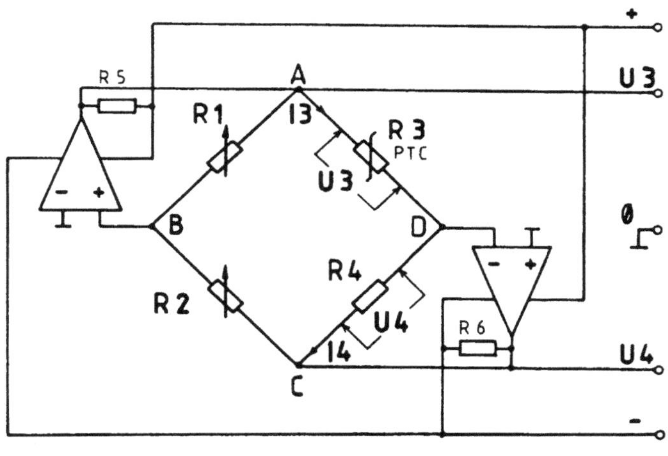

Fig. 2. Briding circuit of the heat flow calorimeter (*PTC*, probe temperature element)

The thermal conductivity coefficient of basal perfusion (blood circulation of perfusion at rest), the basal perfusion index (BPI), is determined when the sensor temperature is below 40°C. The maximum perfusion index (MPI) is determined after hyperemization of the skin by applying local hyperthermy (48°C for 5 min). Dividing MPI by BPI results in the quotient IPI (increased perfusion index: MPI/BPI = IPI) which indicates the blood supply reserve and therefore the extent to which the skin can regulate its circulation. This method is described in more detail by Niepel [5].

Altogether 58 people were examined: (a) 20 healthy subjects with no indication of peripheral occlusive disease (PAOD). Of these 12 were under 40 years of age, eight were over; (b) 20 patients who had at least one risk factor for some years: hypertension, hypercholesterolemia, diabetes mellitus, serious nicotine abuse. Of these, six were under 40 years of age, 14 were over; (c) 18 hospitalized patients who had manifest PAOD, diagnosed by digital subtraction angiography (DSA), and three who were aged between 39 and 77 years old. Of these, seven patients were stage II, eight were stage

III, and three were stage IV (according to Fontaine). Of these 18 patients, 12 were examined before and after surgical recanalization of the large artery in the leg and/or pelvis, and two were examined before and after sympathectomy.

Results

Figure 3 is the heat flow graph of a 20-year-old healthy female's results and is a good example of the linear relationship of sensor temperature and thermal flow in the skin during basal perfusion (represented by the unshaded rectangles) and after hyperemization by means of local hyperthermy (shaded rectangles). The thermal conductivity coefficient – here, called the perfusion index – corresponds to the gradient of the degrees of regression. It is represented by the sensor temperature in Fig. 4. Basal perfusion is determined through the average gradient of BPI = dQ'/dT when the sensor

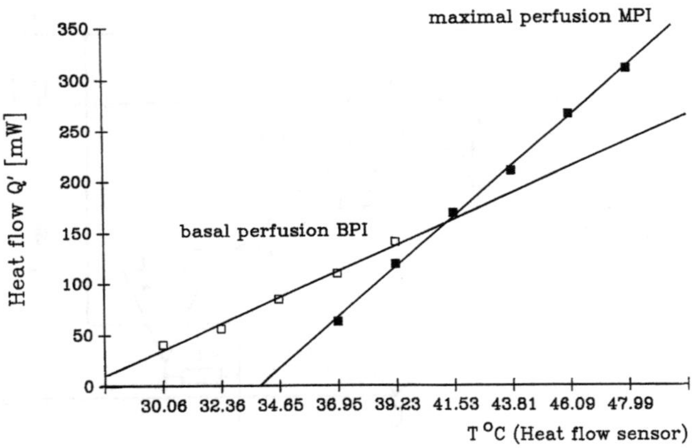

Fig. 3. Heat flow diagram of healthy female subject

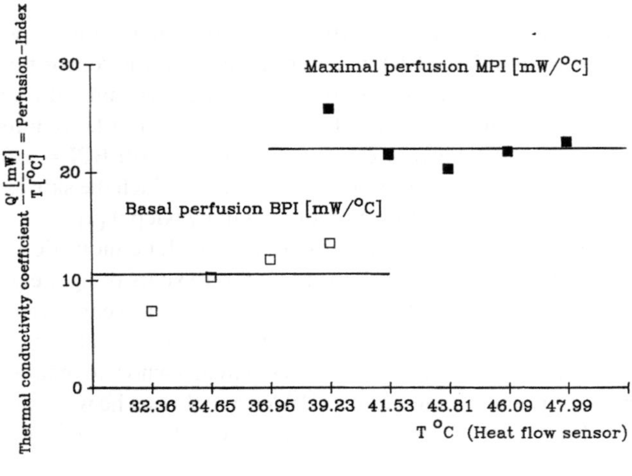

Fig. 4. Heat flow diagram (f prime x) of a healthy female subject

temperature is below 40° C, and maximum perfusion through the average gradient of MPI = dQ'/dT after stimulation by heat.

The separate entries in Table 1 are of the mean value and standard deviation of BPI and MPI after stimulation by heat, and the IPI for the different groups.

The remarkable thing is that the *lowest* BPI values, which means the weakest basal perfusion, are to be found among the *healthy* people younger than 40 (on average 14.5 mW/° C) (Fig. 5). The greater the vascular risk and PAOD stage, the stronger the basal perfusion; the thermal conductivity coefficient (BPI) is at its highest (on average 24.1 ± 1.7 mW/° C) in patients who are in stage IV, as described by Fontaine. Those patients who had disobliteration surgery showed values 1 week after the operation which corresponded to values for risk group patients in stage II, who had fewer symptoms. As far as the circulation of the skin is concerned, this is an optimal surgical result.

Table 1. Basal perfusion (BPI), maximum perfusion (MPI) and increased perfusion (IPI, blood supply reserve) among the test subjects

Subject (*n*)	BPI (mW/°C)	MPI (mW/°C)	IPI
Healthy subjects under 40 (12)	14.5 ± 2.7	26.3 ± 1.2	1.87 ± 0.35
Healthy subjects over 40 (8)	16.6 ± 1.6	23.4 ± 0.9	1.42 ± 0.14
Risk patients (20)	18.1 ± 2.4	23.0 ± 1.6	1.3 ± 0.19
Diabetics under 40 (3)	19.2 ± 1.8	23.2 ± 1.1	1.21 ± 0.09
PAOD patients (18)	20.3 ± 2.5	22.9 ± 1.6	1.14 ± 0.12
Stage II (7)	18.5 ± 2.1	22.5 ± 1.5	1.23 ± 0.10
Stage III (8)	20.5 ± 1.0	23.5 ± 1.4	1.12 ± 0.03
Stage IV (3)	24.1 ± 1.7	23.2 ± 2.9	0.96 ± 0.10
Operation patients (12)			
Before	20.5 ± 2.9	22.8 ± 1.9	1.13 ± 0.13
After	18.9 ± 1.9	24.1 ± 1.3	1.28 ± 0.12
Patients after sympathectomy (2)	23.0 ± 0.1	23.0 ± 0.6	1.00 ± 0.03

PAOD, peripheral arterial occlusion disease

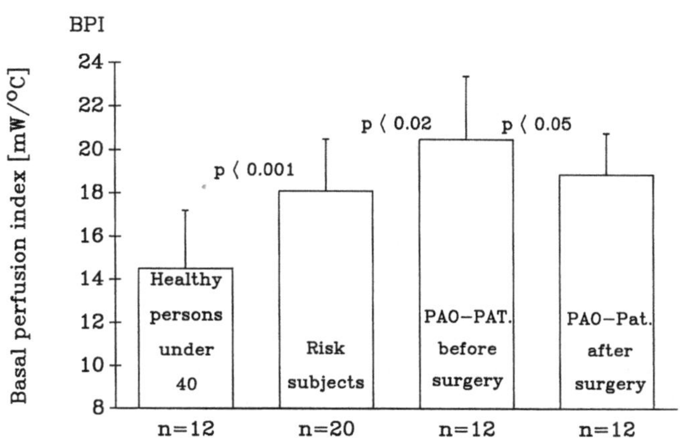

Fig. 5. Mean values and standard deviations for basal perfusion index (BPI). BPI = dQ'/dT, where Q' is heat flow (W) and T is the temperature (°C). *PAO*, peripheral arterial occlusion

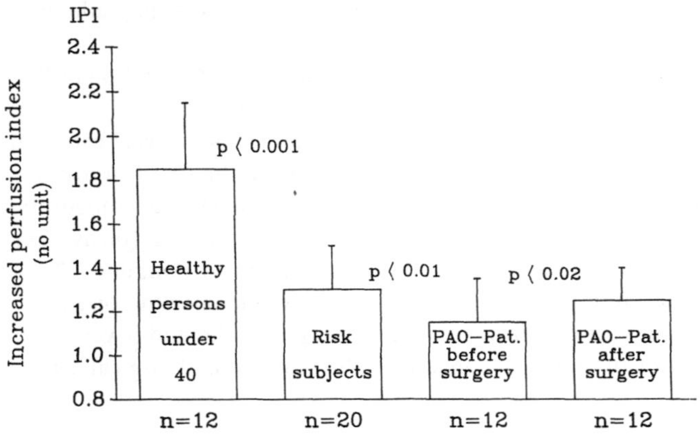

Fig. 6. Increased perfusion index (IPI; blood supply reserve) in 12 patients with peripheral arterial occlusion before and after recanalization surgery. IPI = MPI/BPI, where MPI is the maximum perfusion index (mW/°C) and BPI is the basal perfusion index (mW/°C)

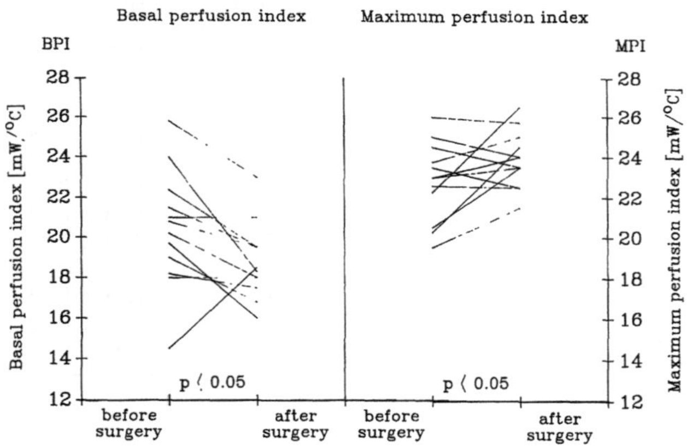

Fig. 7. Basal perfusion (BPI; heat conductivity coefficient) and maximal perfusion (MPI; thermal conductivity coefficient after heat stimulation) in 12 patients with peripheral arterial occlusion before and after recanalization surgery

The quotient of MPI and BPI is IPI, which is a measure of the extent to which the skin can regulate its circulation or the blood supply reserve. As can be seen from the significant differences between the individual groups, IPI is a more reliable parameter with which to assess how severe any impairment of the capillary system is. Some values over 2.0 were registered for young healthy persons: this means that the thermal conductivity of the skin is double that of basal perfusion because the heat stimulation sends a greater flow of blood into the microvessels. Such a large regulation range, due to low basal perfusion and an ability to increase considerably after heat has been applied, could not be found in any other groups under investigation. On the contrary, the IPI mean values for healthy persons over 40 were 1.42 ± 0.14 (In comparison, healthy persons under 40 had IPI values of 1.87 ± 0.35; significantly variable $p < 0.5$). The blood supply reserve reduces to half its amount under physiological conditions with age.

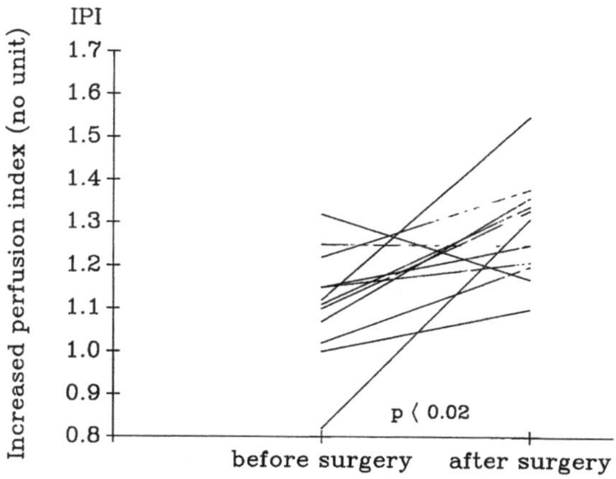

Fig. 8. Increased perfusion index (IPI, blood supply reserve) in 12 patients with peripheral arterial occlusion before and after recanalization surgery. IPI = MPI/ BPI, where MPI is the maximum perfusion index (mW/°C) and BPI is the basal perfusion index (mW/°C)

Likewise, patients from the risk groups with vascular diseases had a smaller regulation range than healthy people (Fig. 6). The difference in the IPI between risk patients and the control group of corresponding age is particularly great in young diabetics (1.21 ± 0.09, $n = 3$, in contrast to 1.87 ± 0.35, $n = 12$ with $p < 0.01$). This is not a surprise since vascular lesions of the skin are typical complications in diabetic angiopathy and can appear relatively soon after the condition has started. If there is trophic impairment of the skin, as in the case of PAOD in stage IV, then there is practically no more range of vascular regulation (Fig. 6). This can be seen from the IPI values in stage IV that are about 1.0 (0.96 ± 0.10, $n = 3$). The high BPI is not sufficient to supply the tissue; increased perfusion, however, cannot be achieved by additional heat stimulation. Similar, but on average slightly better values were recorded in the other stages of PAOD Figures 7 and 8 show, respectively, the mean BPI and IPI values of all the patients with PAOD who had later had disobliteration surgery. The blood supply reserve increases markedly after recanalization (IPI; Fig. 8). This is because while the maximum blood supply increases due to the disobliteration (MPI increases slightly, Fig. 7), the blood supply necessary for the skin at rest clearly decreases (BPI, Fig. 7). The postoperative values for BPI and IPI are similar to those of the risk group patients (Figs. 5, 6). It is worth mentioning the completely different picture after sympathectomy. The aim of the operation is the constant and maximum dilatation of the restistance vessels. Accordingly, the perfusion index remains unaffected by heat stimulation, and this is the reason why the IPI was 1,0 ± 0.03 in the two investigated cases (not shown).

Discussion

The function of the feedback mechanism of the microcirculation of the skin assumes that if precapillary sphincters are dilated, blood supply is increased and this leads to better nourishment of the tissue. This relationship between the width of resistance vessels and nutritive supply to tissue is correct only to a certain degree. Available data show that in PAOD patients, sufficient or poor nourishment is combined with increased basal perfusion, but in young, healthy people, good nourishment is combined with a comparatively low basal perfusion. This could not be deduced purely from the relationship described above and needs some additional explanation.

In all the groups that were examined, there was the described relationship between the degree of vascular disease and basal perfusion. Basal perfusion is anyway lower in young and healthy people than in old or risk patients, and after disobliteration it is lower than previously. Understandably, patients with high basal perfusion do not have increased tissue nourishment, as PAOD patients in stage IV demonstrate (with impaired skin nutrition). On the contrary, angiopathic patients apparently have hyperperfusion of the skin because of impaired economy of the microcirculation [2]. The feedback mechanism tries to compensate for the reduced effectiveness by enlarging the resistance vessels so as to maintain nourishment. This succeeds as long as there is scope for regulation (IPI > 1.0).

A number of pathophysiological mechanisms which probably also reinforce each other could be put forward as the reason for the poor economy of the microcirculation. Here, the insufficient circulation is bound to be especially significant: if all the precapillary sphincters are open to their maximum, only the short capillaries will be supplied with blood because they offer less perfusion resistance than longer capillaries which have a considerably larger diffusion surface. Therefore, with a smaller diffusion surface and, consequently, diminished circulatory effectiveness, nourishment is reduced despite increased circulation [1, 6].

Furthermore, increased plasma viscosity which arises in PAOD can impede circulation, especially in long capillaries. The stenosis causes the blood flow to slow down and this, together with a typically raised fibrinogen level, promotes the formation of erythrocytic aggregates, hindering the release of 0_2.

After disobliteration of vascular stenosis, the blood supply to the muscles increases again and the raised basal perfusion of the skin deceases correspondingly, whereby the skin is better nourished and all the symptoms improve. Verification for this comes from vascular surgery: primarily it aims to improve the blood supply to the muscle, but, as expected, it has a significant effect on the microcirculation of the skin.

The improved nourishment is not only due to the increased volume of blood flow once the vascular stenosis has been removed, but also to the improvement in the economy of the microcirculation, brought about by the higher differential pressure between the arteriole and venule in the peripheral tissues.

References

1. Doermer C, Schroeder W (1975) Blood flow and tissue-pO_2 in the trained and untrained gastrocnemius muscle of the anesthetized guinea pig. Eur 5 Appl Physiol 34: 33
2. Ehrly AM (1986) Heißt bessere Durchblutung auch immer bessere Versorgung? Fortschr Med 25: 492
3. Gibbs FA (1933) A thermoelectric blood flow recorder in the form of a needle. Proc Soc Exp Biol Med 31: 141

4. Hensel H, Bender F (1956) Fortlaufende Bestimmung der Hautdurchblutung am Menschen mit einem elektrischen Wärmeleitmesser. Pflügers Archiv 263: 603
5. Niepel G (1986) Wärmeflußkalorimetrische Untersuchung der Thermoregulationsprozesse in der Haut bei geringer örtlicher Hyperthermie. Thesis, Aachen Medical Faculty
6. Renkin EM, Hudlická O, Sheehan RM (1986) Influence of metabolic vasodilatation on blood tissue diffusion in skeletal muscle. Am J Physiol 211: 87

Transcutaneous Oxygen Pressure Measurement: Methods, Implementation, and Possible Applications

V. WIENERT AND A. LENTNER*

Introduction

Measurement of transcutaneous oxygen pressure ($tcpO_2$) has become widely used in recent years as a noninvasive method to examine the microcirculation of the skin. The method was introduced by R. Huch at the beginning of the 1970s [21], described theoretically in the following years by R. Huch, A. Huch, and D.W. Lübbers, and first used in perinatal supervision of newborn babies [22, 23, 26–28]. Soon other medical departments, such as intensive care (for continuous monitoring of patients on breathing apparatus), surgery (to assess limbs that might have to be amputated), plastic surgery (to monitor the viability of skin transplants), dermatology (to diagnose and observe the course of dermatoses), and, particularly, angiology (for any questions concerning the microcirculation of the skin), became interested in measuring $tcpO_2$. Once commercial equipment for this technique had been developed, the method was also used in routine examination by angiology departments and microcirculation laboratories.

Methods

The TCM3 (Radiometer, Copenhagen, Denmark, Fig. 1) will be described here as an example of the various commercial systems for $tcpO_2$ measurement. The products of other manufacturers are basically the same. Measurement is carried out by applying a sensor about 1 cm in diameter to the skin (Fig. 2). The sensor is held in place by a special adhesive ring that holds the electrolyte solution in which the sensor head is immersed. There is a Clark electrode inside the sensor to determine the oxygen pressure and an element that can be regulated to warm up the liquid under the electrode. The Clark sensor is made up of a central platinum cathode and a ring-shaped silver anode and is separated from the electrolyte solution by a polypropylene membrane (Fig. 3). The oxygen rising from the subpapillary plexus, moving through the epidermis, and diffusing at the surface of the skin is measured polarographically. It is necessary to apply heat under the electrode in order to induce local hyperemia, for it is only then that enough oxygen diffuses at the skin. Without hyperemia there would be practically no oxygen pressure on the epidermis.

* Department of Dermatology of the RWTH Aachen, Dermatological Phlebology, 5100 Aachen, FRG

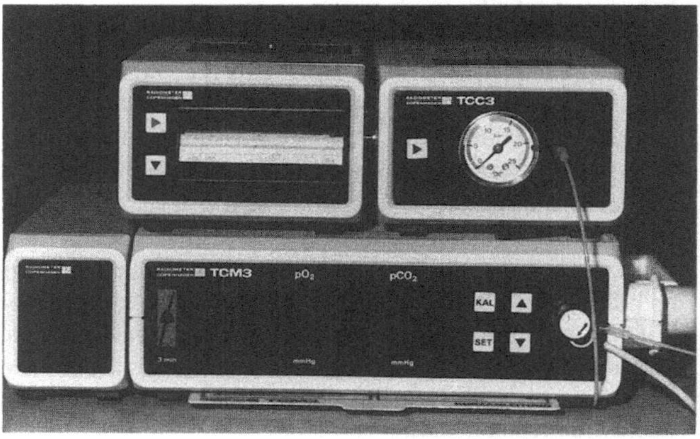

Fig. 1. TCM3, radiometer

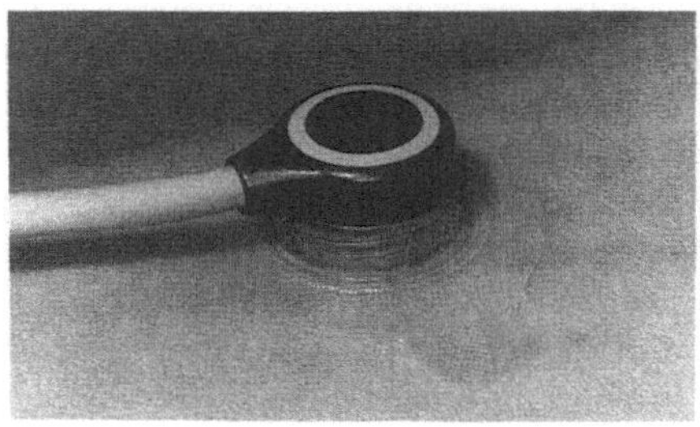

Fig. 2. $TcpO_2$ sensor fixed at the skin

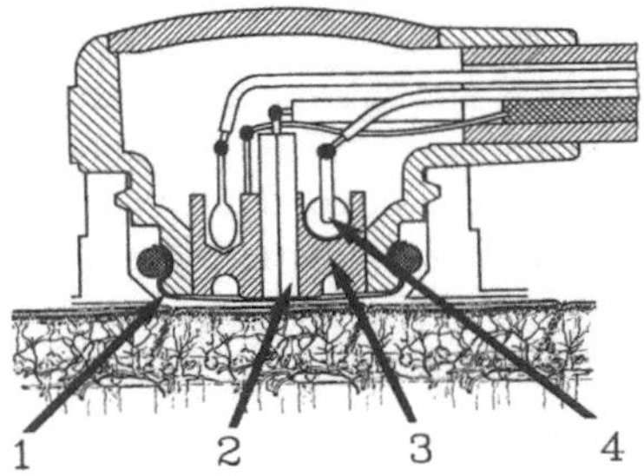

Fig. 3. $TcpO_2$ sensor: *1* polypropylene membrane; *2* platin cathode; *3* silver anode; *4* heating element (Modified from [3])

Factors Influencing Measurement

Although the system is easy to operate, the measurement itself depends on a number of individual parameters. Knowledge of their influence and how to evaluate them is needed to interpret the measured values correctly. The factors can be divided roughly into three groups: (1) the parameters set by the choice of electrode; (2) those caused by the patient under examination; and (3) influences caused by the circumstances in which the examination is carried out.

Influences of the Electrode

Although the principle of measurements is comparable between various commercial types of electrodes, each system has its differences in the construction of the sensor head and the materials used. Before measurement is started, the system is calibrated by means of a standardized calibration gas, with the aim, at least, of comparability of measurement with the same equipment at different times. The membranes used to separate the area of skin from the Clark electrode also differ from each other: some systems use polypropylene, others use Teflon. There are reports that problems arise with Teflon membranes when the transcutaneous oxygen pressure is low.

The core temperature of the electrode is particularly significant. We have already mentioned that without local hyperemia induced by heating there is practically no $tcpO_2$, or, more exactly, it fluctuates between 0 and 2 mm Hg. Small values like these and fluctuations cannot, however, be interpreted properly by the equipment available to date. Therefore, hyperemia is induced in the area of skin under examination and this is usually done by heating electrodes which are fitted in the sensor head (Fig. 4). A general optimal temperature for measurement cannot be specified: the temperature depends first and foremost on the aim of the examination. Two temperature areas have generally gained acceptance: that is, measurements at 37° C and at 44°–45° C. The first value has the advantage that self-regulatory mechanisms can still influence the measurement, whereas autoregulatory influences are largely eliminated at 44°–45° C. It is also more practical to carry out dynamic procedures and stimulation tests at 37° C. The disadvantage of this temperature is, however, that it is much more difficult to reproduce the results when the measurements are repeated on the same patient and skin area at different times. Furthermore, problems in interpreting the results can arise since it is scarcely possible to monitor completely all the parameters which influence measurement. When recording measurements at a core temperature of 44°–45° C, it is assumed that at this temperature there will be maximum dilatation of the subpapillary plexus and this dilatation can hardly influence the self-regulatory parameters. The advantage of this temperature ought to be better reproducibility of measurement results, with the consequence, of course, that this electrode temperature does not seem so suitable for dynamic examinations.

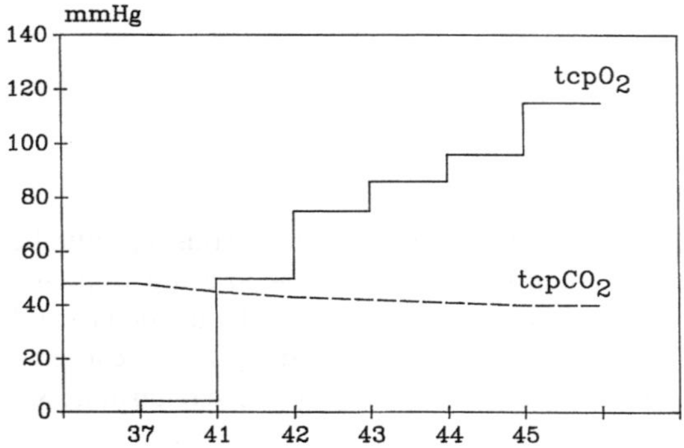

Fig. 4. Electrode's temperature dependency of $tcpO_2$ and $tcpCO_2$ values

Influences Caused by the Patient

We can deal with only a few of the numerous influences caused by the patient. Firstly, there is the patient's age: after more than 100 $tcpO_2$ measurements, it is our experience that the average oxygen pressure decreases with age [39] (Fig. 5).

There were significantly lower values recorded from smokers (whose clinical examination showed no pathological findings) in comparison to nonsmokers. However there were no significant differences between the sexes, although we must wait for investigations into the amount and duration of nicotine intake before any final statement can be made about smokers.

It is also surprising that our own investigations show there is no correlation between artery pressures in the ankle, recorded by Doppler sonography, and $tcpO_2$ values measured at the same time in the forefoot. Other investigators confirm this finding [11]. From this we can draw the conclusion that, when oxygen pressure is measured, there is first and foremost an assessment of the microcirculation, even though it is nonetheless understood that there cannot be an intact microcirculation when the macrocirculation is severely impaired. Patients with anemia caused by the kidneys had clearly lower $tcpO_2$ values. The findings returned to normal if the anemia could be

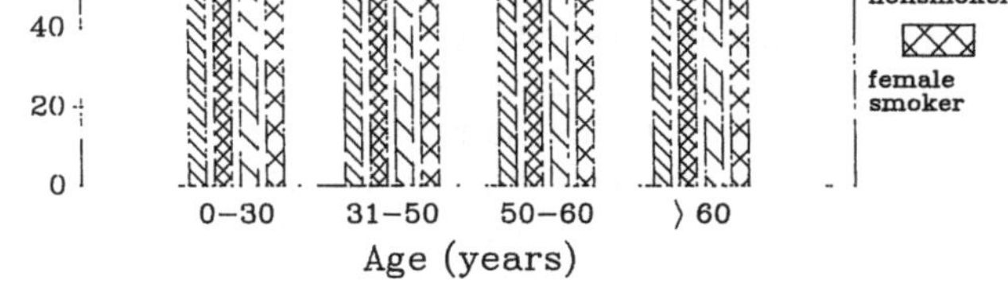

Fig. 5. Influence of age, sex, and smoking habits on $tcpO_2$ values. Instrument, TCM_3; measured area fore foot; electrode temperature, 45° C; water bath temperature, 42° C. (From 25, 39])

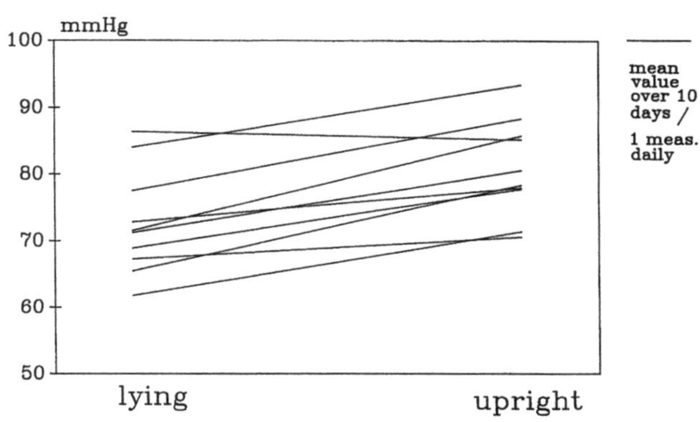

Fig. 6. Influence of body position on $tcpO_2$ values: mean of daily measurement, once daily for 10 days. TCM_3; electrode temperature, 44° C, measurement area, lower leg; n = 10. (From [31])

improved or cured [13]. The part of the body where measurements are taken is also relevant for the measured values (Fig. 6). The density of capillaries per area unit differs greatly in various parts of the body. When capillaroscopic findings and $tcpO_2$ values were compared, a correlation was found: there were higher values in areas with a greater density of capillaries [33]. In addition, hydrostatic pressure influences the measurements: in the transition from lying to standing, the $tcpO_2$ values increase considerably due to the increase in hydrostatic pressure [24].

Influences Caused by the Circumstances of the Examination

Since $tcpO_2$ measurement depends, to a large extent, on capillary blood flow and since the skin is able to adapt its circulation over a large area to the surroundings, great attention must be paid to the circumstances in which each measurement is taken. As will be shown below (Reproducibility of Measured Values) parameters such as ambient temperature and humidity of the room must be monitored and optimized not only when the electrode core temperature is 37° C, but also when the temperature is 44° C. At the same time, it is advisable to carry out measurements in a quiet place, without acoustic or visual distractions for the patient; the opening and shutting of a door, for example, has often had an effect on the sensitive measurement procedure.

Reproducibility of Measured Values

There is no unanimous opinion about reproducibility. It is generally said that it is poor at an electrode temperature of 37° C, while some investigators found reproducibility good at 44° C [12]. After repeated measurements were carried out on the same part of the anatomy at 2 week intervals on healthy volunteers, the investigators came to the conclusion that diagnoses and decisions about therapy (for example, deciding on how much to amputate in severe cases of arterial occlusive disease) should not depend on single measurements but on the average values of repeated $tcpO_2$ measurements [30]. Contrary to these findings, other examiners observed only slight deviations of an average of 4.7 mm Hg in repeated measurements within 30 min [17]. Values were measured in both legs of a healthy control group and compared, and a considerable intraindividual variation was ascertained [29].

We carried out $tcpO_2$ measurements on healthy volunteers at the same site, same time of day, with an electrode core temperature of 44° C and a room temperature of 23° C, on 10 consecutive days. We obtained a wide range of values, namely, between 38 and 98 mm Hg. The problem with this wide range is, however, the fact that there is a large overlap of $tcpO_2$ values between those with vascular disease and those who are healthy. This means one single measurement is limited in its interpretation [25, 31] (Fig. 7).

If some ambient conditions are modified, particularly the temperature, it is possible to improve reproducibility. Thus, all the volunteers had $tcpO_2$ values of more than 90 mm Hg in each investigation; the electrode core temperature was 44° C and the water in the bath for their legs was a constant 40° C. The complete range of measured values was only between 92 and 110 mm Hg [25, 31] (Fig. 8).

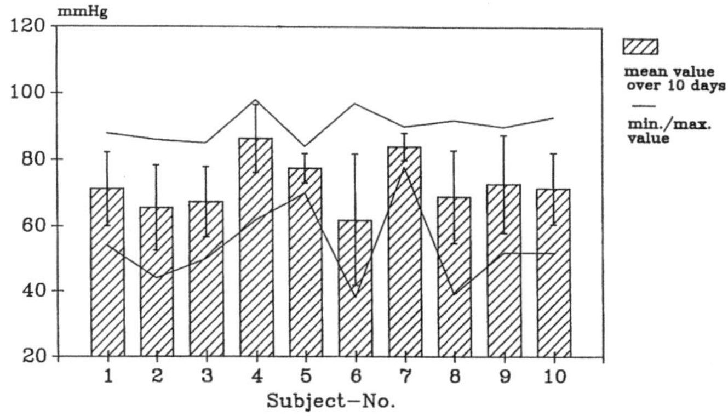

Fig. 7. Reproducibility of $tcpO_2$ measurements at room temperature (23° C). TCM3; electrode temperature, 44° C; measurement area, lower leg; 1 measurement/day; $n = 10$. (From [25, 39])

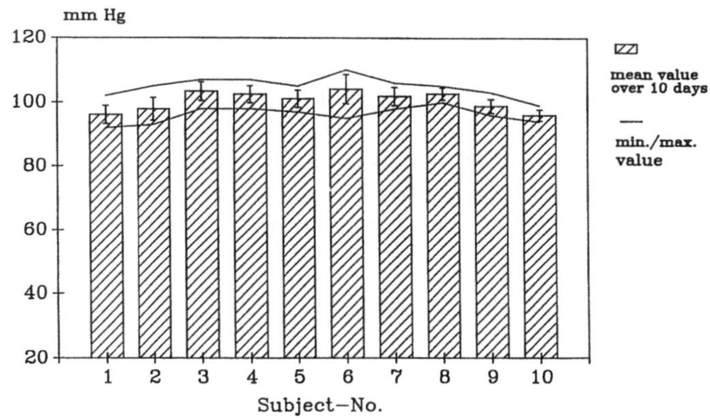

Fig. 8. Reproducibility of $tcpO_2$ measurements in a waterbath (40° C). TCM3; electrode temperature, 44° C; measurement area, forefoot; 1 measurement/day; $n = 10$; (From [25, 39])

These results suggest that heating merely the small area of skin under the electrode is not sufficient for satisfactory reproducibility of individual measured values. Clearly, ambient temperature and probably humidity, too, are also important parameters which have to be monitored and optimized in order to achieve reproducible and meaningful values from $tcpO_2$ measurement. At least it is necessary to keep these parameters constant during each measurement and to quote them in the results so that comparisons can be made with later measured values. Simply stating the electrode core temperature used (37° C or 44° C) is, according to our experiments, not enough. There are, however, few procedures for measurement under controlled conditions. We used a warm water bath, but this is not possible with every part of the body and also not completely safe, considering the use of electricity. An alternative is a room kept at a constant temperature, but this is not always available.

Due to these difficulties, researchers quickly tried to switch from static test conditions, in which absolute $tcpO_2$ values are considered, to dynamic examination. In dynamic examination, it is not the absolute values that are crucial, but the changes in the values under certain stimulation or exercise tests. The various conventional stimulation and exercise tests and their typical findings will be outlined below.

Stimulation and Exercise Test

Basically, such tests have three phases: first of all, the patient is left to rest until a "steady state" is reached, usually within 10 to 20 min after the desired electrode temperature has been reached. As a rule, a temperature of 37° C is chosen for stimulation tests since autoregulative responses of the organism to the stimulants are to be measured. In the second phase, a stimulus of a definite strength and duration is given, and in the third phase the course of the $tcpO_2$ values is observed until an equilibrium is regained.

Postocclusive Reactive Hyperemia

When an inflatable cuff is put on with suprasystolic pressure proximal to the point of measurement, the oxygen pressure of a healthy person rapidly drops to 0 mm Hg. The pressure of the cuff is maintained over a defined period, usually 3–4 min, and then quickly and completely released. After that, reactive hyperemia induces an increase in $tcpO_2$. This reactive hyperemia is the physiological vascular reaction to a temporary hypoxia of the tissue, caused by vasodilators which are released locally, especially prostaglandins [35]. The degree of postischemic hyperemia depends on the patient's age and is greater in younger people [35]. The time until half the initial value is reached can be taken as a diagnostic criterion for the microcirculation [17], as can the maximum value that $tcpO_2$ reaches due to postischemic hyperemia. The time taken to reach the initial value is significantly longer for patients with microcirculation disorders.

Increasing Hydrostatic Pressure

When a patient moves from a lying position to a sitting position and, consequently, the hydrostatic pressure increases, there is a significant increase $tcpO_2$ [17]. This test may be helpful in the diagnosis of venous disorders for example, chronic venous insufficiency, but until yet there are no precise studies regarding this test in venous insufficiency.

Increasing Venous Pressure

When venous pressure is increased by putting on an inflatable cuff and inflating it to 40 mm Hg, the increase in $tcpO_2$ in a healthy person is, on an average, about 10% [17, 25] (Fig. 6).

Giving Oxygen

When oxygen is given via a nasal tube or a mask, there is usually an increase in the $tcpO_2$, depending on the amount given. On the whole, the standard amount of either 5 or 10 liters per minute is given until equlibrium has been regained. The proportion of initial value to maximum value can be calculated and used in the evaluation. Care must be taken when treating a patient with pulmonary emphysema since a so-called CO_2 narcosis can occur.

Exercise Tests

With commercial $tcpO_2$ equipment which is now available, it is possible to record continuously during defined exercise tests. The exercise can be, for example, a treadmill at a set speed and slope, or bending and stretching the foot in time to a metronome. It is in exercise tests that pathological $tcpO_2$ values can be detected early, particularly in patients with incipient arterial occlusive vascular disease (Fontaine stages I and II) [2, 36].

Hyperemia Due To Application of Rubefacients

Hyperemia can be induced by locally applying a skin irritant. After the desired area of skin has been rubbed with, for example, Finalgon the skin becomes distinctly red within 10–15 Min. Measurements can be made before and after the application and the values compared in order to draw conclusions about how the vessels react. Significantly smaller $tcpO_2$ increases were evident in diabetics on insulin than in a control group [27, 38]. In our own investigations into the reproducibility of this stimulation test, there were problems in two respects: (1) the application of ointment to induce hyperemia lost its effect when it was carried out on the same volunteer, on the same area of skin, over a number of consecutive days. We judged this phenomenon to be most likely due to the skin getting used to the ointment. (2) The degree of hyperemia depended on the amount of ointment rubbed in. If the ointment was applied thickly, its effect was greater than when only a little ointment was used. Therefore, this stimulation test needs, among other things, to be standardized to a larger extent if it is to produce meaningful results.

A Selection of Results, and Possible Uses of $tcpO_2$ Measurement

Dermatoses

Examinations with an electrode core temperature of 42° C, carried out on the hands of patients with progressive systemic scleroderma, showed that the half-times of the decrease and renewed increase in the postischemic hyperemia stimulation test were about twice as long as in healthy people [20]. One can deduce much about the course of the disease and the supervision of therapy for patients with progressive systemic scleroderma.

When a skin irritant was applied to patients with necrobiosis lipoidica, a typical finding was an almost complete lack of $tcpO_2$ increase that normally occurs. This phenomenon was observed not only in the area of the necrobiosis lipoidica lesion, but also in the surrounding area [38]. Furthermore, the values were significantly lower in both the lesion and beyond it. When oxygen was breathed in, (10 l/min) there was indeed an increase in the $tcpO_2$ in and around the lesion but the values of the healthy skin could not be achieved [8].

Other Syndromes

A particular characteristic of the microangiopathic impairment of the skin in diabetic children was a reduction in the postocclusive $tcpO_2$ increase [15, 32]. In addition, the increase was also reduced by the application of substances irritating to the skin [37].

No significant differences in the resting value could be detected in patients with primary varicosis either before and after varices exeresis or during various stimulation tests [12]. However, the follow-up period of only 8 weeks was probably too short. Also patients with ulceration of the lower leg (caused by a venous condition) did not show any typical pathological deviation from a control group after various stimulation tests [2]. One or two investigators have found distinctly lower $tcpO_2$ in venous ulceration of the lower leg, even though the findings in arterial ulceration were even lower [5]. It is exactly in this purely venous trophic condition of the lower leg that the usefulness of the $tcpO_2$ method in diagnosis and supervision of therapy has to be proved [1, 9].

There is often no clear decrease in the $tcpO_2$ resting value in incipient arterial occlusive vascular disease (Fontaine stages I and II). However, with the defined exercise on the treadmill there is a significant decrease in the $tcpO_2$ values, so that the state of this disease can be seen objectively by means of this measuring method [36]. However, in more advanced stages of occlusive vascular disease, there is a large decrease in the $tcpO_2$ values, depending, of course, on the severity of the impairment in perfusion.

Discussion

Measurement of $tcpO_2$ has achieved wide use in the last 20 years, especially in angiology and dermatology. Since there has been a diversity of experience with this method, used with a great variety of indications, it has emerged that the value of the results of $tcpO_2$ measurement is very dependent on the suitable choice of examination conditions. While resting values determined at various points on the skin and at various times are only slightly meaningful because of relatively poor reproducibility, suitable and standardized stimulation and exercise tests in certain syndromes produce by far the more reliable information about the degree of impairment and the involvement of microcirculation in the disorder. Consequently, $tcpO_2$ measurement will, in the future, represent a possibility to enhance diagnosis and supervision of therapy. Moreover, due to $tcpO_2$ findings, we can expect further understanding of the etiology of various syndromes.

References

1. Allegra C, Antonini V, Carlizza A, Inglese A, Mari A, Tonelli V (1989) $TCPCO_2$–$TCPO_2$ et RLR dans l'insuffisance veineuse chronique. In: Davy A, Stemmer R (eds) Phlébologie 89, vol 1. Libbey, London pp 384–386
2. Antignani PL, Paolucci A, Perna AM, Ricci A, Ricci G, Bartolo M (1989) Transcutaneous oxygen tension measurements in the valutation of trophic lesions of the lower limbs. In: Davy A, Stemmer R (eds) Phlébologie 89, vol 1. Libbey, London pp 395–398

3. Baumbach P (1988) Verständnis transkutaner pO_2- und pCO_2-Messungen. Radiometer, Kopenhagen
4. Beran AV, Tolle CD, Huxtable RF (1981) Cutaneous blood flow and its relationship to transcutaneous O_2/CO_2 measurements. Crit Care Med 9: 736–741
5. Borzykowski M, Krahenbuhl B (1981) Mesure non invasive de l'oxygénation cutanée en cas d'ulcères chroniques des membres inférieurs. Schweiz Med Wochenschr 111: 1972–1974
6. Breuer HWM, Berger M, Schlaghecken U, Dienel M, Breuer J, Loogen F (1986) The value of different transcutaneous oxygen parameters in studying microcirculation. In: Maurer PC et al (eds) What is new in angiology? Zuckschwerdt, München, pp 48–49
7. Breuer HWM, Breuer J, Berger M (1988) Transcutaneous oxygen pressure measurements in type I diabetic patients for early detection of functional diabetic microangiopathy. Eur J Clin Invest 18: 454–459
8. Brüngger A (1989) Transkutane Sauerstoff- und Kohlendioxiddruckmessung bei Necrobiosis lipoidica. Hautarzt 40: 231–232
9. Caspary L, Creutzig A, Helberg T, Borgmann J, Alexander K (1989) Transcutaneous pO_2 measurements in primary varicosis and postthrombotic syndrome. In: Davy A, Stemmer R (eds) Phlébologie 89, Vol 1. Libbey, London, pp 387–388
10. Creutzig A, Caspary L, Lieth H, Alexander K (1983) Veränderungen des $tcpO_2$ und LDF bei Patienten mit primärer Varikose vor und nach Varizenexhairese. Vasa Suppl 23: 57–58
11. Creutzig A, Dau D, Caspary L, Alexander K (1987) Transcutaneous oxygen pressure at two different electrode core temperature in healthy volunteers and patients with arterial occlusive disease. Int J Microcirc Clin Exp 5: 373–380
12. Creutzig A (1988) Transkutane O_2-Druckmessung. In: Kriessmann A (ed) Aktuelle Diagnostik und Therapie in der Angiologie. Thieme, Stuttgart, pp 52–55
13. Creutzig A, Nonnast-Daniel B, Kühn K, Reimers E, Brunkhorst B, Caspary L, Koch KM (1988) Anstieg des Hautsauerstoffdruckes und des peripheren Gefäßwiderstandes bei der Behandlung der renalen Anämie mit rekombinantem humanem Erythropoientin (rh–Ep). Klin Wochenschr Suppl 13: 189
14. Eickhoff JH, Engel HC (1981) Transcutaneous oxygen tension ($tcpO_2$) measurements on the foot in normal subjects and in patients with peripheral arterial disease admitted for vascular surgery. Scand J Clin Lab Invest 41: 743–748
15. Ewald U, Turemo T, Rooth G (1981) Early reduction of vascular reactivity in diabetic children detected by transcutaneous oxygen electrode. Lancet I: 1287
16. Falstie-Jensen N, Spaune E, Brochner-Mortensen J, Falstie-Jensen S (1988) The influence of epidermal thickness on transcutaneous oxygen pressure in normal persons. Scand J Clin Lab Invest 48: 519–523
17. Franzeck UK, Talke P, Bernstein EF, Goldbranson FL, Fronek A (1982) Transcutaneous pO_2-measurements in health and peripheral arterial occlusive disease. Surgery 91: 156–163
18. Franzeck UK (1991) Transkutaner Sauerstoffpartialdruck in der Klinischen Mikrozirkulation. Huber, Bern
19. Fronek A (1988) Transcutaneous pO_2 determination – its potential and limits – in angiology. In: Kriessmann A (ed) Aktuelle Diagnostik und Therapie in der Angiologie. Thieme, Stuttgart, pp 50–55
20. Hiller D, Kessler M, Hornstein OP (1986) Vergleichende kutane Sauerstoffdruckmessung ($pCUO_2$) bei Gesunden und bei Patienten mit progressiver Sklerodermie. Hautarzt 37: 83–89
21. Huch R (1971) Quantitative kontinuierliche polarographische Sauerstoffdruckmessung aus der hyperämisierten Erwachsenenhaut. Dissertation, University of Marburg
22. Huch A, Huch R (1979) The development of the transcutaneous pO_2 technique into a clinical tool. Birth Defects 15: 5–12
23. Huch R, Lübbers DW, Huch A (1981) Transcutaneous pO_2. Thieme, Stuttgart
24. Kooman JP, Jacobs MJH, Beckers RCY, Jörning PJG, Slaaf DW, Reneman RS (1988) The influence of hydrostatic pressure on transcutaneous pO_2. Vasa Suppl 23: 138
25. Lentner A, Younossi H, Planz S, Wienert V (1991) Der Einfluß von hydrostatischem Druck, Umgebungstemperatur sowie Alter, Geschlecht und Rauchgewohnheiten auf die transkutane Sauerstoffpartialdruckmessung. Vasa Suppl 32: 243–246

26. Lübbers DW (1979) Cutaneous and transcutaneous pO_2 and pCO_2 and their measuring conditions. Birth Defects 15: 13–31
27. Lübbers DW (1981) Theoretical basis of the transcutaneous blood gas measurements. Crit Care Med 9: 721–733
28. Lübbers DW (1987) Possibilities and limitations of the transcutaneous measuring technique. A theoretical analysis. In: Huch A, Huch R, Rooth G (eds) Continuous transcutaneous monitoring. Plenum, New York, pp 9–17
29. Lusiani L, Visona A, Nicolin P, Papesso B, Pagnan A (1988) Transcutaneous oxygen tension ($TcpO_2$) measurement as a diagnostic tool in patients with peripheral vascular disease. Angiology 39: 873–880
30. Olerud JE, Pecoraro RE, Burgess EM, McKnight B, Wyss CR, Reiber GE, Matsen FA (1987) Reliability of transcutaneous oxygen tension ($TcpO_2$) measurements in elderly normal subjects. Scand. J Clin Lab Invest 47: 535–541
31. Planz S (1992) Transkutane Sauerstoffpartialdruckmessungen in der Angiologie: Möglichkeiten zur Verbesserung der Reproduzierbarkeit des Verfahrens. Thesis, RWTH Aachen
32. Railton R, Neumann P, Hislop J, Harrower ADB (1983) Reduced transcutaneous oxygen tension and impaired vascular response in the typ 1 (insulin-dependent) diabetes. Diabetologica 25: 340–342
33. Ranft J, Peters A, Heidrich H (1987) Korrelationsuntersuchungen von vitalkapillarmikroskopischen Befunden und transkutanem Sauerstoffpartialdruck bei Patienten mit peripher-arterieller Verschlußkrankheit (Fontaine-Stad, II–IV). Vasa 16: 1–12
34. Ranft J, Heidrich H, Hirche H (1988) Variabilität des $TcpO_2$ bei wiederholter Messung an Patienten mit peripherer arterieller Verschlußkrankheit. Vasa Suppl. 23: 51–53
35. Rooth G, Ewald U, Caligara F (1987) Transcutaneous pO_2 and pCO_2 monitoring at 37° C cutaneous pO_2 and pCO_2. In: Huch A, Huch R, Rooth G (eds) Continuous transcutaneous monitoring. Plenum, New York, pp 23–32
36. Schmidt JA, Leyhe A, Wichert PV (1989) Transkutaner Sauerstoffdruck unter Belastung bei Patienten mit arterieller Verschlußkrankheit der Beine im Stadium I und IIa. Inn. Med. 16: 41–45
37. Weindorf N, Schultz-Ehrenburg U (1988) Diagnostik der diabetischen Mikroangiopathie durch transkutane Sauerstoffdruck ($tcpO_2$)-Messung. Phlebol Proktol 17: 131–133
38. Weindorf N, Schultz-Ehrenburg U (1989) Vascular aspects in necrobiosis lipoidica, results of transcutaneous oxygen pressure measurements. In: Davy A, Stemmer R (eds) Phlébologie 89, vol 1. Libbey, London pp 389–391
39. Younossi H (1991) Transkutane Sauerstoffpartialdruckmessungen unter konstanter Umfeldtemperatur bei gesunden Männern und Frauen unterschiedlichen Alters. Thesis, RWTH Aachen

Methodology and Application of Fluorescence Techniques in Dermatology

V. WIENERT, A. LENTNER, and U. BÖHLER*

Historical Background

Fluorescein was first made synthetically by the German chemist, Adolf Ritter von Baeyer in 1871 [1]. Baeyer (1835–1917) won the Nobel prize for chemistry in 1905. It was only 10 years after this discovery that the German physician Paul Ehrlich (1854–1915, winner of the Nobel prize for medicine in 1908) introduced fluorescein into diagnostic medicine [14]. Ehrlich injected fluorescein and examined the dependence of the production of aqueous humour in the eye on intraocular pressure. Since then, the use of fluorescent dyes has spread to many fields of medicine.

In 1913, fluorescein was used by Strauss in urology to diagnose kidney function, and in 1953 it was used by Cipolla et al. to diagnose rupture of the urinary bladder [8, 40].

In 1959, two students of ophthalmology, Harald Novotny and David Alvis, developed the fundamental principles of fluorescence angiography of the ocular fundus. The technique has been much modified and is now routine in ophthalmological diagnostics [36, 43].

In 1934, Kurt Lange and Linn J. Boyd first introduced a filter technique that enabled selective observation of fluorescent light. They used the technique to examine circulation times, permeability of the capillaries, and blood flow through tissue in peripheral occlusive vascular disease [23]. Lange and Krewer developed a device in 1943 to record skin fluorescence quantitatively and called it a dermofluorometer [28]. Since then, this method of dermofluorometry has been written about a number of times and has been applied when assessing how well skin grafts have taken [21, 22, 25–27, 35, 38].

In 1972, Lund introduced dynamic fluorescence angiography, whereby a two-dimensional record of peripheral perfusion of the skin can be made [31]. Further improvements of this method were made in 1989 by Scheffler and Rieger with digital video fluorescence perfusography [37].

Antibodies marked with fluorescein are also used in direct and indirect immunofluorescence to identify specific antibodies and cellular antigens [9].

* Department of Dermatology, Medical Faculty of the University of Aachen, Division of Dermatological Phlebology, Pauwelsstraße 30, 5100 Aachen, FRG

Fluorescence

Luminescence is the collective term for all the luminous phenomena which, in contrast to incandescence, do not depend on the luminous substance being hot. There must, therefore, be an initial supply of energy for the light to be emitted. This energy can take various forms, depending on where luminescence is needed: ionizing radiation (radioluminescence), sound waves (sonoluminescence), electrical alternating Field (electroluminescence), mechanical energy (triboluminescence), chemical energy (chemi- and bioluminescence), and light (fluorescence and phosphorescence).

The term "fluorescence" (= photoluminescence) for a form of luminescence is derived from the mineral fluorite. Its characteristic is that it gives off light almost immediately (10^{-7}–10^{-10} s) after its electrons have been excited by visible or ultraviolet light in a form of light of longer wavelength.

The difference in energy between the normal and excited state of the electrons is characteristic for each fluorescent substance, i.e., that only certain wavelengths, depending on the substance, can be absorbed. As the electrons return to their normal state, the difference in energy is given off in the form of a photon, and, following Stoke' law, the emitted light is of a lower frequency (longer wavelengths) than the energy that is radiated on the substance and absorbed.

Chemical and Physical Characteristics of Fluorescence

Fluorescein is an organic compound, produced by heating phthalic acid anhydride with resorcin in the presence of sulphuric acid. Its chemical formula is 2-(6-hydroxy-3-oxo-[3H]-xanthen-9-yl) benzoic acid (molecular formula $C_{20}H_{12}O_5$, molecular weight 332.32). It is also called resorcinphthalein, uranine, or uranine yellow (Fig. 1). Fluorescein, together with rhodamines and rosamines, belongs to the xanthene dyes, also sometimes known as phthaleins. The reddish-brown crystals of the stable pure substance do not dissolve well in water, but dissolve quickly in alcohol, ether, or alkalis. The more easily soluble alkaline salts, especially the sodium derivate, are therefore used in medical diagnosis (molecular formula $C_{20}H_{10}O_5Na_2$, molecular weight 376.27).

This fluorescein-Na (soluble fluorescein) has a yellowish-red color when in a hydrous solution and is characterized by its intensive fluorescence which is still perceptible even when diluted by 1:100 000 000 in sunlight. This fluorescence shows up only when the fluorescein is in a dissociated state. The absorbed excitation radiation has a maximum of between 485 and 500 nm in a aqueous solution, which is the blue area of the visible spectrum. Following Stoke's law, the emitted fluorescent light has a spectrum of longer wavelength, whose maximum of extinction is about 530 nm, the green-yellow area of the spectrum (Fig. 2).

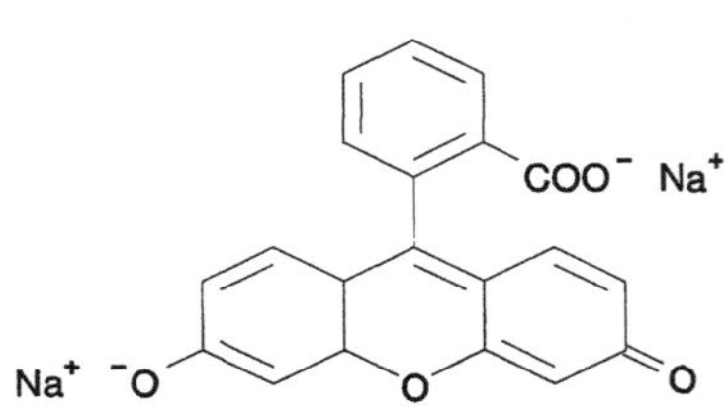

Fig. 1. Structure of fluorescein sodium

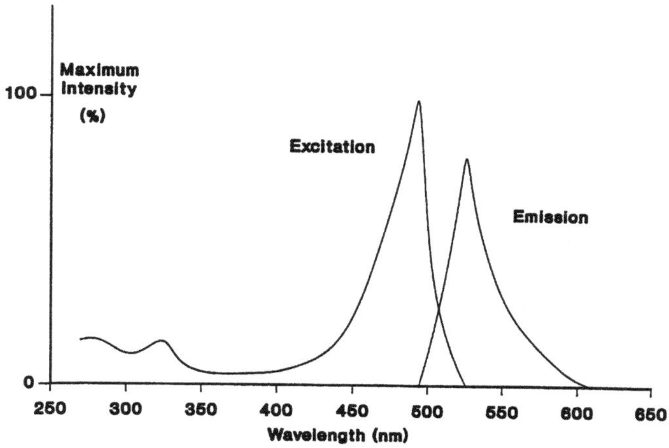

Fig. 2. Excitation and emission spectra of fluorescein sodium in aqueous solution

The intensity of fluorescence in a hydrous solution depends on a number of factors. The most important factors for the fluorescent effect are the pH value and the concentration of the fluorescein. Its dependence on the pH value comes from the fact that, in a hydrous solution, the sodium salt of fluorescein is a conjugated base in chemical balance with the nondissociated organic acid fluorescein:

$$C_{20}H_{10}O_5^{2-} + 2Na^+ + 2H_20 \rightleftharpoons C_{20}\,H_{12}\,O_5 + 2Na^+ + 2HO^-$$

As the H^+ concentration increases (decreasing pH), this equilibrium shifts to the right in the direction of the undissociated fluorescein, which is not fluorescent. Fluorescence appears only in alkaline solutions above pH 6, solutions between pH 6.1 and 3.8 are colorless.

The concentration of the dye also greatly influences the intensity of the fluorescence. When the concentration is weak (up to 10^{-4} g%) the amount of radiated light increases according to the Bouguer-Lambert-Beer law: proportionally to the number of dye molecules that are dissolved. At 10^{-3} g%, the fluorescence reaches its maximum and thereafter decreases as the concentration increases. This phenomenon, called quenching, is caused by the fact that, as the density of the dye molecules in the solution increases, the excitation energy is lost in the form of kinetic energy as it collides with other molecules [34].

Furthermore, the intensity of fluorescence is directly proportional to the intensity of the absorbed light. There is also considerable influence on fluorescence from the composition of the carrier and the presence of impurities and foreign matter which can suppress the fluorescence. This effect, quenching by foreign substances, is caused particularly by heavy metal ions, halogens, or oxygen. Moreover, in vivo the absorption spectra of fluorescein is superimposed by the absorption spectrum of hemoglobin. The maximum values for absorption of hemoglobin are 445 nm and 577 nm (oxygenated Hb) or 555 nm (deoxygenated Hb), whereby a large amount of the emitted and excitation light is absorbed. The extent of this influence was made clear by Dollery et al., who found that the best results came from fluorescence angiography of the retina in anemic patients [12, 13].

The variety of influences through absorption and quenching in vivo and the superimposition of the various absorption spectra also led to different statements about the absorption and emission spectrum of fluorescein in the blood.

Pharmacological Characteristics of Fluorescein

Statements about the distribution and bond conditions of fluorescein sodium given intravenously are still controversial. A large part of the compound probably bonds with plasma proteins, chiefly albumin. The total fraction of bonded fluorescein is between 50% and 85%. The degree of protein bonding depends on the concentration of the substance in the substance in the blood. When the fluorescein concentration is low, about 7×10^{-5} *M*, the plasma protein bond is over 80%, but it falls to just over 50% when the concentration is higher, about 6×10^{-3} *M*[42]. A smaller amount, about 10%, is supposed to attach itself to the red blood corpuscles [11]. The remaining fluorescein sodium is unattached in the plasma. The bond conditions are important, considering that the absorption spectrum of fluorescein sodium bonded to albumin shifts towards longer wavelengths [11]. The maximum absorption and emission of fluorescein sodium in plasma occurs at an excitation wavelength of 500 nm, whereas it occurs at 487 nm when the same concentration is dissolved in water [11].

Fluorescein sodium is eliminated from the body in two ways: most of it is passed out in the urine, with only a small amount being excreted via the gall and bowels. The fraction eliminated via the urine is between 60% and 70% of the original amount of fluorescein sodium that was administered, but there are no conclusive figures yet about the amount from the gall [2]. It depends on the degree of halogenation as to whether more fluorescein sodium is eliminated via the gall or the urine: with increasing halogenation of the molecule, greater amounts leave the body via the gall, whereas the amount leaving via the kidneys decreases [41]. Elimination through the kidneys is quick: 50% of the total amount is in the urine in the first 2 h, and after about 24 h no more fluorescein sodium can be detected in the urine [2]. In general, the metabolite fluorescein glucuronide is eliminated, but there is also a certain amount of the metabolites fluorescein and fluorescein monoglucuronide [7].

Although fundamentally no examinations using fluorescein sodium should be made during pregnancy, the teratogenic risk of this substance is judged to be very low. Controlled animal experiments, for example on pregnant rabbits, produced no indication of an increased teratogenic risk. The rabbits were given large amounts of fluorescein sodium intravenously in the first and second trimesters, which corresponded to three or four diagnostic interventions [32].

The interesting question, whether fluorescein is also absorbed into cells, cannot yet be conclusively answered. Experiments on the human eye indicate that the dye does not get into the cytoplasm but is carried through by cytopempsis [30].

Basic Principles of the Fluorescence Technique

Basically, the technical and physical principles are similar for the various macroscopic and microscopic procedures of fluorescence. An excitation light is shone through a suitable filter onto the area of skin to be examined and causes the dye released from the

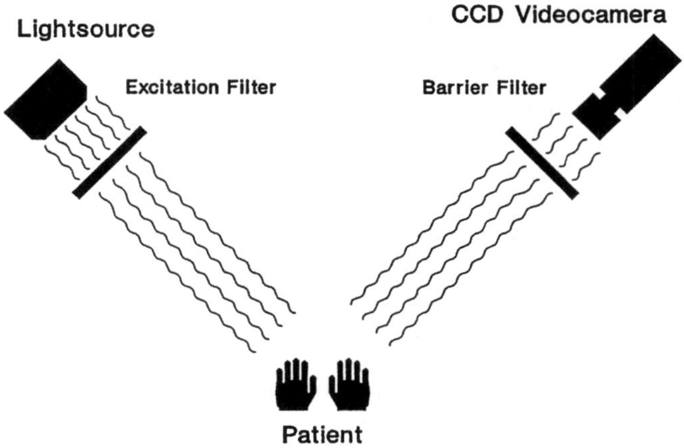

Fig. 3. The principle of the filter technique for selectively detecting the fluorescent light emitted from fluorescein sodium as applied to dermofluorography

capillaries to fluoresce. The fluorescence radiation can pass selectively through a second filter, the so-called barrier filter, but the excitation light is absorbed. The radiation is then picked up behind the filter either by a video camera or a photedetector (Fig. 3).

The main source of light for video fluorescence microscopy is a high-pressure mercury lamp. To date, xenon ring flashes, such as those found in conventional photography, have been used in dermofluorography. The inexpensive tungsten halogen cold lights are usually used in dermofluorography as sources of excitation, but they radiate so much heat there are often problems with cooling the filter. Fluorescence examinations have occasionally been carried out using xenon lamps, an obvious choice due to their continuous emission spectrum in the whole, visible spectrum range. However, they have not been used widely because of their expense.

In theory, there are numerous filter combinations which could be used in fluorescence examinations. Which kind of filter is used depends above all on the absorption and emission spectrum of the dye. For our examinations with the most frequently used dye, fluorescein sodium, we take stained glass filters made by the Schott company: BG 12 for the excitation filter and OG 495 or GG 515 for the barrier filter. The degree of pseudofluorescence is greater when OG 495 is used, which can be desirable for some examinations. FITC filter combinations from conventional fluorescence microscopy are frequently used in capillary fluorescence microscopy. The drawback of these filters, however, is that there is practically no pseudofluorescence, which occasionally leads to difficulties with field adjustment and focusing. Besides the above-mentioned filters, which have proved their worth in our daily routine work, further combinations are, of course, possible.

The fluorescent signal thus obtained can then be recorded and further processed by means of a photodetector, as in dermofluorometry, or a video camera, as in video fluorescence microscopy and dermofluorography. The charge coupled device (CCD) systems of video cameras are now generally accepted because of their excellent light sensitivity and reasonable cost, rather than the tube cameras that were used earlier.

Carrying out the Examination

General Examination

After the examination has been described to the patient and he has been informed of possible risks and side effects, he is made comfortable on an examination couch.

Since the pictures taken at various intervals in dermofluorography are processed digitally (digital subtraction), any movement of the part of the body that is under examination must be avoided during the 10 min observation period. The patient's extremities are therefore rested on a special pad from which the air can be evacuated and which is filled with plastic granules.

In capillary fluorescence microscopy, the patient's hand is laid in a specially made plastic mold, whereas there is no special positioning needed for dermofluorography. The room temperature is kept at about 30° C so as to avoid vascular constriction caused by the cold. Acclimatization takes about 15 min from the time the patient is settled down.

After the acclimatization period and after the camera has been set up and focused, 1.0 ml of a 10% solution of fluorescein sodium per 10 kg body weight is injected into the forearm by means of an indwelling cannula in the vein (fluorescein-sodium 10% Braun injection solution, Braun Melsungen). This corresponds to a dose of 10 mg/kg body weight. The kind of injection is decisive for a high-contrast picture: it should be carried out as a bolus injection in about 3–4 s, thus stopping the fluorescein from spreading into a larger volume of blood, at least during the first circulation time. The indwelling cannula is kept in the vein up to 1 h after the examination has been finished so that there is immediate access to a vein in an emergency. As a prevention against any possible intolerance reactions 2 mg clemastine hydrogen fumarate (Tavegil injection solution, Sandoz) are given intravenously 5 min before the dye is injected.

Complications

In texts on the subject there are descriptions of a number of possible side effects after an intravenous fluorescein sodium injection, but they are mainly of a harmless nature or occur only rarely. Likely pathogenetic mechanisms put forward are psychic factors, irritation of the brain stem by the bolus injection, and anaphylactoid and allergic reactions.

The most frequent side effects observed are mild and pass quickly, such as dizziness and nausea, and they occur from a few seconds to a few minutes after the injection. Their incidence rates, mentioned in papers on the subject, range from 5% to 20%.

Moderate side effects, such as vomiting, thrombophlebitis, syncope, or local necrosis of the tissue, are described as having an occurrence rate of 0.5%–1.5% [15, 20, 33, 39, 44].

Severe side effects, such as anaphylaxis, bronchial spasm, circulatory failure, myocardial infarction, or asystole, have been mentioned mainly as isolated cases, so that their exact rate of incidence is not clear. In the Fluorescein Angiography Complication Survey (FACS) of 1986 in which reports of side effects from 221781 fluorescence angiographies of the retina in 1984 were collected) the rate is given as 1:1900 (0.05%) [44]. Those who produce the injection solution claim there is one potentially fatal incident for every 20000 injections (Braun Melsungen).

Death as a result of a fluorescein sodium injection is exceedingly rare. In the FACS, one death in 221781 injections was reported. Karhunen et al. describe one case of death in 9909 fluorescence angiographies [20, 44].

Contraindications

Any likely contraindications arise from the pharmacokinetics of fluorescein sodium. Since it is mainly passed out of the body via the kidneys, a fluorescein sodium injection should not be given to patients with limited renal function who do not have to have dialysis. Since the dye is dialyzable, patients on dialysis can be examined shortly before a dialysis session. Although to date there are no definite indications of a teratogenic effect of Fluorescein sodium, to be on the safe side, it is better not to administer it during pregnancy or lactation. Further contraindications are an earlier intolerance to fluorescein sodium, a poor state of health and severe angiocardiopathy.

Methods

Dermofluorography

Typical Procedure

The principle of dermoflurography (DFG) is simple (Fig. 3). A 1200 W HMI lamp is shone on the hands or legs to be examined and a CCD camera with a fast lens is trained on them. A Schott glass filter BG 12 (3.0 mm thick) is placed in the path of the source of light as an excitation filter. It only lets blue light through, which excites fluorescein. A Schott filter OG 515 (1.0 mm thick) is placed before the CCD camera lens. This barrier filter makes sure that only the yellow fluorescent light emitted by the fluorescein reaches the camera, whereas reflected blue excitation light is stopped. The quality of the fluorescence pictures is very dependent on the correct choice of filters. The most selective imaging and maximum efficiency of the emitted fluorescent light together with the smallest possible loss of excitation light is what is wanted. However, since the transmission curves of the filters in use have a certain width and overlap at the base, some reflected excitation light always reaches the camera (Fig. 2). This pseudofluorescence reduces the contrast of the fluorescence image, but is not exactly unwanted since it enables adjustment and focusing of the camera at its widest aperture.

Digital Image Processing

The signal received by the CCD camera is first of all transmitted to a black-and-white monitor, then a time signal and, optionally, text are added. The signal is then sent through a U-matic video recorder and further processed by an IBM-compatible AT computer. The real-time digitization of the analogue picture signal is carried out on a video digitization card with 1 megabyte usual storage and a resolution of 512 x 512 pixels with an image depth of 256 gray levels.

Immediately after the injection has been given, the image processing algorithm and video timer are started at the same time. During the examination, the computer controls the taking of one picture at a time at defined intervals: namely, after 0, 10, 13, 15, 18, 21, 25, 30, 35, 40, 50, 60, 90, 120, 300, and 600 s. The computer provides a difference image for each interval between two pictures by subtracting the previous image from the current image each time. Next, every pixel in each difference image that exceeds an arbitrarily determined intensity is colored with a defined gray tone. Finally, each interval is given a defined pseudocolor and the difference images processed in this way are fit together to form a summation image.

The entire image processing is carried out on-line during the 10 min examination, so that the completed, color-coded summation image is available immediately after the examination has ended, when it can be evaluated and further assessed. The fluorescence and summation images are shown on an RGB color monitor. The finished summation images can also be stored on a 120 megabyte hard-disk and can be printed out on a color video printer (Fig. 4).

Evaluation

The color-coded summation image enables direct evaluation of the arrival of the dye and the topographical distribution of the fluorescence. A scale of colors is shown at the edge of the picture to show the time each color appeared. Areas that were first dis-

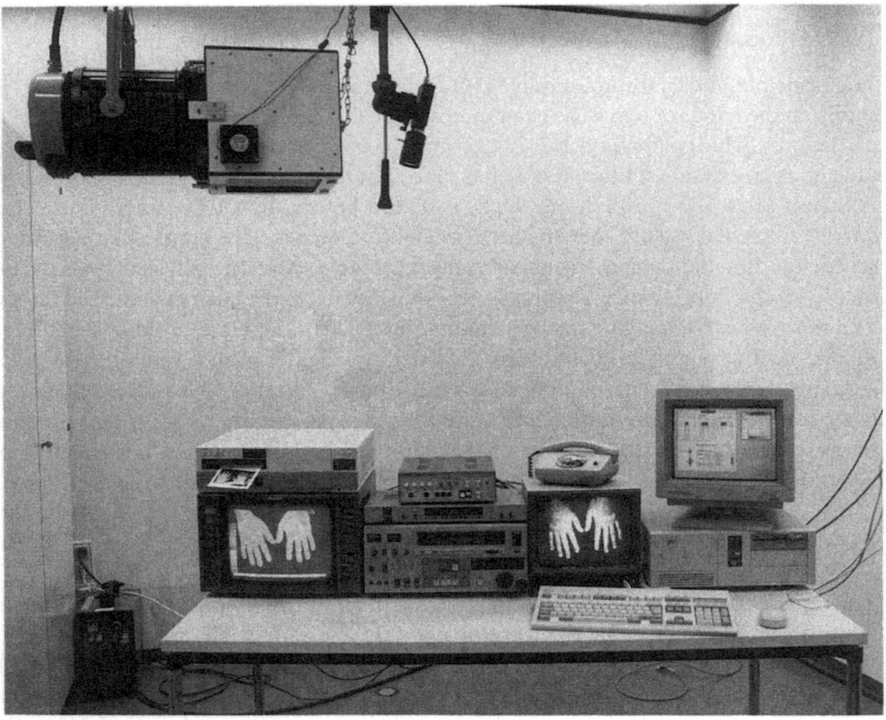

Fig. 4. The dermofluorography equipment. Top left can be seen the lighting unit (1200-W HMI lamp with filter) and the CCD video camera with zoom objective. On the table is the equipment for digital image processing

played are reproduced in shades of red and those displayed later are in blue. Areas where no fluorescence at all occurred remain black.

For further quantitative evaluation, the average time of appearance is automatically computed into "regions of interest" (ROI) that can be freely selected. The dynamics of the arrival of the fluorescence can be produced in a histogram with the aid of a spreadsheet routine. This means, for example, that the arrival of the dye in both sides of the body can be directly compared. Figure 5 shows the completed summation image of typical normal findings with the average appearance times of the ROIs which are outlined in white. Figure 6 shows these areas in their corresponding flow histograms and with the sides in comparison.

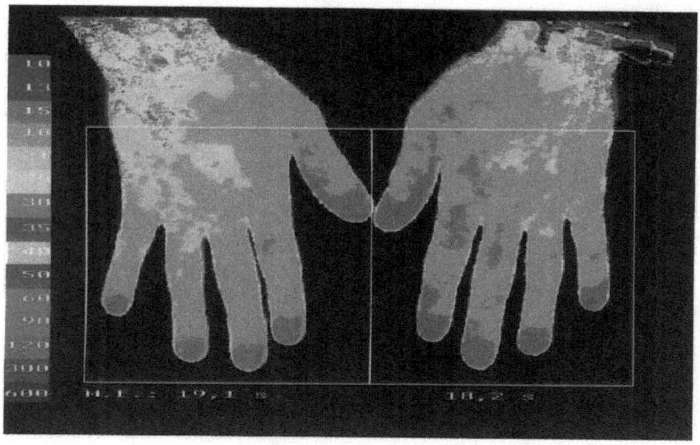

Fig. 5. Dermofluorography image from a normal person. All 15 individual images have been summated to produce this image, in which each point has been assigned a pseudocolor on the basis of the time of its appearance. The color scale on the left indicates the time of appearance in seconds. Red indicates early and blue late fluorescence. In addition, the mean times of appearance of the white-bordered regions of interest are also given

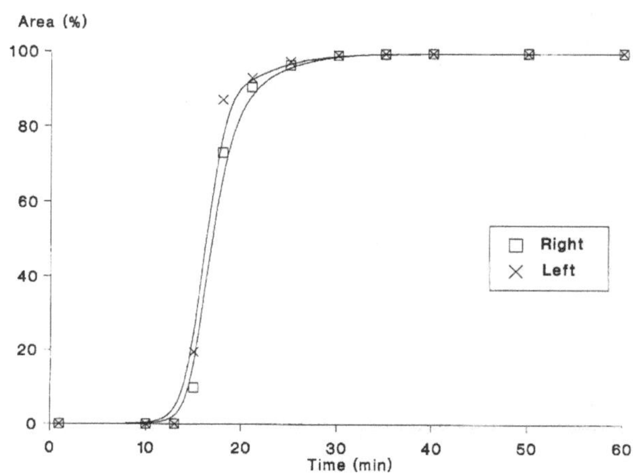

Fig. 6. Time course of the build-up of fluorescence in the regions of interest from Fig. 5

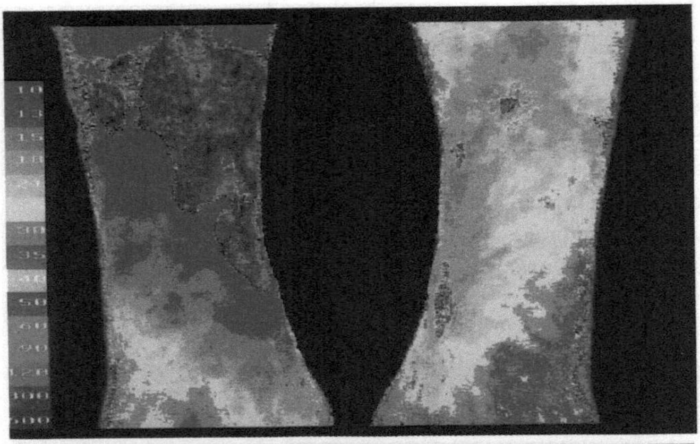

Fig. 7. Dermofluorography image in grade III chronic venous insufficiency. Fluorescence appeared late in the ulcers, while in the periulcer area a wide zone of marked hyperfluorescence can be seen

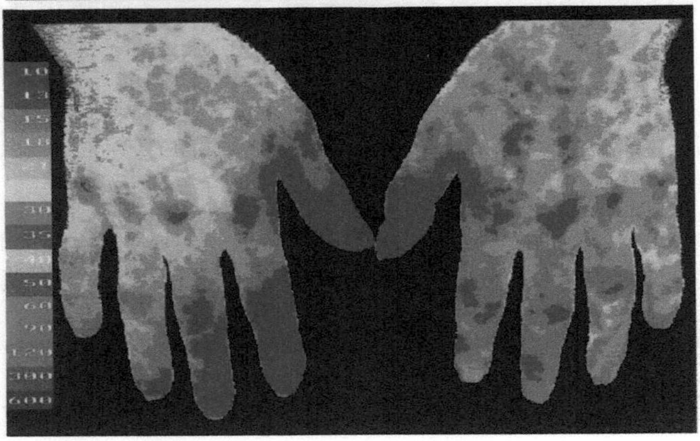

Fig. 8. Dermofluorography image from a patient with CREST syndrome and acroscleroses. Fluorescence appeared early in the acroscleroses

Clinical Results

Arterial Occlusive Vascular Disease

Altogether, there is a delayed arrival of fluorescence in patients with severe AOVD. In patients in stage IV (according to Fontaine) with ulcerations, there is always a periulcer zone with a relatively early appearance of fluorescence. The ulcers themselves appear very late or not at all.

Venous Ulcerations

In patients with ulcerations as part of chronic venous insufficiency or postthrombotic syndrome, there is, as expected, a late arrival of dye in the ulcerations and there is also always a conspicuously periculcerous area with marked hyperfluorescence and an earlier appearance of the fluorescene (Fig. 7).

Scleroderma

Initial examinations of patients with sclerodactylia as part of a CREST syndrome or a progressive systemic scleroderma showed marked hyperfluorescence with premature arrival in the area of the acrosclerosis (Fig. 8). These findings possibly arise from the pathological changes in the interstices which occur in this syndrome. They confirm what Bollinger et al. reported from their video fluorescence microscopy examinations. They, too, found significantly increased intensities of fluorescence in the interstices when the transcapillary diffusion of individual capillaries was raised [4, 6].

When patients with progressive systemic scleroderma and Raynaud's disease in the fingers were compared with healthy subjects, a heterogeneous pattern of appearance was noticed, with localized damage in early flow phases. Figure 9 is a DFG image of the hands of such a patient, who has already lost part of the middle finger on his right hand due to Raynaud's disease. Around the proximal stump of this middle finger there is a clearly delayed appearance of fluorescence. In the histogram of the arrival of the dye on the other side (Fig. 10), this delay is confirmed.

In a period of respite from Raynaud's disease, the DFG image of a female patient's hand shows a compensatory hyperperfusion with a correspondingly earlier arrival of fluorescence in all her fingers (Fig. 11).

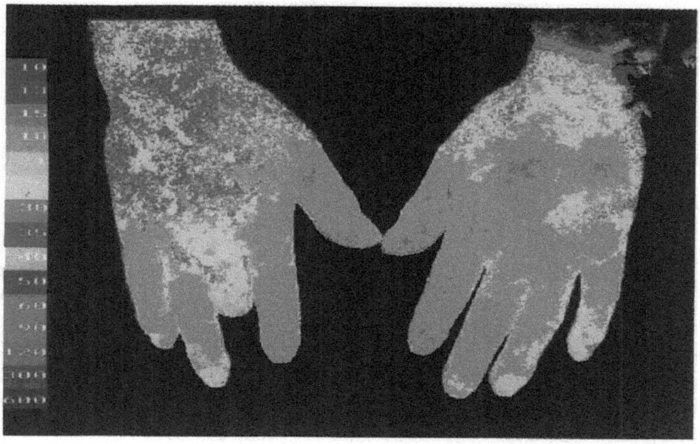

Fig. 9. Dermofluorography image from a patient with systemic scleroderma and Raynaud's phenomenon. In the region of the stump of the right third digit, which was amputated because of the Raynaud's disease, the clearly delayed appearance of fluorescence can be seen

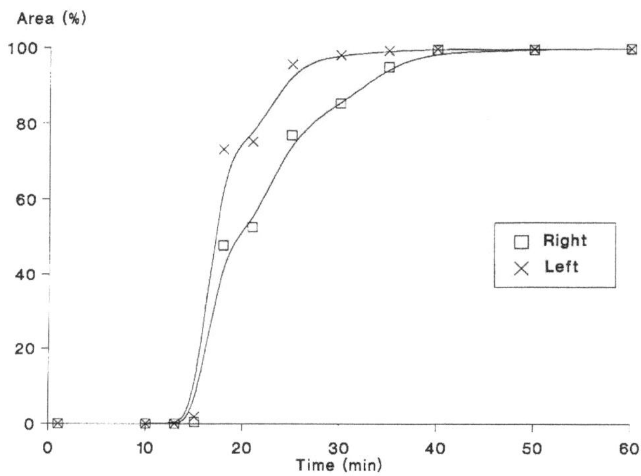

Fig. 10. Time course of the arrival of the fluorescence on the right and left hands

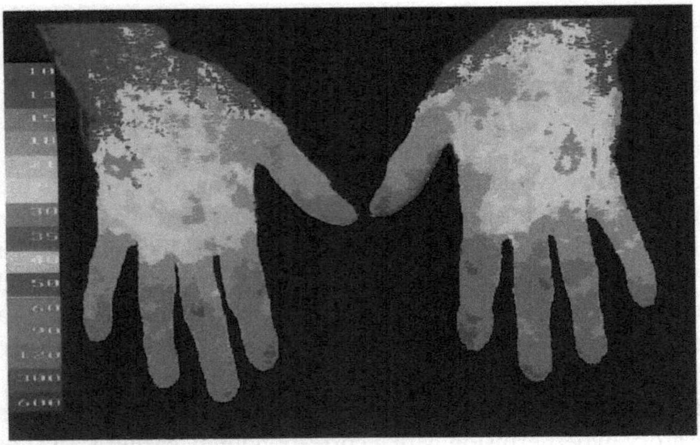

Fig. 11. Dermofluorography image from a patient with Raynaud's phenomenon in a asymptomatic phase. Note the premature appearance of fluorescence in the finger

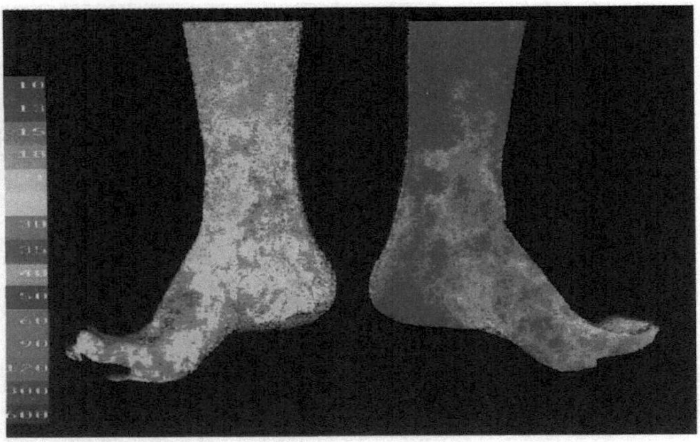

Fig. 12. Dermofluorography image from a patient with pain of unknown origin in the left ankle before lumbar sympathetic blockade

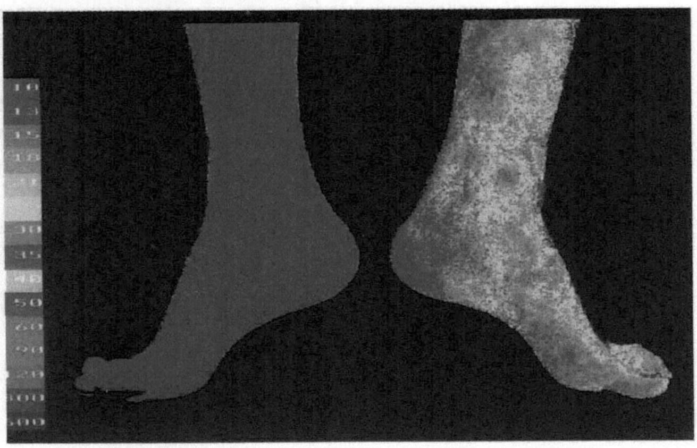

Fig. 13. Dermofluorography image of the patient in Fig. 12 after temporary CT-controlled right sympathetic blockade. The removal of the vasoconstricting effect of the sympathetic system causes extremely early arrival of the fluorescent dye

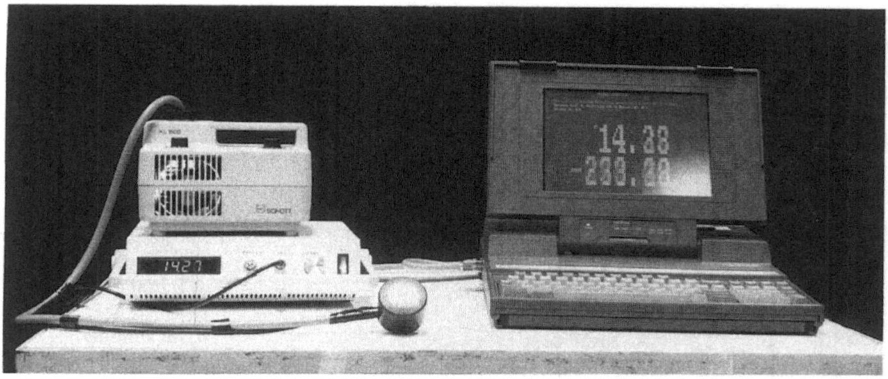

Fig. 14. Dermofluorometry equipment with a cold light source, sensor, amplifier and computer

Monitoring Therapy in Cases of Sympathectomy

Figure 12 is a DFG image of a female patient with symptoms of pain of unknown origin in her right ankle, and Fig. 13 is of the same patient 1 h after temporary lumbar sympathetic blocking on the right. Once the vasospastic components caused by the sympathicus ceased, there was a massive increase in perfusion of the skin of the affected extremity, evident from the early arrival of fluorescence.

The clinical use of DFG is mainly for therapy and follow-ups of the syndromes mentioned. There is not telling yet to what extent prognoses of other diseases can be made with the help of DFG.

Dermofluorometry

In dermofluorometry (DFM), the flow of the fluorescein sodium dye in the interstice of the skin is ascertained densimetrically for any area of skin. The main advantage of this method is that it is easier to use and needs fewer operators than DFG and video fluorescence angiography. In addition, it is possible to determine the reabsorption of the dye and its arrival, and that can be very important in the case of phlebological illnesses and in differential diagnosis of edemas. There is already a commercially available DFM system on the market (Diversatronics, Broomall, PA, USA).

We will now describe the equipment we use (Fig. 14) in order to clarify the principle of DFM.

The light from a 150 W halogen-tungsten lamp with a suitable excitation filter is collimated and connected to an optical fiber. The fiber carries the radiation to a sensor where it is spread and shone onto the skin. The sensor is held on the skin by an adhesive ring.

This beam of excitation energy on the skin causes the fluorescein sodium leaving the capillaries to fluoresce. The fluorescence is picked up by a detector built into the sensor. The necessary barrier filter is connected to the detector.

The signal thus gained is amplified and digitized on-line in a computer, with the sampling frequency remaining adjustable. The sampling frequency depends on the clock pulse frequency of the computer and the digitization card used. Our own tests

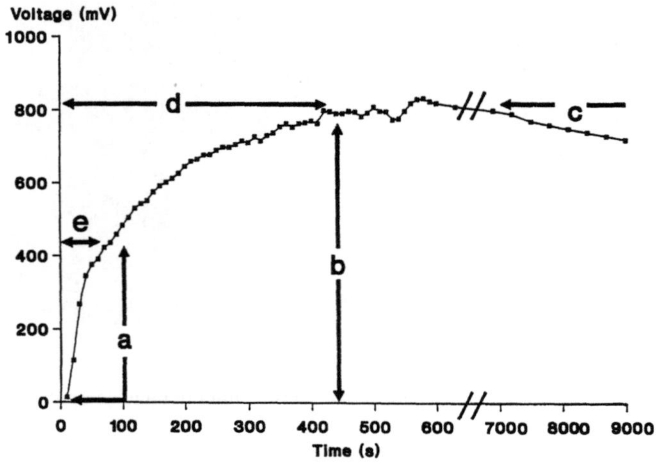

Fig. 15. The dermofluorometry parameters measured. *a*, Initial rise in fluorescence; *b*, maximum; *c*, clearance time; *d*, saturation time; *e*, time to reach half the maximum value

have shown that ten measured values per second are possible without difficulty so that short-term and fast changes are easily detectable.

The examination is evaluated according to which points are under scrutiny: circulation time, initial increase, maximum value, the period before half the maximum value is reached, saturation time, and the time taken for the dye to clear (Fig. 15).

The first examinations with the dermofluorometer were demonstrated by Lange as early as the 1940s [27, 28]. Since the early 1980s, this procedure has also been used frequently in plastic surgery to check how well skin grafts have taken [38]. The method is used clinically to assess impairment in the permeability of the capillaries (for example, in collagenosis and diabetes mellitus) and in angiology in cases of phlebological illnesses, occlusive vascular disease and thromboangiitis obliterans. The descriptions of the assessment of syphilitic ulcerations in the 1940s are now only of historical interest [27].

Fluorescence Capillaroscopy

Fluorescence capillaroscopy is a further development of the clinical capillaroscopy introduced by Müller in the 1920s. It was mostly the team working with Bollinger in the 1970s that worked out the technical and methodological rudiments of video fluorescence microscopy and used it to make images of a series of phenomena and disorders of the microcirculation of the skin.

This method usually uses a conventionally reflected light microscope fixed to a solid tripod, so that the different parts of the anatomy are accessible: for example, foot, calf or fingers (Fig. 16). A high-pressure mercury lamp serves as the source of light, with an excitation filter fixed in its beam. A barrier filter, in front of the video camera which is mounted on the microscope, allows only the fluorescent image to pass. The video fluorescent image can be seen on a monitor, recorded by a video recorder and evaluated by means of densimetry [6] (Fig. 17).

In chronic diabetics, video fluorescence microscopy showed how the fluorescein

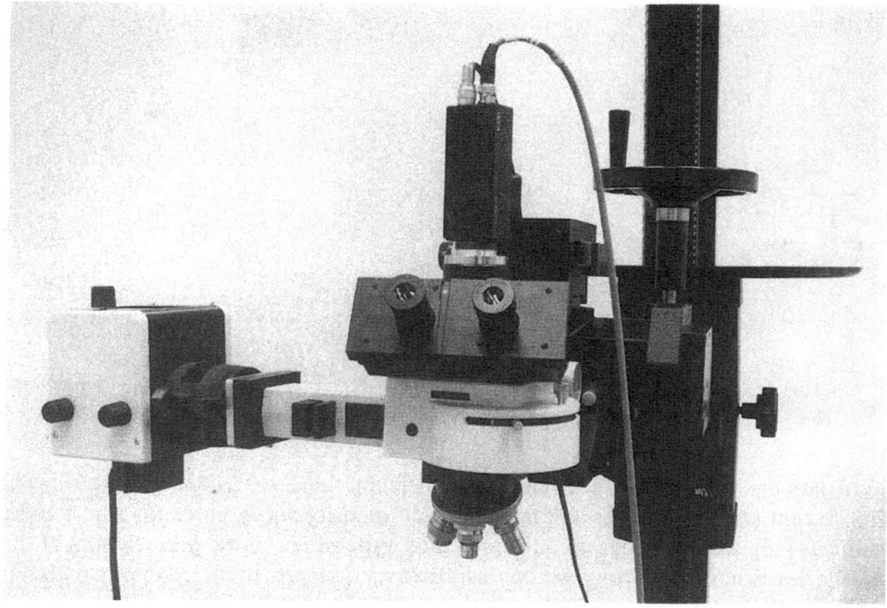

Fig. 16. Capillary microscope with stand and CCD video camera mounted for use in video fluorescence capillary microscopy

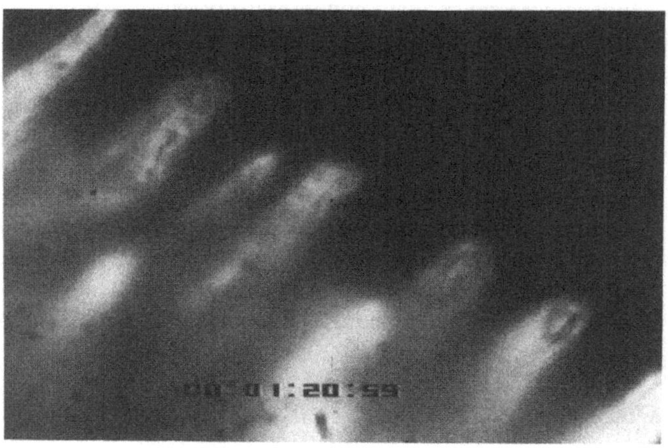

Fig. 17. Image of a normal person taken by video fluorescence capillary microscopy

sodium issued more intensely and rapidly from the capillaries [5]. In scleroderma patients, the intensity of fluorescence in individual capillaries, in the groove of the nail bed, was increased [4]. Also, the fluorescein sodium leaving from along the capillaries of the groove of the nail bed was found to be nonhomogeneous. The clearly delineated pericapillary halo of a healthy person, in whom the fluorescein sodium diffuses first of all, is often missing in scleroderma patients (Fig. 18).

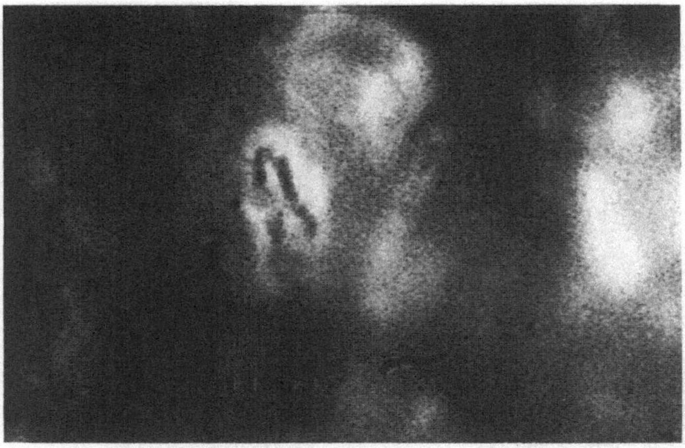

Fig. 18. Image of a patient suffering from scleroderma. In contrast to the normal findings shown in Fig. 17, an inhomogeneous efflux of fluorescein sodium along the capillaries and a practically nonexistent pericapillary halo can be seen

In patients with mild chronic venous insufficiency, there was a homogeneous flow of fluorescein sodium into the interstice but its intensity was greater than in healthy subjects [18]. Such findings are interpreted as impairment of the permeability of the capillaries. Where the chronic venous insufficiency is severe, there are some capillaries full of erythrocytes and often in clusters that show no coloration by dye even a long time after fluorescein sodium has been injected. It remains to be seen whether this is microthrombosis.

Video fluorescence microscopy is used not only to assess the capillary vessels but also to examine the course of initial lymph flow. The method is called fluorescence microlymphography. A microinjection of 0.00–0.01 ml dextran marked with FITC is administered. The initial lymph capillaries take on some of the dye and can then be studied under the video fluorescence microscope [19]. This method is used to distinguish hereditary lymphedema from secondary edema in which the small lymph vessels are aplastic and cannot be imaged [6].

Recently, it has been possible to show with fluorescence microlymphography that not only capillary vessels but also lymph vessels are impaired when there is severe chronic venous insufficiency. When compared with healthy subjects, it was discovered that these patients had an increased permeability of the lymph vessels [18].

Outlook

We have described methods of clinical fluorescence examination that can be used to assess the microcirculation of the skin. Since this field of clinical research has gained in importance over recent years, we can expect these fluorescence methods to be used even more widely in dermatological departments and surgeries. They will also probably become more significant in the prognosis of dermatological and angiological illnesses since they can detect impairment in the microcirculation of the skin before it becomes clinically evident. Seen from this point of view, fluorescence examination could be of crucial importance in the prevention and timely therapy of many disorders.

References

1. von Baeyer A (1900) Zur Geschichte der Indigosynthese. Ber Dtsch Chem Ges 33 [Sonderheft]
2. Barry RE. Behrendt WA (1985) Studies on the pharmacokinetics of fluorescein and its dilaurate ester under the conditions of the fluorescein dilaurate test. Arzneimittel Forschung 35: 644–648
3. Baumann HR, Cottier P (1960) Natriumfluorescein zur Bestimmung des Herzminutenvolumens mit Hilfe der Dilutionsmethode nach Hamilton-Stewart. Helv Med Acta 27: 18–36
4. Bollinger A, Jäger K (1981) Trans- and pericapillary diffusion of Na-fluorescein in scleroderma and chronic venous insufficiency. Bibl Anat 20: 679–683
5. Bollinger A, Jakob F, Jäger K (1982) Pattern of diffusion through skin capillaries in patients with long-term diabetes. New Engl J Med 307: 1305–1310
6. Bollinger A, Franzeck UK, Jäger K (1983) Fluoreszenz-Videomikroskopie zur quantitativen Analyse dynamischer Phänomene in der menschlichen Mikrozirkulation. In: Meßmer K, Hammersen F (eds) Vasomotion und quantitative Kapillaroskopie: Berichte des 2. Bodensee-Symposiums über Mikrozirkulation, Karger, Basel pp 111–133
7. Chen SC, Nakumura H, Zenzo T (1980) Studies on the metabolites of fluorescein in rabbit and human urine. Chem Pharm Bull (Tokyo) 28: 1403–1407
8. Cipolla A, Khedroo L, Casella P (1953) Fluorescein test for intraperitoneal rupture of the urinary bladder. Surgery 33: 102–106
9. Coons AH, Creech HJ, Jones R N, Berliner E (1942) The demonstration of pneumococcal antigen in tissues by the use of fluorescent antibody. J Immunol 45: 159–170
10. Crismon JM, Fuhrman FA (1947) Studies on gangrene following cold injury. IV. The use of fluorescein as an indicator of local blood flow. Distribution of fluorescein in body fluids after intravenous injection. J Clin Invest 26: 259–267
11. Delori FC, Castany MA, Webb RH (1978) Flurescence characteristics of sodium fluorescein in plasma and whole blood. Exp Eye Res 27: 417–425
12. Dollery CT, Hodge JV, Engel M (1962) Studies of the retinal circulation with fluorescein. Br MJ 2: 1210–1215
13. Dollery CT, Hodge JV, Engel M (1963) Retinal photography using fluorescein. Med Biol III 13: 4–14
14. Ehrlich P (1882) Über provozierte Fluoreszenzerscheinungen am Auge. Dtsch Med Wochenschr 8: 21–22, 35–37, 54–55
15. Enzmann V, Ruprecht KW (1982) Zwischenfälle bei der Fluoreszenzangiographie der Retina. Symptomatik, Prophylaxe und Therapie. Klin Monatsbl Augenheilk 181: 235–236
16. De Haan J, van Creveld S (1921) Über die Wechselwirkungen zwischen Blutplasma und Gewebeflüssigkeiten, insbesondere Kammerwasser und Cerebrospinalflüssigkeit: II. Durchlässigkeit für Fluorescein und Jodsalze. Biochem Z 124: 172–184
17. Hantke U (1986) Chemilumineszente organische Verbindungen. Mechanistische Vorstellungen zur Chemilumineszenzreaktion und mögliche Einflußgrößen auf die Chemilumineszenz dieser Verbindungen. Ärztl Lab 32: 1–10
18. Hoffmann U, Franzeck UK, Speiser D, Bollinger A (1990) Mikroangiopathie bei chronischer Veneninsuffizienz. Phlebol Proktol 19: 10–15
19. Isenring G, Franzeck UK, Bollinger A (1982) Lymphatische Mikroangiopathie bei chronisch venöser Insuffizienz (CVI). Vasa 11: 104–110
20. Karhunen U, Raitta C, Kala R (1986) Adverse reactions to fluorescein angiography. Acta Ophthalmol 64: 282–286
21. Kramer DW, Abramson EB (1947) Fluorescein studies in peripheral vascular disorders Am J Med Sci 214: 368–371
22. Lange K (1944) The vascular prerequisites to successful skin grafting. Surgery 15: 85–89
23. Lange K, Boyd LJ (1934) The technique of the fluorescein test to determine the adequacy of circulation in peripheral vascular diseases, the circulation time and capillary permeability. Bull New York Med Coll 6: 78–81
24. Lange K, Boyd LJ (1942) The use of fluorescein to determine the adequacy of the circulation. Med Clin North Am 26: 943–952

25. Lange K, Boyd LJ (1943) The technique of the fluorescein test to determine the adequacy of circulation in peripheral vascular diseases, the circulation time and capillary permeability. Bull NY Med Coll 6: 78–81
26. Lange K, Boyd LJ (1943) Objective methods of determine the speed of blood flow and their results. (Flurescein and acetylene). Am J Med Sci 206: 438–448
27. Lange K, Boyd LJ (1944) Use of fluorescein method in establishment of diagnosis and prognosis of peripheral vascular diseases. Arch Intern Med 74: 175–184
28. Lange K, Krewer SE (1943) The dermofluorometer. J Lab Clin Med 28: 1746–1750
29. Laurence DJR (1952) A study of the adsorption of dyes on bovine serum albumin by the method of polarization of fluorescence. Biochem J 51: 168–180
30. Liegl O, Mehring M (1970) Der Weg des Fluoreszeinnatriums durch die Hornhaut. Klin Monatsbl Augenheilk 159: 219–221
31. Lund F, Lund S (1973) Dynamic fluorescein angiography. A new method for assessment of skin circulation of the limbs in peripheral arterial disease. In: Shimamoto T et al (eds) Atherogenesis II. Proceedings of the 2nd international symposium on: thrombogenesis and pyridionalcarbamate treatment, Tokyo 1972. Excerpta Med Int Congr Ser 269: 336–346
32. McEnerney JK, Wong WP, Peyman GA (1977) Evaluation of the teratogenicity of fluorescein sodium. Am J Ophthalmol 84. 847–850
33. Marcus DF, Bovino JA, Williams D (1984) Adverse reactions during intravenous fluorescein angiography. Arch Ophthalmol 102: 825
34. Mecklenburg W, Valentiner S (1914) Über die Abhängigkeit der Fluoreszenz von der Konzentration. Physikal Z 15: 267–274
35. Neller JL, Schmidt ER (1945) Wheal-fluorescence. A new method of evaluating peripheral vascular diseases. Ann Surg 121: 328–337
36. Novotny HR, Alvis DL (1961) A method of photographing fluorescence in circulating blood of the human retina. Circulation 24: 82–86
37. Scheffler A, Rieger H (1989) Ein Bildverarbeitungssystem für den klinischen Einsatz der digitalen Videofluoreszenzperfusographie. Vasa Suppl 27: 86–87
38. Silverman DG, Larossa DD, Barlow CH, Bering TG, Popky LM, Smith TC (1980) Quantification of tissue fluorescein delivery and prediction of flap viability with the fiberoptic dermofluorometer. Plast Reconstr Surg 66: 545–553
39. Stein MR, Parker CW (1971) Reactions following intravenous fluorescein. Am J Ophthalmol 72: 861–868
40. Strauss H (1913) Fluorescein als Indikator für die Nierenfunktion. Berl Klin Woschenschr 50: 2226–2227
41. Webb JM, Fonda M, Brouwer EA (1962) Metabolism and excretion patterns of fluorescein and certain halogenated fluorescein dyes in rats. J Pharmacol Exp Ther 137: 141–147
42. Weiye L, Rockey JH (1982) Fluorescein binding to normal human serum proteins demonstrated by equlibrium dialysis. Arch Ophthalmol 100: 484–487
43. Wessing A (1968) Fluoreszenzangiographie der Retina. Lehrbuch und Atlas. Thieme, Stuttgart, pp 8–9
44. Yannuzzi LA, Rohrer KT, Tindel LJ, Sobel RS, Costanza MA, Shields W, Zang E (1986) Fluorescein angiography complication survey. Ophthalmology 93: 611–617

Quantitative Assessment of Scaling in Winter Xerosis Using Image Analysis of Adhesive-Coated Disks (D-Squames)

A. M. KLIGMAN[1], H. SCHATZ[1], S. MANNING[2], and T. STOUDEMAYER[2]

Indroduction

Xerosis is the term dermatologists use to describe rough scaling skin which is not classifiable as one of the hereditary hyperkeratotic ichythotic disorders.

Xerosis, otherwise known to the laity as dry skin, is a family of conditions which arises in different ways, e.g., cold, dry, wintery weather (winter xerosis), excessive washing with soaps, old age, and photodamage from sunlight.

Winter xerosis, which mainly affects the face and extremities, is the most common of the dry skin syndromes. An extraordinary variety of emollient substances, generally known as moisturizers, are commercially offered to ameliorate the signs and symptoms of dry skin.

The pathogenesis of dry skin is poorly understood. While it is appreciated that defective desquamation of the horny layer is the central feature of xerosis, investigators have been unable to explain the fundamental structural and biochemical changes which result in a dry, chapped, rough, scaly surface.

The lack of a reliable method to assess the degree of dryness quantitatively is a troublesome problem in comparing of the efficacy of different moisturizers.

Clinical grading of xerosis by sight and touch, the traditional method of assessment, is useful but has serious limitations. How the skin looks and feels is strongly dependent on ambient meteorologic conditions. A day or two of warm, humid weather obliterates scaling owing to hydration of the horny layer. This is purely an optical effect unaccompanied by any structural change in the quality of the horny layer.

Skin care specialists are familiar with these vagaries, which are a source of frustration in otherwise well-conducted assessments of moisturizers based on the regression model [1].

Previous attempts to estimate scaling by application of adhesive-coated slides (sticky slides) have been a technical improvement but are difficult to standardize and have not come into general use [2, 3]. A further refinement has been reported by Serup et al., who collected scales on adhesive disks (D-Squames) and estimated their quantity by attenuation of transmitted light [4].

We used D-Squames to develop a technique of image analysis which enables quantification of scaling utilizing image analysis.

[1] University of Pennsylvania, School of Medicine, Department of Dermatology, Philadelphia, PA 19104–6142, USA

[2] Biosearch Inc., 3408-50 B Street, Philadelphia, PA 19134, USA

Procedure

Sampling by D-Squames

The sampling device was a 22 mm, clear, adhesive-coated disk (D-Squames, Cuderm Corporation, Dallas, Texas). Serup's account provides practical information on the proper use of D-Squames [4]. After peeling off the protective seal, the D-Squame was briefly and firmly pressed with the fingers to the skin surface, gently lifted off with tweezers, and placed on a black storage card included in the D-Squame kit.

Illumination

We built a white light box utilizing halogen lamps and coordinated fiber optic light carriers. Since scales scatter and reflect light, they appear white against the black storage card. Brightness is a function of the thickness of the scales.

Video Imaging

The image analysis system consisted of four components: (1) a live image source through a video camera, (2) display of the image on a video screen (3), a video digitizing board frame grabber, and (4) a computer to run the software.

The images were obtained by a high-resolution black and white CCD video camera (Dage-MTI CCD72, Michigan City, IN, USA) connected to a stereomicroscope (OPMI 1-FC, Zeiss, Germany). A separate video control panel with manual gain and black level controls guaranteed consistent video processing under identical conditions.

The image was captured by an image analysis program (Java, Jandel Scientific, CA, USA) using a frame grabber board (Truevision Targa-M8 Frame Grabber), both installed in a Unisys personal computer. The frame grabber translates the image into 512 × 480 picture elements (pixels). Each pixel is given a numerical value according to its intensity on a gray scale from 0 to 255.

Image Analysis

An electronic mask was used to define a measurement area of 200 mm^2. We then used a look-up table to rate gray levels on a 1–5 scale. Each pixel was assigned to one of these levels, corresponding to one of five arbitrary thickness levels of the scales. We calculated the number of pixels in each thickness group as a percent value. Additionally, we determined the percentage area occupied by the scales. These two functions were integrated to yield the desquamation index (D.I.) according to the following formula:

$$\text{D.I.} = \frac{2A + \sum_{n=1}^{5} T_n \times (n-1)}{6}$$

where
A is the percent area covered by scales;
T_n is the percentage of scales in relation to thickness; and
n is the thickness level (1–5).

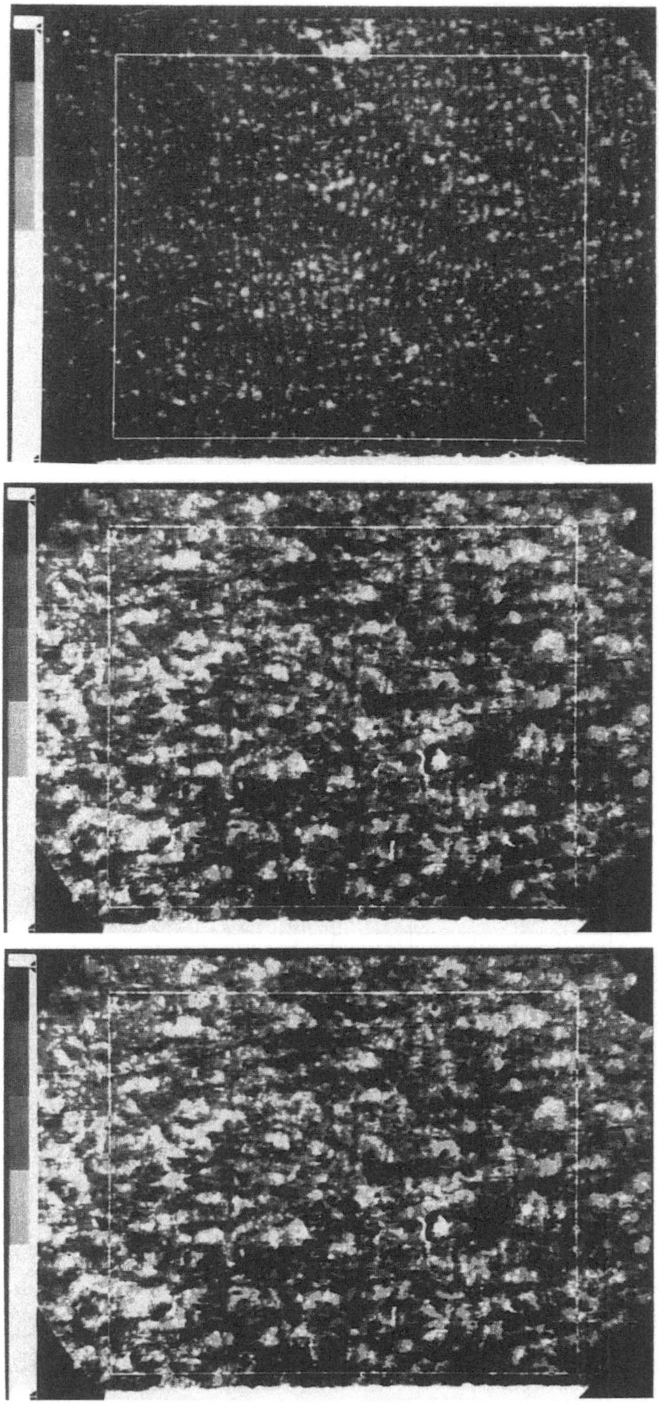

Fig. 1. **a** D-Squame sample from a non-dry leg. The scales cover only 15% of the surface and are very thin. **b** D-Squame from subject with moderately dry leg. Scales cover most of the surface and are thicker and larger. **c** D-Squame from a subject with severely dry leg. The scales are large and very thick, covering the entire surface except where interrupted by furrows

Results

Assessment of Leg Dryness by the D-Squame Method

D-Squames from non-dry, moderately dry, and severely dry midlateral legs of adult women were captured by the video camera and processed by image analysis.

Figure 1 illustrates the gross appearance of D-Squames against a black background for non-dry, moderately dry, and several dry legs. The differences are very striking to the naked eye.

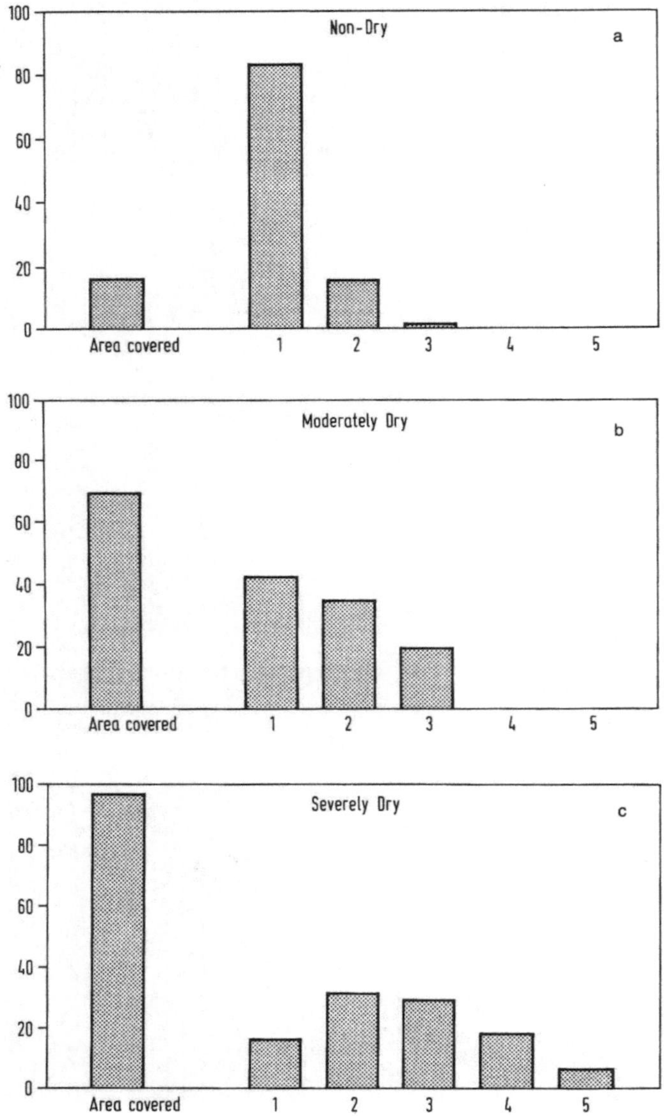

Fig. 2. a Non-dry skin; 16% of the surface is covered with scales and almost all of the scales are very thin (thickness level = 1). **b** Moderately dry skin. Scales over 69% of the surface and about 50% comprise thickness levels 2 and 3. **c** Severely dry skin. The scales cover the entire surface, 85% comprise thickness levels of 2 or greater

Figure 2 illustrates the scale distribution generated by image analysis of these same three specimens. The differences between non-dry and dry skin are dramatic, both in regard to the area covered by scales and the larger proportion of thick scales.

Table 1 shows the desquamation indices in relation to the distribution of scales for the three levels of clinical dryness and the area covered by scales. The thickness of the scales increased proportionately to the area covered, always accompanied by a sharp increase in the desquamation index.

Table 1. Quantitative comparisons among non-dry, moderately dry and severely dry skin

		Non-dry	*Moderately dry*	*Severely dry*
Area occupied by scales (%)		16	69	97
Thickness levels (% of total)	1	83,2	42,2	16,0
	2	15,9	34,4	30,9
	3	0,9	19,4	28,8
	4	0,0	0,1	17,9
	5	0,0	0,0	6,4
Desquamation index		8,1	37,2	60,3

In the progression from nondry to severely dry skin, the scales cover more of the surface, they increase in thickness, and are accompanied by a substantial increase in the desquamation index

Comparative Efficacy of Three Moisturizers

We compared the efficacy of three proprietary cream-type moisturizers on a group of 25 women, ages 28–55 years, who suffered rather severely from dry skin in the winter (winter xerosis). We modified the routine regression method [5, 6] by applying more than one moisturizer to each leg. We marked out circular areas 25 mm in diameter on the midlateral legs.

Eight test sites on each leg were delineated with ink allowing three duplicate sites for each moisturizer. The two remaining sites served as untreated controls. The treatment sites were randomized to avoid position effects. The test was conducted in January in Philadelphia, PA.

A total of 10 μl of the test moisturizer was applied to each site by a micropipette and evenly spread with a glass rod. Applications were made twice daily every week for 2 weeks.

The posttreatment evaluations (regression phase) were made on Monday, 3 days after the last application (to avoid interference from residues of the moisturizers) and on the following Monday, 10 days after the last treatment.

At the same time, trained monitors graded dryness on the following scale:

0 = no dryness
1+ = slightly dry, powdery, ashy appearance
2+ = moderately dry, small, uplifting scales
3+ = severely dry, large scales with marked flaking

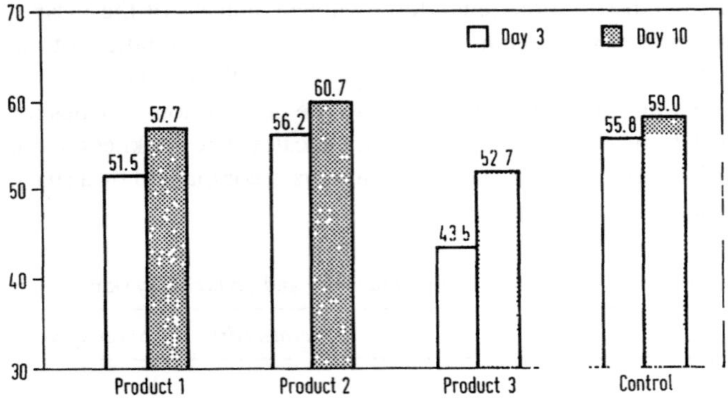

Fig. 3. Desquamation indexes for the three moisturizers on days 3 and 10 of the regression phase. Product 2 is ineffective and does not differ from the control. Product 3 is clearly the most effective product. Product 1 is slightly effective compared to the control

Figure 3 shows the desquamation indices for the three test creams at days 3 and 10 of the regression phase. Statistical significance was assessed by the paired t test. As expected, efficacy ratings on post-3 day were greater than at day 10. Product 3 was the most effective, being significantly different from both the untreated control and the other two creams at days 3 and 10 ($p = < 0.005$).

Product 1 was the next most effective and was statistically different from the control and from product 3 at days 3 and 10 ($p = < 0.005$). Product 2 was ineffective, with values very similar to the untreated control. However, by clinical grades, product 2 was estimated to be statistically more effective than the untreated control at day 3 (Mann-Whitney *U* test). Our explanation for this seeming paradox relates to the relatively high viscosity of this particular moisturizer, which thickly coats the surface without spreading. This reduces the scattering of light, masking the true situation in the desquamating portion of the horny layer. As it happily turns out, this special instance demonstrates the greater reliability of the D-Squame method, which does not depend on appearance.

We mention here some recent refinements which are now standard operating procedure.

Sampling errors have been further reduced by delipidizing the skin with 2 ml of ether: acetone (1:1) in a glass cylinder for 1 min. After evaporation, scales become bright white and conspicuous to the eye. Delipidization often reveals small scales which are not evident clinically. Greater amounts are removed after delipidization. Additionally, sampling by D-Squames is more uniform and reproducible.

We see two practical applications for this D-Squame model: (1) to select matching subjects for studies of moisturizers. Clinical grading alone is often faulty so that not all the subjects initially given maximum score at 3 are equally xerotic. (2) Manufacturers of moisturizers often quarrel with each other by making claims of efficacy which are then disputed by others. The D-Squame method helps to resolve such conflicts by supplying numeric ratings amenable to statistical analysis.

Of course, determination of the desquamation index by image analysis is something of a technological luxury. Simpler methods may be adequate for routine work, especially for screening moisturizers. Serups'optical attenuation method has merit even though information on the distribution of thickness levels is not retrievable [5]. We have modified that technique by placing the D-Squame in an ordinary 35 mm slide mount which is viewed by a slide file projector (Model H-I, Slidex, Slidex Corp., Tokyo, Japan). Optical transmission can then be measured from the projected image using a Mavolux digital light meter (Gossen GMBH, Erlangen, Germany) mounted to a shield fitted to the screen.

References

1. Kligman AM, Lavker RM, Grove GL, Stoudemayer T (1982) Some aspects of dry skin and its treatment. In: Safety and efficacy of topical drugs and cosmetics. Kligman A M, Leyden J J (eds), Grune, and Stratton, New York, pp 221–238
2. Goldschmidt H, Kligman AM (1967) Exfoliative cytology of human horny layer. Arch Dermatol 96: 572–576
3. Grove GL, Exfoliative cytology procedures as a nonintrusive method for dermatogerontological studies. J. Invest. Dermatol. 73: 67–69
4. Serup J, Winther A, Blichmann C (1989) A simple method for the study of scale pattern and effect of a moisturizer – qualitative and quantitative evaluation by D'Squame tape compared with parameters of epidermal hydration. Clin Exp Dermatol 14: 277–282
5. Boisits EK, Nole GE, Cheney MC (1990) The refined regression method. J. Cut. Aging Cosmet Dermatol 1: 155–163
6. Kligman AM (1978) Regression method for assessing the efficacy of moisturizers. Cosmet. Toil 93: 27–35

Subject Index

Springer-Verlag and the Environment

We at Springer-Verlag firmly believe that an international science publisher has a special obligation to the environment, and our corporate policies consistently reflect this conviction.

We also expect our business partners – paper mills, printers, packaging manufacturers, etc. – to commit themselves to using environmentally friendly materials and production processes.

The paper in this book is made from low- or no-chlorine pulp and is acid free, in conformance with international standards for paper permanency.

MIX
Papier aus verantwortungsvollen Quellen
Paper from responsible sources
FSC® C105338

If you have any concerns about our products,
you can contact us on
ProductSafety@springernature.com

In case Publisher is established outside the EU,
the EU authorized representative is:
Springer Nature Customer Service Center GmbH
Europaplatz 3, 69115 Heidelberg, Germany

Printed by Libri Plureos GmbH
in Hamburg, Germany